CIRCULATORY
PHYSIOLOGY
—*the essentials*
SECOND EDITION

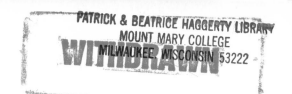

CIRCULATORY PHYSIOLOGY
—the essentials
SECOND EDITION

James J. Smith, M.D., Ph.D.

Professor of Physiology and Medicine
The Medical College of Wisconsin
Milwaukee, Wisconsin
Deputy Director, Cardiopulmonary Rehabilitation Center
Veterans Administration Medical Center
Wood, Wisconsin

John P. Kampine, M.D., Ph.D.

Professor of Anesthesiology and Physiology
Chairman, Department of Anesthesiology
The Medical College of Wisconsin
Milwaukee, Wisconsin
Director of Anesthesiology
Milwaukee County Medical Center
Wauwatosa, Wisconsin

WILLIAMS & WILKINS
Baltimore/London

Editor: Maureen K. Vardoulakis
Copy Editor: Leilani Cochran
Design: Robert Och
Illustration Planning: Lorraine Wrozsek
Production: Raymond E. Reter

Made in the United States of America

First Edition, 1980

Reprinted 1980, 1981, 1983

Second Edition, 1984

Library of Congress Cataloging in Publication Data

Smith, James John, 1914-

   Circulatory physiology.
   Includes bibliographies and index.
   1. Cardiovascular system. 2. Blood—Circulation. 3. Cardiovascular system—Diseases. I. Kampine, John P. II. Title. [DNLM: 1. Blood circulation. WG 103 S651c]
QP102.S64   1984   612'.1   83-10475
ISBN 0-683-07886-0

Composed and printed at the
Waverly Press, Inc.
Mt. Royal and Guilford Aves.
Baltimore, Md. 21202, U.S.A.

Dedicated to our parents

James W. and   and   Dr. Clifford and
Catherine Smith   Florence Kampine

They showed us the way.

Preface to the Second Edition

Our primary purpose in this second edition remains the same, *i.e.* to provide for medical and other health professional students a text that presents the basics of circulatory physiology in a stepwise and, we hope, understandable manner. We have, in addition, emphasized the pathophysiological aspects for those who are (or will be) charged with the diagnosis and care of cardiovascular patients. In accord with the latter objective we have again noted clinical applications throughout the text and have also included two chapters dealing specifically with the pathophysiology of some of the more common circulatory disorders. Sections on the physiology of exercise, physical training, responses to non-exercise stress and aging might also be useful to physicians involved with circulatory stress testing, coronary care units or cardiac rehabilitation.

The comments and suggestions we have received from medical students, nurses, exercise physiologists, technicians and physical therapists have been both helpful and encouraging. Our continued objective is to make the text broadly applicable to all professionals in the health sciences. We would very much welcome comments and criticisms of this revision.

In fashioning the chapters on pathophysiology some license has been exercised in the matter of adding material from other disciplines. In the consideration of disease processes, academic boundaries are largely artificial. We have therefore included brief accounts of the epidemiological, biochemical, anatomical, pathological, and pharmacological aspects where it seemed appropriate. We thought that this approach might put the physiology into a broader setting and perhaps provide a fuller understanding of the clinical problems. We are very grateful to our colleagues in these allied fields who reviewed these aspects of the book and prevented us from going too far astray.

In various parts of the text, we have pointed out some fields of current investigation that we believe are particularly significant and have noted certain research and diagnostic methods that seem especially promising. New methods are often the springboard from which great advances are made; furthermore, intelligent evaluation of information is hardly possible without an understanding of how such information was obtained. These accounts, albeit brief, might also provide some indication of the future directions of cardiovascular research.

While the basic objectives and approach are the same as in our original text, this edition represents an extensive updating and revision. Alterations with some expansion have been made in sections on electrical and ionic events of cardiac contraction, myocardial contractility, physiology of the venous system, autonomic transmitters, cardiovascular reflexes, physiology of exercise, physical training and ischemic heart disease. New sections on renal circulation and splanchnic circulation have been added and 38 figures have been redrawn or added.

James J. Smith   **John P. Kampine**

Preface to the First Edition

This book—which is intended for medical students—has evolved from our lectures in cardiovascular physiology to the medical and graduate classes. However, we have also been influenced in the method of presentation by our teaching sessions with nurses and allied health students as well as with residents and physician groups. It seems that all of us share the perennial problem of the increasing volume of material and the pressing need to cull out the relevant in the time allotted. As a consequence we have tried to confine ourselves to the essentials.

We have two primary aims in the preparation of this book; the first was to present the basics of circulatory physiology mainly for those who are (or will be) charged with the diagnosis and care of cardiovascular patients. As a result, many interesting topics dealing with fundamental mechanisms have usually been omitted or treated only briefly. In further accord with this objective, clinical applications have been emphasized throughout the text and two chapters on the pathophysiology of certain cardiovascular disorders have been included. Physicians and others involved with coronary care units and circulatory stress testing may find this approach useful.

A second objective has been to develop some of the more difficult concepts in an orderly, stepwise and hopefully intelligible manner. Diagrams have been liberally used and physical, chemical and biological principles and analogies incorporated when they seemed useful.

In developing topics rather briefly and bypassing some of the complex issues, the danger is that the student may feel that the subject is straightforward and that most problems are resolved, which of course is far from the truth. Not only on questions of diagnosis and treatment but on a number of basic concepts, there is still intensive investigation and considerable controversy.

But it is sometimes helpful to have a small-scale map of the battlefield,

ix

which is why we undertook to write this book. And, in any event, for the student, the classroom and the laboratory may be better places to air the unsolved problems. We also hope that the references we have included, many of them reviews by leading authorities, will help to focus attention on current research in this field.

We wish to acknowledge, with very real gratitude, our many colleagues and our own students who have made helpful comments and valuable suggestions. However, in the final analysis, the selection of content and method of presentation must be our own responsibility; such selection is a highly individual process and no doubt others would have made different choices. we would, therefore, very much welcome comments, not only regarding specific errors or omissions but also general impressions and suggestions.

James J. Smith   **John P. Kampine**

Acknowledgments

Circulatory physiology is without question one of the fastest growing fields in science, and research advances since the first edition have been notable. We have made a serious effort in this second edition to incorporate what we believe to be the more important of these advances, as well as an estimate of their possible impact on the care and treatment of cardiovascular patients. This book would not have been possible without the helpful advice of a number of our colleagues in physiology and other disciplines who checked various parts of the manuscript and made comments and recommendations. We were fortunate to have reviewers who were not only first-class scientists with extensive research skills, but also experienced teachers in their respective disciplines. The latter factor is important since it undoubtedly influenced these men and women in their judgment of concepts and material which would be most relevant for teaching purposes.

From the faculty of other universities it is a pleasure to acknowledge the help of the following: Dr. Francis L. Abel, Professor and Chairman, Department of Physiology, University of South Carolina School of Medicine; Dr. Carleton H. Baker, Professor and Chairman, Department of Physiology, University of South Florida School of Medicine; Dr. Jerry B. Critz, Division of Heart and Vascular Diseases, National Institutes of Health; Dr. David A. Cunningham, Professor of Physiology and Physical Education, University of Western Ontario; Dr. Peter A. Farrell, Associate Professor and Director of Exercise Physiology, University of Wisconsin-Milwaukee; Dr. James P. Filkins, Professor and Chairman, Dr. Walter C. Randall, Professor, and Dr. John X. Thomas, Assistant Professor, all of the Department of Physiology, Loyola University, Stritch School of Medicine; Dr. Irwin J. Fox, Professor of Physiology, University of Minnesota; Dr. Joseph P. Gilmore, Professor and Chairman, Department of Physiology, University of Nebraska; Dr.

Dean C. Jeutter, Professor of Biomedical Engineering, Marquette University; and Dr. Carl F. Rothe, Professor of Physiology, Indiana University School of Medicine.

Members of our own faculty at the Medical College of Wisconsin contributed notably with advice on specific chapters. Among these were Dr. Harold L. Brooks, Chief, Dr. Felix E. Tristani, Dr. Virinderjit S. Bamrah, Dr. H. Sidney Klopfenstein and Dr. Michael J. Ptacin of the Cardiology Section, Department of Medicine; Dr. Chesley P. Erwin and Dr. Karl Pintar, Department of Pathology; Dr. Garrett J. Gross, Department of Pharmacology; Dr. Mahendra S. Kochar, Chief, Hypertension Section, Department of Medicine; Dr. William J. Willems, Department of Neurology; and Dr. Lyle H. Hamilton, Dr. William J. Stekiel, Dr. Jeffrey L. Osborn, Dr. Jeanne L. Seagard, Dr. David F. Stowe, Dr. Carol J. Porth and Dr. Thomas J. Ebert of the Department of Physiology.

We would like to extend special thanks to several physiologists who critically reviewed large portions of the manuscript and who made very valuable suggestions. These were Dr. Robert F. Bond, Professor and Chairman of Physiology, Oral Roberts University; Dr. Peter H. Kot, Professor of Physiology and Biophysics, Georgetown University; Dr. Joel A. Michael, Professor of Physiology, Rush Medical College; and Dr. V. Thomas Wiedmeier, Associate Professor of Physiology, Medical College of Georgia. While we take pleasure in acknowledging the assistance of our colleagues, we, of course, take full responsibility for any errors or omissions in the text.

It is a particular pleasure to acknowledge the skill and assistance of DeWayne Risley, medical illustrator, David Wimmer, Mary Raddatz, Douglas Bode, photographers, and Mr. Carl Henderson, Chief, Medical Media Service, Veterans Administration Medical Center. We also wish to thank Carole Hilmer, medical illustrator, for medical art services rendered in both editions.

A special tribute goes to our own staff who never failed or flinched no matter how long the road; in this tribute we include Susan Sommer, who did a superb job of typing the manuscript, Mavis E. Baurle, who lent valuable assistance when and where it was most needed, and above all, our special thanks to Jill A. Barney, the Chief Technician of our stress testing laboratory who coordinated and masterminded the production of the entire manuscript. It is also a pleasure to acknowledge the unfailing help and encouragement of the publishers, Williams & Wilkins.

Contents

CHAPTER 5. CONTRACTILE PROPERTIES OF
THE HEART

CHAPTER 6. PRESSURE AND FLOW IN THE
ARTERIAL AND VENOUS SYSTEMS

CHAPTER 8. THE MICROCIRCULATION AND
THE LYMPHATIC SYSTEM

CHAPTER 9. THE PERIPHERAL CIRCULATION
AND ITS REGULATION

CHAPTER 12. PHYSIOLOGY OF EXERCISE
AND THE EFFECT OF AGING

CHAPTER 13. CIRCULATORY RESPONSE TO NONEXERCISE STRESS

CHAPTER 14. PATHOPHYSIOLOGY: ISCHEMIC HEART DISEASE AND CONGESTIVE HEART FAILURE

chapter 1

Blood and the Circulation: General Features

General Characteristics

Because the circulatory system is the sole agent for delivery of oxygen to and the removal of carbon dioxide from all tissues of the body, it is indispensable for the survival of the organism. The circulation also delivers nutrients from the gastrointestinal tract to all the body parts, carries waste products of cellular metabolism to the kidney and other excretory organs, transports electrolytes and important chemical regulators called hormones, and serves to maintain body temperature. In addition, it transports various activator and immune substances which are concerned with body defense mechanisms.

Because of the very limited storage capacity of tissues for oxygen, the survival times of the "vital organs," *i.e.*, the brain and heart, without oxygen, are only a few minutes, so that even a brief failure of the circulatory or respiratory system may have a serious or fatal outcome.

Another significant characteristic of the circulatory system is its

1

vulnerability to disease. The incidence of cardiovascular disorders is particularly high in the so-called "developed" nations of the western world. While rheumatic and coronary heart disease as well as cerebro-vascular accidents (stroke) have become prevalent, the most common of all circulatory disorders is hypertension; it is estimated that in the United States 35 million have the disease and require therapy and an additional 25 million have borderline hypertension which warrants surveillance.

Of the current annual two million deaths in the United States, 52% are the result of cardiovascular disease—more than cancer (20%), trauma (6%) and all other causes combined. The majority of these deaths are associated with atherosclerosis of the coronary, cerebral or renal arteries. Although the specific cause of atherosclerotic disease is unknown, major "risk factors" such as high blood pressure, cigarette smoking and increased blood cholesterol are known to predispose to its development. A world-wide research and educational effort has been mounted in recent years in an attempt to deal with the immense problem of cardiovascular disease.

Functional Divisions of the Circulation

The two main components of the circulation are the smaller pulmo-nary division consisting of the pulmonary artery, capillaries and pul-monary veins, and a much larger systemic division, consisting of the aorta, arterial branches, capillaries, veins and vena cavae. The systemic vessels supply and drain all the organs and tissues of the body. These two divisions are series-connected, hydraulic circuits and form a closed system. Each division consists of a pump, a distributing system, an exchange system and a collecting system (Fig. 1.1). Whereas the two divisions function in a generally similar manner they have some impor-tant differences; the pulmonary division has a much smaller volume, its vessels are shorter and thinner walled and it operates under lower pressure and with less resistance to flow.

The heart, which propels the blood through both divisions, has four chambers, a right and left atrium and a right and left ventricle. The atria are, in essence, auxiliary pumps which assist the flow of blood into the ventricles and help fill these chambers properly so they will be better primed for the subsequent power stroke. The ventricles are the main pump elements. The right ventricle propels blood through the pulmo-nary artery to the lungs (pulmonary circulation) and the left ventricle through the aorta and systemic arteries to the remainder of the body (systemic circulation). Each ventricular chamber has inlet and outlet valves which act reciprocally, that is, one closes before the other opens, thus preventing backflow (Fig. 1.2).

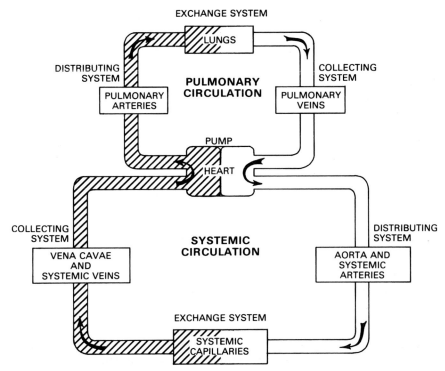

Figure 1.1. Functional divisions of the circulation. The pulmonary circulation delivers blood to the lungs for the elimination of carbon dioxide and the acquisition of oxygen. The systemic circulation transports oxygen (as well as nutrients and other substances) to all tissues of the body.

During ventricular contraction (*i.e.*, systole) the internal ventricular pressures rise rapidly to a peak; the ventricles then relax, the internal pressures fall quickly to near zero followed immediately by the ventricular filling phase (*i.e.*, diastole). In the ventricles and large arteries, the pressures continually fluctuate between the higher levels which prevail during contraction (systole) and the lower levels during relaxation (diastole). Clinically, however, systolic pressures in the ventricles and large arteries are usually designated as the highest (during systole) and diastolic pressures as the lowest (during diastole), expressed in millimeters of mercury. Thus in the left ventricle, which is a high pressure pump, typical pressures would be 120/0, while in the right ventricle, which is a low pressure pump, the corresponding pressures would be about 25/0. Normally the two ventricles are in almost identical phase and rhythm because they are compressed simultaneously by the muscular myocardium which envelops both chambers. The myocardium of the left ventricle is usually 8 to 10 mm thick, that of the right ventricle

Figure 1.2. Right and left side of the heart (semidiagrammatic). When the right and left atria (RA and LA) contract, they propel blood into the respective ventricles. When the latter contract, the right ventricle (RV) forces blood toward the lungs and the left (LV) toward the periphery. All the valves—the right and left atrioventricular (AV) valves and the pulmonary and aortic valves—are unidirectional. With the onset of systole, both ventricles contract simultaneously, the AV valves close, the aortic and pulmonary valves open and blood is ejected. Note the greater wall thickness of the left ventricle.

about 2 to 3 mm. Since the overlying muscle mass is an important factor in determining the internal pressure developed in a hollow organ, it is logical that the ratio of the peak internal pressures of the two ventricles would be similar to the ratio of their muscle thicknesses.

Distributing System. The arteries are branched, hollow cylindrical tubes. In the systemic division the largest artery (the aorta) and its arterial branches are long, rather thick-walled, high pressure conduits which transport blood over the systemic circuit to the small arteries and arterioles. Their internal pressure diminishes from about 120 mm Hg (systolic) and 80 mm Hg (diastolic) at the beginning of the aorta to a constant mean pressure of about 25 mm Hg at the arteriolar end of the capillaries. The pulmonary artery pressure, normally about 25/10 mm Hg, decreases to a mean pressure of about 10 mm Hg at the entrance to the lung capillaries. Aside from blood distribution, the arterial systems have two additional important functions; the large arteries serve a pressure-storing or "windkessel" function while the terminal arterioles provide a resistance or "stopcock" function. These aspects are described later in this chapter.

Exchange System. Capillaries are numerous, tiny, highly branched, microscopic tubes. Their very large surface area facilitates the transfer of oxygen, carbon dioxide, water, nutrients and electrolytes through their walls. The internal pressures in the capillaries range from values of approximately 25 mm Hg on the arterial side to about 10 mm Hg at their confluence on the venous side. The combined volume of the capillaries is small but their surface and cross-sectional areas are immense.

Collecting System. The collecting system, which extends from the smallest venules to the largest terminal veins in the chest (vena cavae), drains blood back to the atria. Veins are large capacity, very thin-walled cylindrical vessels; veins below the heart have one-way valves which prevent reflux and thereby assist in the transport of blood back to the heart. Their internal pressure is low, ranging from about 10 mm Hg near the capillaries to about 0 mm Hg at their entrance to the heart. In the erect subject, the vascular pressures in the lower extremities are increased due to the effect of gravity as will be discussed in Chapter 6.

Blood

Formed Elements

Blood is essentially a two-phase fluid consisting of formed cellular elements suspended in a liquid medium, the plasma. The formed elements are red cells (erythrocytes), white cells (leukocytes) and platelets. If a blood sample from a normal adult is centrifuged in a graduated test tube of uniform bore, the relative volume of the packed red blood cells, termed "hematocrit," will be about 40 to 45% of the total, as shown by the height of the packed cell column (Fig. 1.3). Thus, the red cells occupy about 40 to 45% of the total volume of blood in the body. The white cells, being less dense, will settle on top of the red cells in a thin so-called "buffy" layer. The remaining 55 to 60% is plasma, sometimes called the "plasmacrit."

The erythrocytes are biconcave discs about 2.4 μm in thickness and 8 μm in diameter which are produced in the bone marrow through a process known as erythropoiesis. Their biconcave shape increases the total surface area available for diffusion. The red cells owe their characteristic color to the presence of the pigment hemoglobin, which has a remarkable capacity to combine with and transport oxygen. In the normal adult there are about 4.5 to 5.5 million red blood cells per cubic millimeter of peripheral blood. A greater than normal red cell volume in the blood is called polycythemia. A deficiency of red blood cells is known as anemia which has pathophysiological consequences because of the accompanying hemoglobin deficiency (Fig. 1.3).

In the normal individual, there are 5,000 to 7,000 white blood cells per cubic millimeter in the peripheral blood; an excess is usually termed leukocytosis and a deficiency, leukopenia. The white cells are mainly concerned with combating bacterial infections, with immune processes

Figure 1.3. Hematocrit and red blood cells (RBCs). *Left*, The percentage of packed RBCs in the centrifuged blood samples, termed the hematocrit, is increased in polycythemia and decreased in anemia. The corresponding changes in hemoglobin content alter the oxygen carrying capacity of the blood. *Right*, Surface and cut views of red cells. RBCs sometimes gather into stacks called rouleaux which tend to offer increased resistance to flow.

and with bodily defense. Platelets are vital elements for blood coagulation; there are about 150,000 to 300,000 platelets per cubic millimeter in normal peripheral blood but because of their small size (2–3 μm) they occupy only an insignificant fraction of the blood volume.

Plasma

The plasma or fluid fraction of the blood normally occupies about 55% of the blood volume and carries a variety of substances including plasma proteins (which are the major portion of the plasma solids), nonprotein nitrogen, electrolytes, hormones, enzymes and blood gases. The normal concentrations of some of the more important constituents of plasma are given in Table 1.1.

Blood Volume

The total blood volume is the sum of the volume of the cells and plasma, both of which are usually determined by dilution methods. This involves (in the case of plasma) the injection of an amount (A) of a test

Table 1.1.
Normal Concentration of Plasma Constituents

Per dl (deciliter) plasma	
Total protein	6.0–7.8 g
Albumin	3.2–4.5 g
Globulin	2.3–3.6 g
Fibrinogen	0.2–0.4 g
Glucose (fasting)	70–110 mg
Total lipids	400–1,000 mg
Cholesterol	150–300 mg
Triglycerides	50–150 mg
Non-protein nitrogen (NPN)	20–45 mg
Blood urea nitrogen (BUN)	10–25 mg
Uric acid	3–7 mg
Creatinine	0.9–1.5 mg
Electrolytes (serum)	
Na^+	136–145 Meq/L
K^+	3.5–5.0 Meq/L
Ca^{++}	4.5–5.5 Meq/L
Cl^-	98–110 Meq/L

substance such as ^{125}I-labeled human serum albumin (HSA). After about a 10-minute mixing period, a sample of blood is withdrawn, the red cells removed by centrifugation and the plasma concentration (C) of the test substance determined. The total plasma volume (V) is then determined as: V (ml) $= A$ (mg)$/C$ (mg/ml).

The red blood cell volume can similarly be estimated with red cells labeled with radioactive chromium (^{51}Cr) using the same principle. The plasma volume, at any particular moment, represents a temporary balance between the intake of fluid and its output via kidneys, gastrointestinal tract, etc.; while it may temporarily fluctuate over a period of time, in a relatively steady state, an individual's total blood volume usually remains remarkably constant. Since values in the normal adult generally range from 70 to 75 ml/kg of body weight, a 70-kg adult might therefore have a total blood volume of about 5000 ml with about 55% or 2,750 ml of the total as plasma volume and about 45% or 2,250 ml as total red cell mass.

The dilution principle assumes that none of the indicator material is lost and that perfect mixing occurs. This is not entirely true since some of the plasma protein (with indicator attached) is slowly eliminated during the test period and some ^{51}Cr is sequestered in the spleen and other reticuloendothelial organs. For more accurate determinations of cell and plasma volumes, the blood concentrations of the indicator material are followed over a 30- or 60-minute period, plotted against time on log graph paper and the original concentration estimated by extrapolating backward to zero time.

Volume and Pressure

Volume and Pressure Distribution

The most important physical characteristics of the circulation are volume, pressure and flow. Volume and volume-pressure relations comprise the *statics* of the system and define the basic qualities which distinguish important functional properties of arteries and veins. Pressure and flow relate to the moving stream of blood and so characterize the *dynamics* of the circulation.

In the circulatory system, about two-thirds of the blood, *i.e.*, about 3,300 ml, is on the venous side (Fig. 1.4). Because the lungs (very vascular organs) and many large capacity vessels are in the chest, about a quarter of the total blood volume, or approximately 1,250 ml, is in the thorax and comprises the thoracic blood volume (TBV).

It has been estimated that in a normal 70-kg adult with a TBV of 1,250 ml, about 350 ml are contained in the vena cavae and right heart and serve, in a sense, as immediate right heart reserve. This means that in case of stress, when more cardiac output may be needed, this volume can be drawn upon to increase right ventricular filling and filling pressure. About 900 ml are contained in the pulmonary artery, lungs, pulmonary veins and left heart and similarly serve as immediate reserve

Figure 1.4.   Distribution of blood volume in the systemic circulation. Not shown is the 8% fraction in the pulmonary vessels.

for the left ventricle. TBV, which is frequently referred to as central blood volume (CBV), thus constitutes an immediate source of filling pressure and volume for the two ventricles. This ready reserve is highly important since ventricular filling is a critical determinant of stroke volume and cardiac output (see Chapter 5, Intrinsic Regulation of Heart).

The thoracic (or central) blood volume, being at low pressure, is easily dislocated. About half of the TBV (500–700 ml) gravitates to the lower extremities when in the upright position as described in the section on postural effects (Chapter 13). Although this blood remains within the circulatory system, it is less readily available to the heart. Its dislocation, therefore, reduces both the volume and the pressure of the central venous reservoir for cardiac filling, which will cause about a 20% to 25% reduction in cardiac output. For the normal adult this does not pose a circulatory problem, but in certain cardiovascular disorders this becomes a significant stress (Chapter 13). Similarly, in case of hemorrhage or dehydration, *i.e.*, whenever general venous volume or pressure decreases, TBV is relocated into the general circulation to bolster general venous volume. In the supine position, in overhydration, during water immersion or in congestive heart failure, *i.e.*; whenever extrathoracic venous volume is increased, thoracic blood volume and pressure rise.

Volume-Pressure Relations in Blood Vessels

Although about two-thirds of the blood volume is normally in the venous system and only about one-sixth on the arterial side, the pressure distribution is quite different, being in an almost inverse relation to the volume distribution (Fig. 1.5). This disposition of pressure and volume is due in large part to the structure and relative elasticity of the arteries and veins, that is, to their pressure-volume relations. While it is true that the entire arterial tree serves as a distributing conduit, all arteries are not alike. From an anatomical and functional standpoint they may be divided into two main groups which differ structurally and functionally from each other, and both of which, in turn, differ notably from veins.

1. Aorta and Large Arteries. All blood vessels have an endothelial lining and contain varying proportions of smooth muscle, elastin and collagen; however, the aorta and the large arteries have unusually large amounts of elastin in their walls and thus are capable of considerable expansion and recoil. This quality enables them to store pressure energy as their walls are stretched during ventricular systolic ejection; with subsequent rebound of the vessel wall, this pressure energy can then be released as kinetic energy of flow in the succeeding diastole. This helps

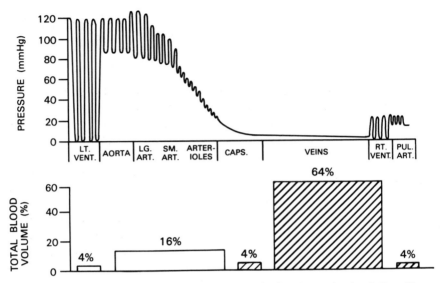

Figure 1.5. Pressure and volume distribution in the systemic circulation. Illustrating the inverse relationship between internal pressure and volume in different portions of the circulatory system.

to propel the blood toward the tissues during the diastolic phase of the cardiac cycle and promotes a more even flow to the capillaries. The large arteries are therefore the "pressure storers" of the circulation. As previously mentioned, the internal pressure in the large arteries is normally about 120/80 mm Hg.

2. Small Arteries and Arterioles. These vessels have fewer elastic fibers and more circular smooth muscle fibers. They have, therefore, contractile capabilities which, when activated, serve to constrict their lumen, dam back the flow, increase the pressure centrally (toward the heart) and decrease the pressure peripherally (toward the capillaries). These vessels thus serve as the "stopcocks" of the circulation and are usually called the "resistance" vessels. Their pressures generally range from 60 to 90 mm Hg in the small arteries to 40 to 60 mm Hg in the arterioles.

3. Veins. The veins are very thin-walled vessels with only small amounts of elastin and limited smooth muscle in their walls. Their pressures are low, ranging from about 10 mm Hg at the venular ends of the capillaries to about 0 mm Hg at the entrance of the vena cavae to the heart. As indicated in Figure 1.5, the venous system normally contains about four times more blood than the arterial system; yet, if more fluid or blood is infused into the vascular system, 90% of the new fluid will be taken up by the veins because of their great distensibility.

Because of this property, the veins are known as the "volume storers" of the circulation.

Distensibility and Compliance of Blood Vessels

In order to compare more precisely the volume and pressure characteristics of blood vessels, their "distensibility," that is, the increase in volume necessary to induce a unit pressure change, may be determined. If a large artery or vein is removed, tied at both ends and blood or fluid injected slowly into the lumen, the internal pressure will increase progressively as volume is added. If the percentage of volume change is plotted against the internal (transmural) pressure, pressure-volume or distensibility curves similar to those in Figure 1.6 will result.

The slope of the curve at any point (ratio of percentage of volume increase to pressure increase), which is a measure of the distensibility, varies with the degree of filling. The normal young aorta has good distensibility and recoil at normal physiological pressures of about 75 to 150 mm Hg (Fig. 1.6*A*), which gives it the important property of a "pressure storer." However, at higher pressures such as 200 mm Hg,

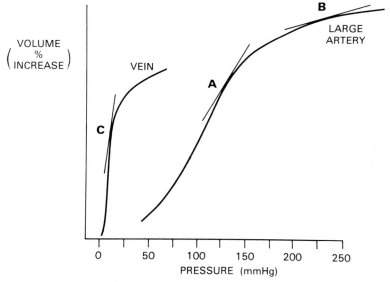

Figure 1.6. Distensibility (percentage of volume increase per unit pressure change) in a normal large artery and vein. Note the decreased slope of the arterial curve at higher pressure (*B*). Also the steep slope and much higher distensibility of the veins (*C*) at their physiological pressures (0–10 mm Hg) compared to the slope and distensibility of arteries (*A*) at their usual pressures (75–150 mm Hg).

when it is "overfilled," (Fig. 1.6*B*), its wall becomes more rigid and has lesser distensibility, a smaller slope and less recoil.

In the latter case, the expandable qualities of elastin in the arterial wall are limited by the less expandable collagen and smooth muscle which, when stretched, reaches its limits and resists further distension. Distensibility is influenced, therefore, not only by the thickness and composition of the vessel wall but also by the degree of filling of the vessel.

As illustrated in Figure 1.6*C*, veins at their physiological pressures (0–10 mm Hg) have a high distensibility, ranging from 6 to 8 times that of arteries. However, vessels do not begin to show distensibility until they are filled. Since the veins have, in addition, about 3 to 4 times more volume than the arteries, the capacity of the venous system for storage of blood is about 25 to 30 times that of the arterial system and accounts for the primary function of veins as "volume storers" of the circulation.

"Compliance" and "capacitance," terms which are similar but not identical with distensibility, may be defined as the volume change per unit pressure change when fluid is added. These terms are commonly used to measure the expandability of vessels or of organ systems such as lungs. However compliance and capacitance have the disadvantage of defining the pressure-volume relationship without reference to the size of the vessel; obviously a given increment of volume will induce a much larger pressure rise in a smaller vessel than a large one so that the smaller vessel may have an apparently lesser compliance. For this reason "distensibility" or the *percentage* of volume change per unit of pressure, permits a more logical comparison of vessels of different sizes and types.

Distensibility may be altered by age, disease, autonomic stimulation and various drugs. In the elderly, the arterial walls become infiltrated with less distensible fibrous tissue which increases their stiffness (Fig. 1.7). This can affect pressure and flow relations in the entire arterial tree. This lesser distensibility at increased age is offset to some extent by the increased volume of the aorta in older individuals since this increased volume enables the aorta to accommodate the ejected left ventricular blood with less increase in pressure. However, the increased rigidity of the aorta coupled with the greater vascular resistance of the arteries constitute a significantly greater impedance to left ventricular ejection in the older subject, which is undoubtedly a considerable factor in increasing cardiac work and limiting left ventricular function in the elderly (see Chapter 12, Aging).

Oxygen Transport

Although the assimilation and transport of oxygen is a definitive part of respiratory physiology, its importance to the normal and abnormal circulation warrants a brief review.

YEARS

20-24

29-31

36-42

47-52

71-78

Figure 1.7. Decrease in aortic distensibility with advancing age. Note particularly the changes in distensibility within the physiological pressure range of 75 to 150 mm Hg and the greater differences at the higher pressures. (Reprinted with permission from P. Hallock and J.C. Benson, *J Clin Invest* 16: 597, 1937.)

The chief constituent of the erythrocyte is hemoglobin (Hb), the primary oxygen carrier, which is normally present in a concentration of 14 to 15 g/dl of whole blood. Hb combines reversibly with oxygen to form oxyhemoglobin (HbO$_2$), the primary oxygen carrier. When exposed to certain drugs and other oxidizing agents, Hb is converted to a darker colored methemoglobin, which is present in only very small amounts in normal blood. Because Hb has a higher affinity for carbon monoxide, it can displace the O$_2$ to form carboxyhemoglobin; thus, exposure to excessive amounts of carbon monoxide can significantly reduce the oxygen-carrying capacity of the blood.

If blood is exposed to a sufficiently high oxygen pressure so that all the Hb is combined with oxygen to form HbO$_2$, it is "fully saturated"; under these circumstances, 1 g of Hb can combine with 1.39 ml of oxygen so that blood with a Hb concentration of 15 g/dl will then have an "oxygen capacity" of 20.8 ml/dl of blood or 20.8 vol %. The amount of oxygen with which each unit of Hb will actually combine is dependent primarily on the partial pressure of oxygen (Po$_2$) to which the Hb is exposed. This relationship is defined by the oxygen dissociation curve (Fig. 1.8).

Figure 1.8. *Left*, Oxygen dissociation curve showing the relationship between the partial pressure of oxygen (Po₂) and the percentage of oxyhemoglobin (HbO₂) saturation of the blood. In the alveoli of the lungs (*A*) the Po₂ is about 100 mm Hg which results in 97% HbO₂ saturation. In the mixed venous blood returning from the tissues, the Po₂ has fallen to about 40 mm Hg and the HbO₂ saturation is approximately 75% (*V*). *Right*, Small shifts of the curve to the right, which occur in the tissues because of the lower pH, higher PCO₂ and higher temperature, tend to lessen the affinity of Hb for oxygen and assist in release of oxygen to the tissues. (Adapted from J.B. West, *Respiratory Physiology*, Baltimore: Williams & Wilkins, 1979, p. 75.)

In the alveoli of the lungs, where the Po₂ is normally at a high level, the blood will be about 97% saturated, *i.e.*, 97% of Hb is combined with O₂ (*A* in Fig. 1.8). In this case arterial blood with a Hb concentration of 15 g/dl will have an oxygen content of 20.2 ml/dl. After the blood has given up some of its oxygen in the tissues and reached the large veins (mixed venous blood) its Po₂ value will have decreased to about 40 mm Hg. As indicated in Figure 1.8, *V*, at this Po₂ the blood will be only about 75% saturated with oxygen and the blood oxygen content will be about 16 ml/dl; therefore, this blood will have released to the tissues about 4 ml of gaseous oxygen for each 100 ml of blood flow through the capillaries.

While oxygen content is determined primarily by the Po₂, it is also influenced to a lesser extent by four other factors: pH, PCO₂, blood temperature and the concentration of 2,3-diphosphoglycerate (2,3-DPG). An increased red cell concentration of the organic phosphate, 2,3-DPG, may occur in chronic hypoxia or chronic lung disease.

A decrease in pH or an increase in any of the other three will produce a "shift to the right" in the oxyhemoglobin dissociation curve (Fig. 1.8); the result is that at the same Po_2, less O_2 will be bound to the Hb and consequently more released to the tissues which results in a lesser affinity of Hb for O_2. Conversely, an increase in pH or a decrease in Pco_2, blood temperature or 2,3-DPG will have the opposite effect, *i.e.*, the dissociation curve will shift to the left, so there is greater affinity of hemoglobin for oxygen.

The shape of the oxygen dissociation curve has other implications; at the upper "plateau" portion of the curve where it is flatter, large changes in Po_2 will have relatively little effect on HbO_2 saturation and content. As a result, moderate decreases in Po_2 encountered at high altitude or other low oxygen environments result in smaller reductions in HbO_2 saturation and content than would ordinarily be the case, so that the hypoxia will be partially "buffered." On the other hand, in the capillaries, where the Po_2 falls sharply, as represented by the steep portion of the curve, the tissues have the advantage of being able to pick up a large supply of oxygen with only a small decrease in Po_2.

References

Bader H. Anatomy and physiology of vascular wall. In: *Handbook of Physiology*, Section 2: *Circulation*, edited by WF Hamilton and P Dow. Washington, D.C.: American Physiological Society, 1963, Vol. II, pp. 865–889.

Burton AC. *Physiology and Biophysics of the Circulation.* Chicago: Year Book Medical Publishers, 1972, pp. 66–67, 119–120.

Honig CR. *Modern Cardiovascular Physiology.* Boston: Little, Brown, 1981, pp. 127–136.

Yu PN. *Pulmonary Blood Volume in Health and Disease.* Philadelphia: Lea & Febiger, 1969.

West JB. *Respiratory Physiology—The Essentials.* Baltimore: Williams & Wilkins, 1979, 2nd ed., pp. 70–74.

chapter 2

Hemodynamics

Poiseuille's Law

In 1846, Poiseuille, a French physician, described the factors governing non-pulsatile flow of a homogeneous fluid through rigid tubes. He stated that if all other factors are held constant, the rate of flow, Q, through a cylindrical tube of length, L, and radius, r, was directly proportional to the driving pressure, ΔP (the difference in pressure between two ends of the tube). In addition, Q was inversely proportional to the length of the tube, L, inversely proportional to the viscosity of the flowing liquid, η, and directly proportional to the fourth power of the radius of the tube, r.

He added two necessary proportionality constants (π and 8) to elaborate "Poiseuille's law": $Q = \Delta P r^4 \pi / \eta L 8$. (Fig. 2.1).

Although blood is a non-homogeneous fluid, which in the body flows through branching, distensible tubes in a pulsatile manner, Poiseuille's law nonetheless gives good approximations and has proven very useful in understanding the *in vivo* circulation. Furthermore most of the factors in his equation are analogous to an ordinary hydraulic system and lend themselves to simplifications which may profitably be applied to basic and clinical cardiovascular problems.

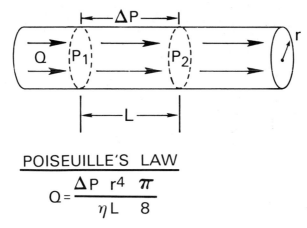

POISEUILLE'S LAW

$$Q = \frac{\Delta P \; r^4 \; \pi}{\eta L \quad 8}$$

Figure 2.1. Poiseuille's law. In an artificial system, flow through a cylindrical tube or any segment of a tube is directly proportional to ΔP, the driving pressure along the tube, and the fourth power of the radius, r. Flow is inversely proportional to L, the length of the segment and to η, the viscosity of the liquid. The proportionality constant is $\pi/8$.

Resistance to Flow

If ΔP in Poiseuille's equation is considered to be the driving pressure, the remaining factors, $r^4/\eta L$, may be considered impediments to flow. If these residual factors are collected together, inverted $\left[\dfrac{\eta L}{r^4}\right]$ and designated R, as resistance to flow, the formula can then be simplified to: Q (flow) $= \Delta P$(driving pressure)$/R$ (resistance to flow), and by transposing: R (resistance to flow) $= \Delta P$ (driving pressure)$/Q$ (flow).

In this very basic and useful hemodynamic generalization, R is defined as that resistance provided by a vessel or circulatory bed, which permits a given pressure differential to produce a unit flow. It will be recalled that this equation is an analogue of Ohm's law, which states that with direct current, the electrical resistance, R (in ohms), is the ratio of electromotive force (in volts) and the current (in amperes).

By generalizing from an isolated cylindrical tube to the intact circulation in an organ or in the entire circulatory system, the vascular resistance to flow may similarly be estimated as the ratio of the pressure gradient across the organ or system and the blood flow through it. When this method of calculation is used, resistance is sometimes expressed in PRU units (pressure-resistance units) which are defined as mm Hg/ml of flow/min. An adult human, for example, with a mean aortic pressure of 100 mm Hg and a mean right atrial pressure of 0 mm Hg, would have a pressure gradient across the systemic circulation of 100 mm Hg

(ΔP). If the cardiac output were 5 L/min, the total peripheral resistance (TPR) of the system would be: TPR = 100 mm Hg/5,000 ml/min or 0.02 mm Hg/ml/min or 0.02 PRU units.

Although the concept of vascular resistance is commonly employed in basic cardiovascular studies, its clinical application has been somewhat limited because measurements of flow, particularly in individual organs and tissues, are still technically rather difficult.

In comparing vascular resistances of different organs and organisms, it should be noted that blood flow (the denominator) is strongly influenced by the size and vascularity of the organ while arterial pressure (the numerator) is not. Thus an infant with a body weight and cardiac output only ½₀ that of an adult will have a calculated total vascular resistance much greater than the adult even though the relative dimensions of vessels and tissues as well as flow per unit mass may be generally similar. For this reason, when comparing organisms, vascular resistance is usually expressed on a weight basis, *e.g.*, per 100 g of tissue.

Components of Vascular Resistance

In the previous discussion of Poiseuille's law, the question of what actually constitutes resistance was temporarily bypassed. In transposing Poiseuille's law, the vascular resistance became $R = \eta L/r^4$.

It is seen that η, the viscosity, is the fluid resistance factor and L/r^4, the blood vessel resistance factor. While it seems reasonable that the viscosity and length of the system would be important in determining resistance to flow, the disproportionate role of the radius—which makes it the predominant factor in the equation—is rather surprising. The fourth power effect is due to the fact that flow in a cylinder is proportional, not to the radius of the tube, but to its cross-sectional area, which is an r^2 factor ($A = \pi r^2$); in addition, flow is a function of the velocity of the moving column; which in turn is proportional to the square of the distance from the axis to the vessel wall. The combination of these two r^2 terms and the consequent magnification of the radius factor has important implications for the control of flow in the intact organism.

Within the same vascular bed over a short period of time, neither length of the circuit nor blood viscosity would ordinarily change appreciably; the most important adjustment of vascular resistance, therefore, is accomplished by alteration of vessel diameter. A decrease in lumen diameter is brought about by contraction of the smooth muscle of the vessel wall (vasoconstriction) which increases resistance to flow; relaxation of the tone of the muscle (vasodilation) increases the lumen size and, therefore, decreases resistance. Thus, alteration of vascular resistance to an organ is almost entirely a function of the adjustment of the caliber of blood vessels. By virtue of this radius effect, large changes in resistance to flow can be brought about quickly with small changes in vessel diameter.

In addition to the calculation of total peripheral resistance (TPR) described above, how can we estimate the resistance (R) of a part of the circuit, *i.e.*, determine the distribution of the resistance? If we assume a constant flow (Q) through all the collective cross sections of the entire circulation (Fig. 2.2), and if $R = \Delta P/Q$, the greatest resistance will lie in that segment in which the pressure fall is the greatest (the arterioles) and the resistance is least where the pressure fall is least (the aorta) (Fig. 2.2).

Series and Parallel Resistances

In a manner analogous to electrical circuits, vascular resistances may be in series or parallel. If in series, the resistances are additive, but when in parallel they are additive as reciprocals so that $1/R_T = 1/R_1 + 1/R_2 + 1/R_3$ (etc.) This means that in a parallel circuit, R_T is less than any of the individual R terms.

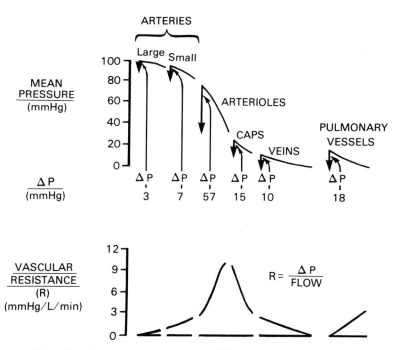

Figure 2.2.   *Top,* Vascular resistances in different segments of the circulation. The pressure fall (ΔP) is shown in different parts of the circulation and is least in the aorta and the greatest at the arteriolar level. *Center,* If the ΔP values are divided by the cardiac output (5 L/min) which will be constant through all the segments, the vascular resistance of the different segments (*bottom*) can be estimated. As expected, it is least in the aorta and highest in the arterioles.

Viewed as a total system, the large majority of the vascular resistances of the organs and tissues of the body are in parallel. For the circulatory system this provides a significant advantage, not only because greater flow can be achieved with small changes of pressure but also because parallel vascular circuits permit greater flexibility in the control of flow to individual beds (Fig. 2.3). Thus, through manipulation of resistances, flow through one circuit can be increased or decreased without necessarily affecting the proximal arterial pressure or flow through other parallel circuits. For example, in Figure 2.3 (parallel resistances), if R_1 is increased, flow through that circuit is decreased without affecting the driving pressure ΔP or the resultant flow across circuits 2 and 3. By contrast, increase in R_1 in the series conduit (Fig. 2.3) will reduce flow to all the downstream circuits. Because of the awkwardness of adding reciprocals, the conductances of parallel circuits ($G = 1/R$) are sometimes used in place of resistances for hemodynamic calculations.

In the above, it was emphasized that a decreasing vessel radius greatly increases vascular resistance; however, it should be recalled that this applies only to a single tube system. In the intact organism, we know that while vessel radii decrease, the number and cross-sectional area of the vessels increase considerably as we move from aorta to capillary and furthermore, as mentioned above, their parallel arrangement decreases

Figure 2.3. Vascular resistances in series and in parallel. *Top,* If across each series resistance, the driving pressure, (ΔP), is 3 mm and the flow (Q) 1 ml/min, then each resistance (R) would be $\Delta P/Q$ or 3 mm Hg/ml/min and R_T (total resistance) = 9 mm Hg/ml/min. *Bottom,* In parallel resistances, if across each resistance the driving pressure (ΔP) were 3 mm Hg and the flow (Q) 1 ml/min, then the total resistance is calculated as $1/R_1 + 1/R_2 + 1/R_3$ or 1 mm Hg/ml/min. Note that when the three resistances are in parallel, the total resistance is only $\frac{1}{9}$ of that which would prevail if the three resistances were in series (*i.e.,* the ratio of $R_p/R_s = \frac{1}{9}$) so that it takes a ΔP of only 1 mm Hg (instead of 9 mm Hg) to produce a flow of 1 ml/min.

their resistance. Theoretical quantitative analyses of these two diverse factors indicate that despite the great increase in the number and cross-sectional area of vessels, there is a net increase in vascular resistance from the aorta down the arterial tree. This is further evidence of the disproportionate resistance effect of the smaller radii on flow. It should also be pointed out that these factors do not negate the empirical usefulness of regional or total resistance calculations done on the same organism, *e.g.*, in pressure-flow studies described below, in which the formula $R = \Delta P/Q$ is used.

Figure 2.4 is a diagrammatic sketch of the main circulatory resistances of the body. Although the great majority of vascular circuits are in parallel, in certain organs such as the kidney and liver, the blood traverses two capillary beds in tandem so that their resistances are in series. The result of this is that the second capillary bed has a lower pressure and lesser ability to increase its flow when such increases are needed.

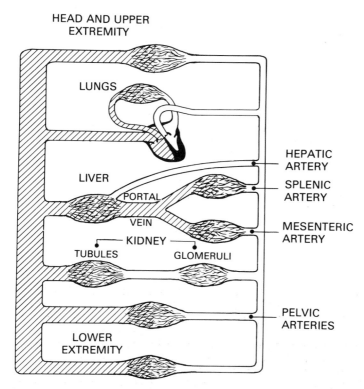

Figure 2.4. Diagrammatic sketch of vascular resistances in the body showing parallel and series circuits. Note the predominance of parallel circuits.

Vascular Impedance

The resistance to flow (R), which was defined above as the ratio of the mean values of $\Delta P/Q$, resides mainly in the arterioles and applies only to a steady-flow system. But what about vascular resistance to pulsatile flow, *e.g.*, in the aorta, where it is most marked? The opposition to this type of flow offered by the aorta and arterial bed is termed "impedance," which may be defined simply as pulsatile resistance or the resistance to phasic flow.

The major determinants of aortic impedance are (a) the viscoelastic properties of the aorta and large arterial vessels, (b) the inertia and viscosity of the blood, (c) the reflection of the flow and pressure waves back through the arterial tree from the periphery and (d) the peripheral vascular resistance. Thus, aortic impedance depends partly on the frequency of the arterial pressure and flow curves and their relationship. Because these are complex waves, the quantitative analysis of aortic impedance depends on precisely timed biophysical measurements of pressure and flow at multiple points in the flow tract.

Such analyses have shown that pulsatile resistance (impedance) is much higher than resistance would be at equivalent steady-flow levels. But in spite of the fact that oscillatory flow is mechanically much less efficient than steady laminar flow, numerous investigators have reported that the mammalian organism apparently functions best when blood flow is pulsatile.

Recent investigators have indicated that in normal aging and in certain circulatory diseases such as hypertension, the decreased compliance of the aorta and large arteries combined with increased peripheral resistance elevate aortic impedance to the point where left ventricular ejection is severely handicapped. Some investigators have proposed that these impedance defects may be the critical factors in the declining ventricular performance in such conditions. Because of the technical difficulty of measuring vascular impedance, relatively few studies of this type have been made thus far in clinical situations. However, the increasing efforts now being expended in this direction will undoubtedly assist in determining more precisely the possible role of vascular impedance in circulatory disease.

Viscosity

As indicated in Poiseuille's equation, the resistance to flow due to the friction of molecules in the moving stream is known as the viscosity. In a homogeneous liquid such as water, in an artificial system, viscosity is a constant. However, in the case of a two-phase medium such as blood flowing in an *in vivo* circulatory system viscosity is not constant but depends on several factors: (a) the concentration of the suspended medium (the cells), (b) the velocity of flow and (c) the radius of the vessel.

If measured with reference to water, as is commonly done, the relative viscosity of plasma is about 1.3. The relative viscosity of whole blood depends mainly on the cell concentration or hematocrit as shown in Figure 2.5. At normal hematocrits of 42 to 45, the relative viscosity of blood is about 3.6 compared to water. However, because the relationship is exponential, an increase of 10 in the hematocrit from the level of 40 will increase the viscosity about 25% and an increase of 20 to the level of 60 will increase viscosity about 60%.

In low hematocrit states such as anemia, viscosity, and therefore vascular resistance, both fall, resulting in increased cardiac output. In high hematocrit conditions such as polycythemia and leukemia in which hematocrit levels may reach 60 to 70%, a profound increase in systemic and pulmonary vascular resistance occurs with a resultant elevation of blood pressure.

Vessel bore and flow rate are two additional factors affecting blood viscosity in a two-phase medium. In tubes less than 200 μm in diameter—which would include arterioles, capillaries and venules—the relative viscosity of the blood decreases and offers less resistance to flow. This phenomenon, for which there is no satisfactory explanation, is sometimes called the Fahraeus-Lindqvist effect.

A further peculiarity of two-phase fluids such as blood is that at low flow rates, the apparent viscosity increases (anomalous viscosity). This

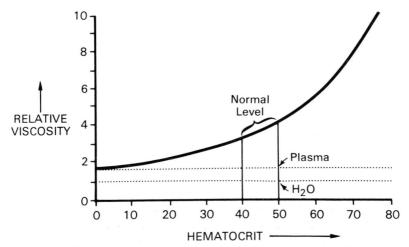

Figure 2.5. Effect of hematocrit on relative viscosity of blood. Note that as hematocrit increases, the relative viscosity increases disproportionately.

phenomenon has been attributed to the disposition of red cells in the flowing stream; at higher velocities the cells accumulate in the axial part of the stream but at low velocities assume a more even distribution and hence offer greater flow resistance. Another factor that is probably involved in anomalous viscosity is the tendency of erythrocytes to aggregate into stacks or "rouleaux" at lower flow velocities (Fig. 1.3). This effect has been found by some investigators to be exaggerated in low flow states such as burns or shock, causing pronounced cell clumping or "sludge" in the microcirculation with severe hindrance to flow and a resultant ischemia of the tissue.

It should also be mentioned that in the capillary bed, the blood hematocrit is usually about 10% less than in the large vessels for reasons which are not well understood at present.

It is evident, therefore, that in different parts of the circulation, there will be significant variations in vessel diameter, flow velocity and hematocrit and that the net effect on viscosity is not always predictable. Present evidence suggests, however, that the hematocrit effect on viscosity is the most important and predominant one.

Under special circumstances, temperature may affect blood viscosity in a significant manner. There is about a 2% rise in viscosity per 1°C fall in temperature. During prolonged exposure to cold and high wind, the extremities will become chilled and the reduced flow effect of vasoconstriction will be enhanced by the increased vascular resistance resulting from the heightened viscosity. In addition, the shift of the HbO_2 dissociation curve to the left and consequent lesser release of O_2 to the tissues at the same Po_2 (Fig. 1.8) will intensify the ischemia and increase the possibility of frostbite and serious damage to the part.

Flow Velocity and Turbulence

The linear velocity of blood flow varies widely in the circulatory system—from a mean value of about 30 to 35 cm/sec in the aorta to about 0.2 to 0.3 mm/sec in the capillaries as illustrated in Figure 2.6. If we assume that equal volumes will be transported through the collective segments of the circulation in equal times, the mean flow velocity ($\bar{V}$) will vary inversely with the cross-sectional area; *i.e.*, $\bar{V}$ (mm/sec) = flow (ml/sec)/cross-sectional area (πr^2 in mm^2).

By transposing the factors in the above equation, the circulation time (CT) between two points (A and B) in a closed circulation can be calculated as the quotient of the volume contained between A and B and the mean rate of flow between the two points, *i.e.*, CT in sec = volume (A to B) in ml/mean flow (A to B) in ml/sec. In states of circulatory failure, an increased CT for the systemic circulation is usually

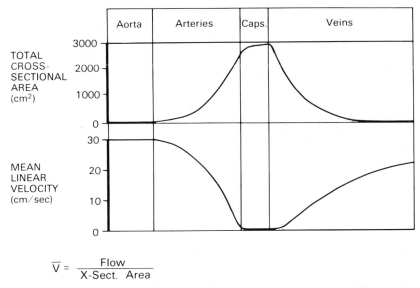

$$\overline{V} = \frac{Flow}{X\text{-Sect. Area}}$$

Figure 2.6. Relation of cross-sectional area and mean velocity of flow in the systemic circulation.

an index of decreased total flow, *i.e.*, of low cardiac output and inadequate circulation.

Poiseuille's law assumes that the different layers of molecules move parallel to each other in longitudinal streamlines, somewhat resembling concentric sleeves. The molecules adjacent to the vessel wall are stationary; each succeeding layer has increasing velocity with the maximum at the axis. Under these circumstances of "streamline" flow, the frictional resistance is independent of the pressure-flow relations and thus in the case of a homogeneous fluid is linear as has been previously described.

However, under certain circumstances, particularly at high velocities, the flow is no longer streamline but becomes turbulent with swirls and eddies (Fig. 2.7). In this case flow is approximately proportional to the square root of the pressure gradient rather than the pressure itself; the turbulent stream now offers a considerable increase in resistance.

Reynolds has defined the factors affecting this phenomenon and stated that turbulence is likely to occur in a moving stream when the Reynolds ratio (R_e) exceeds a value of about 1,000 for blood or 2,000 for homogeneous fluids: $R_e = \sigma \times v \times D/\eta$ in which σ is the density of the fluid (g/cm^3), v is the average velocity (cm/sec), D is the diameter of the vessel (cm) and η is the fluid viscosity (g/sec/cm^2). Since blood density is relatively constant, the factors tending to increase the Reynolds number and cause it to exceed the R_e are increased velocity of flow

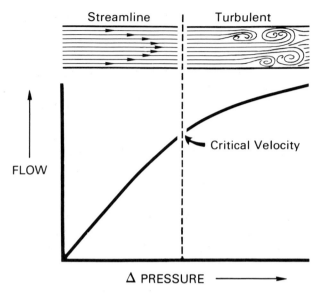

Figure 2.7.   Relationship between velocity of flow and turbulence. (Reprinted with permission from T.C. Ruch and H.D. Patton, *Physiology and Biophysics*, Philadelphia: W.B. Saunders, 1974.)

(such as in larger blood vessels), decrease in viscosity such as in anemia, and a decrease in radius of the vessel such as a stenosis (fixation) of a heart valve or coarctation (fibrotic constriction) of a blood vessel such as the aorta.

From the clinical standpoint, an important factor is that streamline flow is silent but turbulence produces noise which can often be heard with the unaided ear or with a stethoscope. Sounds used in the conventional determination of arterial blood pressure are audible because of the turbulence induced in the flow stream. In circulatory disease, defects in valves and constrictions of orifices will produce additional abnormal sounds which are used in clinical diagnosis (Chapter 3).

Rheology (the study of flow characteristics and deformation) and its application to human disease is an important area of current research. It is known, for example, that atherosclerotic lesions are often localized in the region of orifices, bends and branch points of arteries. Rheological studies now indicate that in these regions, the high pressure, high velocity stream in large arteries may subject the wall to continuous pressure stresses. These local injuries increase the permeability of the endothelium to plasma lipoproteins, thus greatly accelerating the atherosclerotic process at these sites.

Tension in the Blood Vessel Wall—Laplace's Theorem

Consideration has previously been given to the internal volume and pressure of a blood vessel but not to the vessel wall itself, which obviously is a key factor. In a hollow cylindrical tube, the circumferential tension, T, in the wall along the linear axis of a vessel is usually measured in dynes/cm and is calculated as the product of the transmural pressure, P_t (inside pressure minus outside pressure) and the radius, R (Fig. 2.8). This relationship (first defined by Laplace) was later expanded by Frank to include the factor of wall thickness "μ" as follows: $T = P_t R/\mu$. This relationship suggests that in normal vessels in which the radius and wall thickness are in approximate proportion, the wall tension will vary with the transmural pressure and the two will tend to stay in reasonable balance. A capillary, for example, with a small radius and low pressure will require only a thin wall to sustain its lesser tension but a large artery with a greater pressure and radius will have a higher tension and a need for a thicker wall.

Wall tension may be important in certain pathological conditions such as severe arteriosclerotic disease in which an aortic wall may

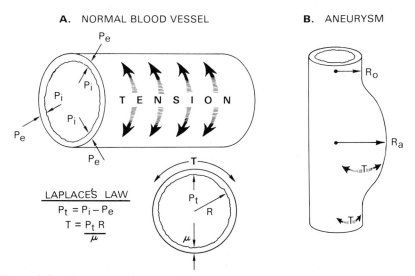

Figure 2.8. Pressure-volume-tension relations in blood vessels (Laplace's law). *Left* (A), P_t, the transmural pressure (dynes/cm^2) is equal to the P_i (internal pressure) minus the P_e (external pressure). R is the radius (cm) and μ, the wall thickness (cm). T is the tension in the vessel wall (dynes/cm of longitudinal length). *Right* (B), Aortic aneurysm is the atherosclerotic weakening of the vessel with resultant bulging. The increased radius R_a at the aneurysm site increases tension at that point and puts further stress on the aortic wall.

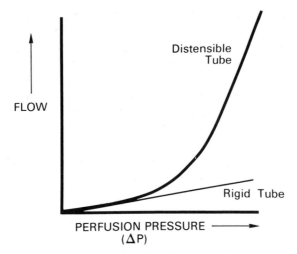

Figure 2.9. Pressure-flow curves in an artificial system using rigid and distensible tubes. Note that with increase in perfusion pressure, there is a large increase in flow in the distensible tube.

weaken, gradually bulge and become thinner at that point. With increasing radius and the progressive thinning, the tension at that site will further increase and the aorta may balloon and develop an "aneurysm" which might require surgical repair to prevent a rupture.

In congestive heart disease, the progressively increasing size of the failing heart may also produce inordinate tension in the wall of the heart. Because myocardial oxygen requirements are partly a function of myocardial tension, a reduction in heart size through medication will often promote increased cardiac efficiency by reducing wall tension and, therefore, reducing oxygen requirements per unit of mechanical work of the heart (see Chapter 14, Congestive Heart Failure).

Pressure-Flow Curves

The vascular resistance of an organ, tissue or entire organism is determined mainly by the caliber of the blood vessels, particularly the arterioles. The caliber of the arterioles is determined by the "tonus" or contraction state of the vascular smooth muscle. The tone of the vascular muscle is, in turn, the result of a balance between the inherent tone due to the muscle itself, the sympathetic efferent vasoconstrictor impulses to the vessel and the effects of humoral agents such as catecholamines, angiotensin and local metabolites (Chapter 9).

In certain experimental and clinical situations, it is advantageous to measure peripheral vascular resistance. In the treatment of hypertension, *e.g.*, it is useful to know whether the high arterial pressure is due to excess vascular resistance or increased cardiac output. In peripheral vascular disease it would be helpful to periodically quantitate the degree of vascular resistance of the region in order to follow the course of the disease or the effectiveness of various types of therapy. In the development of new vasoactive drugs, it is important to assess the ability of the drugs to produce or reverse a state of vasoconstriction. Therefore, attempts are often made to determine the pressure-flow relations of an organ, tissue or entire circulatory system.

If a homogeneous fluid is perfused through a rigid tube and the radius and length of the cylinder and the fluid viscosity kept constant, the flow as predicted by Poiseuille's law will vary directly with the pressure gradient ΔP, so that a straight-line relationship will result (Fig. 2.9). However, if the tube is distensible, the radius of the vessel will increase as the perfusion and the transmural pressure increase; the resultant flow will then increase according to the fourth power of the radius.

With *in vivo* systems, resistance to flow will be influenced not only by the distensibility of the vessels but also, as previously discussed, by the effect of vessel caliber and flow velocity. Flow resistance is also influenced by the type of tissue involved. In lung or skin tissue, for example, if perfusion rates are altered gradually rather than abruptly so that the vessels are permitted to adapt, a pressure-flow curve similar to that shown in Figure 2.10*a* will result.

In the normal resting tissue (Fig. 2.10*a*) the curve is exponential and convex to the pressure axis; thus, the flow through the tissue rises disproportionately with increasing perfusion pressure (ΔP) due to the increased distension of the vessels as described above. This is a "passive" type of pressure-flow curve. In other tissues which show "autoregulation" the pressure-flow curve will have a different configuration (Chapter 9).

A pressure-flow perfusion system similar to this is frequently used to test the pharmacological effects of drugs on vascular smooth muscle. Injection of a constrictor agent such as norepinephrine will reduce the caliber of vessels and shift the curve to the right (Fig. 2.10*c*), *i.e.*, there will be less flow per unit pressure and the resistance of the bed will be increased. Similarly if a vasodilating drug such as histamine is injected (Fig. 2.10*d*) there will be a reduction in the pressure-flow ratio and lesser resistance to flow.

It will be noted that these pressure-flow curves do not go through the origin, that is, flow goes to zero while there is still positive pressure in the perfusion system. The reason that this phenomenon occurs in certain tissues is not known. One theory is that as the vascular smooth muscle contracts, its inherent constrictive force and the resultant tension of the

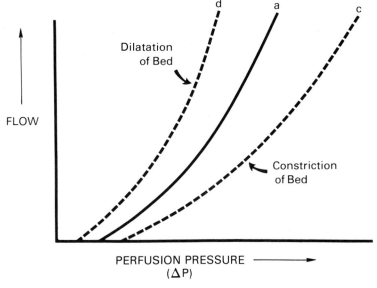

Figure 2.10. Pressure-flow curve of cutaneous vascular bed. As perfusion pressure is increased, the flow to the vascular bed increases disproportionately, *i.e.*, the peripheral resistance decreases. If a vasoconstrictor drug is injected, the pressure-flow curve changes from *a* to *c* indicating a general increase in vascular resistance. After a vasodilator drug, the pressure-flow curve will resemble that shown at *d*.

wall become greater than the distending force of the internal pressure; as the lumen becomes smaller, the tension becomes disproportionately greater than the distending pressure and the tension "wins," closing the vessel before the pressure has dropped to zero. The internal pressure which still exists when the vessel closes is known as the "critical closing pressure." Regardless of the explanation, the phenomenon is a potential hazard in low flow states such as shock in which tissues already ischemic are further threatened with sudden complete cessation of flow to certain capillary beds.

References

Burton AC. *Physiology and Biophysics of the Circulation.* Chicago: Year Book Medical Publishers, 1972.
Cokelet GR. Rheology and hemodynamics. *Annu Rev Physiol* 42:311–324, 1980.
Folkow B and Neil E. *Circulation.* London: Oxford University Press, 1971, pp. 4–56.
Green HD, Rapela CA and Conrad MC. Resistance and capacitance phenomena in terminal vascular beds. In: *Handbook of Physiology*, Section 2: *Circulation*, edited by WF Hamilton and P Dow. Washington, D.C.: American Physiological Society, 1963, Vol. II, pp. 935–960.
Milnor WR. *Hemodynamics.* Baltimore: Williams & Wilkins, 1982.

Patel DJ and Vaishnav RN. *Basic Hemodynamics and Its Role in Disease Processes.* Baltimore: University Park Press, 1980.

Saari JT and Stinnett HO. Diameter vs number in diameter of vessel resistance. *Physiol Teacher* 24:51–56, 1981.

Strandness DE and Sumner DS. *Hemodynamics for Surgeons.* New York: Grune & Stratton, 1975.

chapter 3

The Heart: Structure and Function

Functional Anatomy

The atria, whose walls consist mainly of two thin, overlying muscular sheaths arranged at right angles to each other, serve as blood reservoirs as well as pumps. The two thicker-walled ventricles pump blood from the low-pressure venous systems into the higher-pressure arterial systems.

In the pulmonary circuit, the right ventricle receives venous blood at about zero pressure and propels it into the pulmonary artery to a peak systolic pressure of about 25 mm Hg. The blood is oxygenated in the pulmonary capillaries and returned to the left heart. The left ventricle takes oxygenated blood, again at about zero pressure, and pumps it at a peak pressure of about 120 mm Hg into the aorta and systemic circuit and then to all the tissues of the body. The pulmonary circuit, because of its lower pressure and its shorter, wider-bore vessels with thinner walls, is characterized as a low-pressure, low-resistance system.

The ventricles generate pressure energy by ejecting blood against arterial resistance, and kinetic energy by imparting velocity to the blood. Pressure work—which usually comprises more than 95% of the mechanical energy expended by the heart—can be estimated as the product of the stroke volume and mean arterial pressure against which the ventricle works. Since the two ventricles eject similar volumes at identical heart rates, the left ventricle, because of its higher ejection pressure, performs about five to seven times as much pressure work as the right.

Myocardial Contraction

The myocardial muscle of each ventricle consists of three interdigitating layers (Fig. 3.1). The two outer muscle layers are oriented obliquely from the base of the heart (superior portion), which is the area of attachment to the aorta and other great vessels, to the apex, which is the tapered free portion. Upon contraction, the oblique fibers shorten the ventricular wall and pull the apex anteriorly and toward the base. The circumferential fibers constrict the ventricular diameter.

Right Ventricle

X-ray studies of the heart chambers have shown that the right ventricle has a concave outer wall and during contraction moves toward the

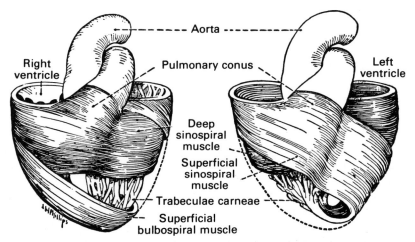

Figure 3.1. Components of the myocardium. The outer muscle layers pull the apex of the heart toward the base; the inner circumferential fibers constrict the lumen, particularly of the left ventricle. (Reprinted with permission from R.F. Rushmer, *Cardiovascular Dynamics*, Philadelphia: W.B. Saunders, 1976.)

interventricular septum with a bellowslike action, while the atrioventricular (AV) groove, or external depression, separating the right atrium and right ventricle, shortens toward the apex (Fig. 3.2). This anatomical configuration permits the thin and flexible wall of the right ventricle to eject a large volume of blood with a minimal amount of shortening against a low outflow pressure. However, if the pulmonary valve becomes thickened and stenotic, the resistance against which the right ventricle contracts will be much increased and flow into the pulmonary artery impeded. The right ventricular muscle then hypertrophies and may gradually approach the left ventricle in wall thickness.

Left Ventricle

As indicated above, left ventricular contraction involves both a decrease in diameter and a shortening of the axis between the base and apex of the heart; the net result is a movement of the apex toward the mitral valve. Simultaneously, the interaction of the various cardiac muscle groups produces a lifting effect on the apex, moving it toward the anterior chest wall and producing a palpable impulse at the left midclavicular line at about the interspace between the fifth and sixth ribs. The left ventricle with its more cylindrical outline (Fig. 3.2) has a mechanical advantage over the right ventricle in generating stroke volume and power, because the volume it ejects through a decrease in the diameter of a cylinder is a function of the square of the radius, rather than a linear function (Laplace's law, Chapter 2). The thick-walled and heavier left ventricle is also thought to provide a type of splint against which the outer wall of the right ventricle is pulled, thus ejecting the right ventricular blood by means of a squeezing, bellowslike action.

After careful anatomical studies, Streeter has proposed that the ventricular muscle fibers are arranged in figure-eight paths similar to an unevenly folded lariat with the smaller loop around the apex and the larger loop around the base of the heart. He suggests that tightening of the lariat simulates ventricular emptying and that it is this unique arrangement that permits the remarkably rapid and energy-efficient ventricular ejection.

Heart Valves

Efficient pumping action of the heart requires a minimum of reflux as the blood is transported. This is achieved through two sets of unidirectional, reciprocating valves. One pair, the aortic and pulmonic (also called semilunar) valves are located at the exits of the right and left ventricles and open and close passively (Fig. 3.3, *right*). When open, the

A. RIGHT VENTRICULAR EJECTION

SHORTENING OF
THE FREE WALL

COMPRESSION OF
THE CHAMBER
(BELLOWS ACTION)

B. LEFT VENTRICULAR EJECTION

CONSTRICTION
OF CHAMBER

SHORTENING
OF CHAMBER

TRACTION ON
RIGHT VENTRICULAR
WALL

Figure 3.2. Right and left ventricles. Contraction characteristics and modes of emptying. (Reprinted with permission from R.F. Rushmer, *Cardiovascular Dynamics*, Philadelphia: W.B. Saunders, 1970.)

three-cusped aortic valve does not flatten against the aortic wall. This is important since it permits blood to flow unimpeded into the left and right main coronary arteries, whose openings are located in the aortic wall directly behind the open valve leaflets.

The two AV valves consist of the "tricuspid" on the right and the "mitral" on the left, which open toward the ventricles, permitting blood to enter from the atria. Both valves are thin walled and attached at the lower or free sides of their leaflets to papillary muscles on the ventricular walls by means of thin, stringy chordae tendineae (Fig. 3.3, *left*). The papillary muscles contract when the ventricles contract and so prevent the valves from bulging too far into the atrial chamber during ventricular contraction. A small amount of blood may occasionally regurgitate through a normal AV valve during ventricular contraction but with little effect on cardiac function. However, if one of the chordae tendineae becomes ruptured, the valve leaflet to which it is attached may bulge significantly. This produces an incompetent valve with regurgitation of a sizeable fraction of the blood backward into the atrium during ventricular systole which results in a marked loss of pumping efficiency.

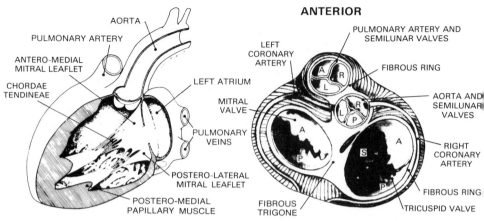

Figure 3.3.   Heart valves. *Left*, Schematic drawing of left lateral view of mitral valve complex showing mitral annulus, the two mitral leaflets, chordae tendineae and papillary muscles. *Right*, A section through the base of the heart at the level of the fibrous ring supporting the cardiac valves. The right coronary artery arises from the anterior aortic sinus and the left coronary from the left posterior aortic sinus. (Adapted from J.W. Hurst, *The Heart, Arteries and Veins*, 5th ed., New York: McGraw-Hill, 1982, and J.T. Shepherd and P.M. Van Houtte, *The Human Cardiovascular System*, New York: Raven Press, 1979.)

This complication, which may follow a "myocardial infarction" or "heart attack," may result in rapid death.

The AV valves have larger cross-sectional areas than the semilunar valves and are subjected to less mechanical force during valve opening and closure.

Methods of Studying Cardiac Function

The pressure changes described in the following section were determined in the human subject with high-fidelity pressure transducers. The transducers were attached to long, thin tubes (catheters) threaded into the heart chambers and the large vessels through a peripheral vein or artery (cardiac catheterization). If a radioopaque contrast material is injected, the outlines of the chambers can be visualized. With high speed fluoroscopy, rapid single or biplane photography, ultrasound and other techniques (Chapter 7), the rate of movement of the cardiac wall, the stroke volume and the emptying characteristics can be studied. These methods are used routinely in many cardiac catheterization laboratories. Methods of recording pressure and flow are further discussed in Chapter 6 and of cardiac output in Chapter 7.

For more precise study of heart sounds and murmurs, a small microphone is placed on the chest wall. The sound vibrations are amplified and recorded on an oscilloscope or polygraph; this *phonocardiogram* records the sounds as oscillations and through use of filters and other special devices, permits an accurate analysis of sound frequency and intensity from which their clinical significance can be determined.

An additional technique of great clinical value is the recording of the electrical changes generated by the heart, *i.e.*, the electrocardiogram (ECG). The development of multiple leads for precise electrical recording at different points on the body has aided considerably in the diagnosis of certain cardiac irregularities (arrhythmias) and in the localization of myocardial damage. Electrical characteristics of the heart are described in Chapter 4.

The Cardiac Cycle

The cardiac cycle represents a combination of mechanical, electrical and valvular events whose interrelationship is complex but essential to the understanding of how the heart functions and how disease processes affect it. At rest, the normal adult heart beats at a rate of about 70 to 75 per minute. Blood flows from the atria to the ventricles and from the ventricles to the large arteries at a velocity which is determined by the pressure differences between the chambers. Normally the valves offer no resistance and open or close as a function of the relative pressures exerted by the flowing stream and the energy imparted by the contractions of the atrial and ventricular musculature.

At a rate of 75 per minute, the complete cycle for filling and emptying of the chamber would occupy 0.8 sec or 800 msec (Fig. 3.4). The cardiac cycle is divided into systole and diastole. Left ventricular systole (*i.e.*, the contractile period of the left heart) extends from the early rise of ventricular pressure and the closure of the AV valve (Fig. 3.4*A*) to the closure of the aortic valve and the beginning of diastole (Fig. 3.4*C*). During most of the period from *B* to *C*, the ventricular pressure is higher than the aortic, the aortic valve is open and the ventricle ejects blood into the arterial system. At *C* the aortic valve closes.

Diastole, which is the period of ventricular relaxation and filling, begins with the closing of the aortic valve (*C*). When the ventricular pressure falls below the atrial, the AV valve opens (*D*) and the ventricle begins to fill. Diastole ends when the ventricle again contracts and the new cycle begins.

At a heart rate of 75 per minute, systole will ordinarily occupy 250 to 300 msec; thus almost two-thirds of the cycle (or about 500–550 msec) is taken up with diastolic filling. However, with an increase in heart rate up to 180 per minute, which can occur in severe exercise, the length of the total cycle is reduced to about 330 msec. At this high heart rate most of the reduction is in diastolic time, which will ultimately restrict ventricular filling and limit cardiac output.

Figure 3.4. Left ventricular systole and diastole, atrial pressure waves and the electrocardiogram (ECG). *Top,* As the ventricle contracts at *A,* the mitral valve closes; as pressure increases and exceeds aortic, the aortic valve opens (*B*). Upon completion of ejection, the pressure falls below aortic and the aortic valve closes (*C*). As ventricular pressure falls below atrial, the mitral valve opens (*D*) and diastolic filling continues until the ventricle contracts again. *Bottom,* The P wave (atrial depolarization), the QRS complex (ventricular depolarization) and the T wave (ventricular repolarization) are shown. Note that depolarization inevitably precedes mechanical contraction.

All cardiac events are normally timed according to systole and diastole of the ventricles, even though this may not always coincide with the state of activity of other parts of the heart. Figure 3.4 and most of the subsequent figures refer only to the left ventricle. It should be emphasized, however, that the events of the right side of the heart are analogous and that the right atrium and ventricle have similar timing of their electrical, mechanical and valvular events. The primary differences in the cardiac cycle between the two sides of the heart are those relating to the lower pressures in the right ventricle and pulmonary artery.

Role of the Atria

From a performance standpoint, the ventricles are necessarily the central factors in the cardiac cycle; the atria, however, play a significant supporting role. The normal atrial pressure curve has three positive deflections (Fig. 3.4). Shortly after the P wave of atrial depolarization (discussed below) the atria contract with a resulting positive *a wave* which occurs late in diastole. With the beginning of systole, the ventricular contraction causes a pressure wave to be transmitted through the thin-walled AV valves to the atria and also to the adjacent large veins resulting in the atrial *c wave*. During the last half of systole, as venous blood returns from the peripheral veins and the AV valves remain closed, atrial filling continues and atrial pressure rises with a resulting positive deflection called the *v wave*.

The atrial contraction, occurring late in ventricular diastole, aids materially in conveying blood to the ventricle and may contribute as much as 25 to 30% of the total ventricular filling. In some disease states, in which atrial contraction is absent, the heart is usually able to compensate for the loss of this atrial pump and can function reasonably well under resting conditions. However, during stress or exercise, the absence of the atrial pump may result in a serious functional impairment of cardiac output with a resultant fatigue and other signs of acute heart failure.

Electrical Events of the Cycle

In order for the cardiac muscle to contract, there must be a preceding action potential which initiates the electrical and ionic events that culminate in ventricular systole. The ECG, which is recorded at the body surface, is a graphic representation of the summed voltage changes produced by electric depolarization and repolarization of the heart. These electrical impulses begin at the sinoatrial (SA) node in the right atrium, spread over the entire heart and initiate the contraction wave. The electrical phase of the cardiac cycle begins with excitation of the atrium (*i.e.*, atrial depolarization), denoted on the ECG by an initial upward positive deflection called the P wave (Fig. 3.4), which triggers atrial contraction.

After completion of the P wave, the ECG trace returns to base level, *i.e.*, the isoelectric line. About 0.16 to 0.22 seconds following the onset of the P wave, a second series of negative and positive waves are seen. A negative Q wave usually precedes a positive R and a negative S wave. This QRS complex is caused by electrical depolarization of the ventricles and is quickly followed by ventricular contraction. After a short interval, a positive T wave appears which corresponds to repolarization of the ventricular muscle mass. The ECG then returns to the isoelectric line and usually there is electrical silence for the remainder of diastole. The S-T segment is an important phase of the record because it is specifically distorted in myocardial ischemia.

It should be emphasized that the action potential is the indispensable forerunner to cardiac contraction. The heart has a spontaneous, intrinsic rhythmicity and automaticity, and contraction is inevitably coupled to excitation. Electrical characteristics of the heart are considered in greater detail in Chapter 4.

Ventricular Systole

It is necessary to examine more closely some of the events associated with the cardiac cycle. Systole is often divided into three parts—an *isovolumic contraction period,* a *rapid ejection period* and a *slower ejection period.*

Isovolumic (Isometric) Contraction Period (ICP). The ICP is the important interval between the closure of the mitral valve and the opening of the aortic valve, so called because there is no change in ventricular volume (Fig. 3.5). Several significant events occur during this period. The rate of rise of ventricular pressure (dP/dt), which is sometimes used to characterize the contractile ability of the heart (Chapter 5), is maximum during this time. In addition, during the ICP, the atrial c wave occurs and the aortic and pulmonary arterial pressures are at their lowest level. This occurs just before the opening of the aortic and pulmonary valves.

Rapid Ejection Period. The first one-third of systole is comprised of the rapid ejection period, during which about two-thirds of the ventricular volume is emptied into the aorta. Toward the end of this period, the aorta begins to distend as it absorbs the impact of the ejected blood and the rate of rise of aortic pressure decreases. The normal end-diastolic volume (EDV) is about 120 ml and the end-systolic volume (ESV) about 40 ml. Thus the average stroke volume (SV) is about 80 ml, and the ejection fraction (EF) about 67%. A decrease in EF is a common sign of a weakened myocardium.

Slower Ejection Period. At the peak of the aortic pressure curve, the ventricles begin to relax slightly, yet blood continues to flow from the ventricle to the aorta, but at a lesser rate. This is called the slower ejection period. Near this phase, the aortic pressure actually exceeds the left ventricular pressure by a few millimeters of mercury, but outflow continues because of the inertia of the blood. This is followed by an even greater reversal of the pressure gradient, causing the flow to reverse briefly and the aortic valve to close producing the second heart sound.

Because the valves and aorta are distensible, they recoil, producing a secondary pressure wave in the aortic curve with a notch between the primary and secondary pressure curve which is referred to as the dicrotic

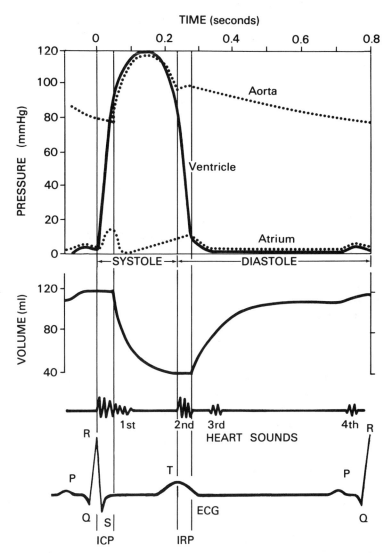

Figure 3.5.   Mechanical and electrical events of the cardiac cycle showing also the ventricular volume curve and the heart sounds. Note the isovolumic contraction period (ICP) and the relaxation period (IRP) during which there is no change in ventricular volume because all valves are closed. The ventricle decreases in volume as it ejects its contents into the aorta. During the first third of systolic ejection—the rapid ejection period—the curve of emptying is steep.

notch. As these events occur in the left side of the heart, a similar sequence of events is occurring in the right ventricle and pulmonary artery resulting in closure of the pulmonary valve.

In practice, the term systole is often referred to as the period between the beginning of the first and the beginning of the second heart sounds although clearly one may refer to atrial systole, right ventricular systole, etc.

Ventricular Diastole

During the period between closing of the semilunar valves and the opening of the AV valves, *i.e.*, the isovolumic relaxation period (IRP), the ventricular pressure falls rapidly while the ventricular volume remains constant. When ventricular pressure falls below atrial pressure, the AV valves again open and the period of ventricular filling begins.

The ventricles become approximately two-thirds filled within the first one-third of ventricular diastole; this is referred to as the passive rapid-filling phase. In late diastole, ventricular filling is again augmented by atrial contraction, a period known as the active rapid-filling phase. The period between these two rapid-filling phases is sometimes called diastasis (a slower filling phase).

Heart Sounds

The two primary heart sounds are usually heard as a "lup-dup," a low-pitched first sound, followed by a quicker, higher-pitched second. The intensity of heart sounds, as heard at the chest wall, depends upon several factors, *i.e.*, the rate of rise of ventricular pressure, the physical characteristics of the ventricles and valves, the volume contained in the heart, the position of the AV valve leaflets at the beginning of ventricular systole and the transmission characteristics of the chest wall. The relationship of the heart sounds to other events of the cardiac cycle is shown in Figure 3.5. The major components of the heart sounds are associated with the abrupt acceleration and deceleration of blood in and near the heart, but there is not full agreement on the relative significance of valve activity and muscle vibration.

The first heart sound (S_1) is associated with the closure of the mitral and tricuspid valves at the start of ventricular systole and the two components can sometimes be distinguished. If so, the first component of S_1 is mitral in origin and the second component tricuspid.

The second heart sound (S_2) is usually of higher frequency and shorter duration than the first. It marks the end of ventricular systole and the beginning of diastole and is associated with the closure of the semilunar valves. It consists of two components, aortic and pulmonic. Normally, the aortic valve closes several milliseconds before the pulmonic and the time difference is accentuated during the inspiratory phase of respiration.

This respiratory delay in closing of the pulmonary valve produces a "physiological" splitting of the second heart sound and is mainly due to the sudden decrease in intrathoracic pressure associated with inspiration. This in turn, causes a temporary increase in venous return, and an increase in right heart volume resulting in increased right ventricular output, a temporary prolongation of ejection time and a delay in pulmonary valve closure. At the same time, pulmonary venous return to the left heart is diminished so that left ventricular stroke volume decreases and the aortic valve closes slightly earlier. Variations in the degree of splitting of the second heart sound occur in certain types of congenital heart disease and in cases of abnormal conduction of the electrical impulses of the heart.

A third heart sound (S$_3$), shown in Figure 3.5, is associated with the passive rapid-filling phase. For reasons which are not clear, a physiological third sound may be present in younger individuals; however, if it occurs after the age of 40 years, it is generally considered abnormal. It may occur in fever, cardiac failure and certain other cardiac disorders.

The fourth heart sound (S$_4$) is associated with the active rapid-filling phase (Fig. 3.5). While it can often be recorded by phonocardiography, it is generally not audible. When it does occur, it is usually recorded at the peak of atrial contraction and may be associated with increased atrial pressures.

Pathophysiology

Heart Murmurs

Disturbances of normal blood flow patterns in the heart and great vessels often result in abnormal sound, producing vibrations in the auditory frequency range known as murmurs. They are classified on the basis of their timing as systolic, diastolic and continuous murmurs. If the aortic or pulmonary valve is diseased or deformed, the increased turbulence through the narrowed or distorted orifice results in the crescendo-decrescendo systolic murmur characteristic of aortic or pulmonary valve disease (Fig. 3.6*I*).

If AV valve closure is incomplete because of disease of the mitral or tricuspid valves, the valve will become incompetent and blood will regurgitate into the atrium producing a blowing "whoosh" noise following the first heart sound. If this systolic murmur persists throughout systole, as indicated in Figure 3.6*II*, it is sometimes referred to as a pansystolic or holosystolic murmur.

Abnormal heart sounds which occur during diastole are associated either with an abnormality of AV valve opening (usually mitral) or an abnormality of semilunar valve closure (usually aortic). A murmur originating at the aortic valve and heard in early diastole may be produced by incomplete closure of the aortic valve at the end of systole. Such an abnormality could be due to fibrosis or stiffening of the valve in the open position or destruction of valve leaflets. The defect causes regurgitation of blood back into the left ventricle at the end of systole through the incompetent valve, producing the diastolic murmur of aortic regurgitation or aortic insufficiency (Fig. 3.7*III*).

Stenosis of the mitral valve may cause abnormal heart sounds during early or late diastole (Fig. 3.6*IV*). The early component of this murmur is often initiated with an opening snap of the mitral valve; the late component may be associated with the atrial systole, just before the onset of ventricular systole, and is referred to as a "presystolic" murmur. See also the following section for a further description of aortic stenosis.

In addition to the preceding, certain types of murmurs may be heard throughout systole and diastole, such as the murmur of the patent ductus arteriosus (Fig. 3.6*V*). This is the result of a constant movement

Figure 3.6. Diagrammatic representation of phonocardiograms of common systolic and diastolic murmurs. S_1 and S_2, 1st and 2nd heart sounds. (Adapted from P. Wood, *Diseases of the Heart and Circulation*, 3rd ed., Philadelphia: J.B. Lippincott, 1968.)

of blood through the patent ductus which occurs during the entire cycle and produces a heart murmur with a continuous machinerylike quality, with a waxing and waning of intensity. Blood flow is continuous through the patent ductus arteriosus during the entire cycle because of a persistent pressure gradient from the aorta to the pulmonary artery during both systole and diastole. This will not occur if there is a reversal in the pressure gradient due to severe pulmonary hypertension.

When present, the fourth heart sound usually indicates a noncompliant ventricle; this commonly occurs in ischemic heart disease, pulmonic or aortic stenosis and pulmonary and systemic hypertension. However, it does not occur in mitral or tricuspid stenosis since the sound is also dependent upon rapid ventricular inflow.

Abnormal Intracardiac Pressures and Oxygen Saturations

In the preceding chapters, it has been pointed out that the circulation is maintained on the basis of pressure, flow and oxygen gradients and normal values in different parts of the circulatory system have been cited. There are, however, variations in the healthy population and even wider variations in disease.

In the following section approximate ranges of normal cardiac pressures and oxygen saturations are given; two examples are also presented to illustrate how deviations in these normal relationships may be produced by cardiac disorders. In later chapters the effects of other vascular diseases will be considered more fully.

While there are phasic changes, mean right atrial pressure in the normal adult varies from about 0 to 6 mm Hg, right ventricular systolic pressure from 25 to 30 mm Hg, and diastolic pressure from 0 to 5 mm Hg. In the pulmonary artery, systolic pressure varies from about 22 to 30 mm Hg and diastolic pressure from about 9 to 12 mm Hg.

The left atrium shows pulsatile fluctuations similar to the right, but with slightly higher mean values ranging from about 4 to 10 mm Hg. Left ventricular pressure ranges from about 120 to 140 mm Hg systolic, and from 0 to 10 mm Hg diastolic. Aortic systolic pressures vary in the young adult from about 120 to 140 mm Hg and diastolic pressures from about 70 to 80 mm Hg.

Aortic stenosis is an obstruction to left ventricular ejection which produces an increased systolic pressure gradient between the left ventricle and aorta (Fig. 3.7, *bottom*). In an effort to maintain adequate flow, the left ventricular systolic pressure begins to rise and may increase to levels above 200 mm Hg with an aortic systolic pressure of 100 mm Hg or less. With progressive stenosis, this abnormal ventricular-aortic pres-

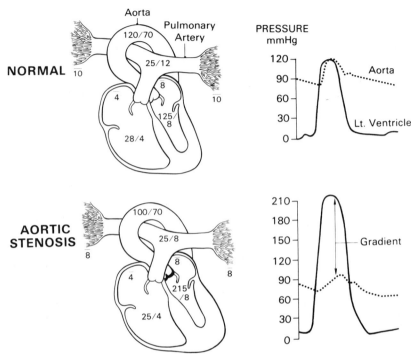

Figure 3.7.   Left ventricular and aortic pressure gradients in a normal adult and in stenosis. Note in aortic stenosis the excessive left ventricular systolic pressure, the large systolic pressure gradient and the abnormally thickened left ventricle. ($\overline{X}$, mean value.) (Adapted from an original painting by F.H. Netter, *Ciba Collection of Medical Illustrations*, Vol. 5. Summit, N.J.: CIBA-Geigy Corp., 1955–1963).

sure gradient (Fig. 3.7, *bottom*) requires increased cardiac work that may result in severe left ventricular hypertrophy (Chapter 14). However, in spite of this hypertrophy, the insufficient output due to the stenosis and inadequate coronary perfusion for the enlarged ventricle may result in cardiac failure.

Oxygen Concentrations in the Cardiac Chambers. The blood oxygen content in the vena cavae, right atrium, right ventricle and pulmonary artery is about 15 to 16 ml/dl of blood, and the oxygen saturation is normally 70 to 80%. Usually there is a slight decrease in oxygen saturation at the level of the right atrium where blood from the coronary sinus, which has a very low oxygen content and saturation, mixes with blood from the vena cavae. On leaving the pulmonary capillary bed, the blood is usually 97 or 98% saturated with an oxygen content of 19 to 20 ml/dl blood. Because of drainage of bronchial venous blood (from

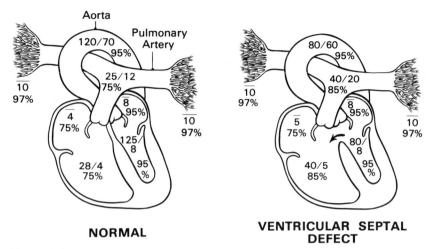

Figure 3.8. Intracardiac pressures and oxygen saturations in a normal adult and in ventricular septal defect. Because of the mixing of the two streams in ventricular septal defect, the left ventricular pressures are decreased and those on the right side of the heart are increased. Right ventricular and pulmonary arterial blood have a higher oxygen saturation. (Adapted from an original painting by F.H. Netter, *Ciba Collection of Medical Illustrations*, Vol. 5. Summit, N.J.: CIBA-Geigy Corp., 1955–1963).

the lungs) and thebesian venous blood (from the myocardium) into the left heart, there is a small decrease in oxygen saturation in the left ventricle to about 95%. Normally, systemic arterial blood has the same oxygen content and saturation as left ventricular blood (Fig. 3.8).

In *ventricular septal defect*, a shunt of oxygenated blood occurs during systole from the left to the right ventricle through the defect, producing an abnormally high oxygen saturation in the right ventricle and frequently an abnormally high right ventricular pressure (Fig. 3.8, *right*). If not repaired, the right ventricle may become hypertrophied and the shunt may reverse to become a right to left shunt with cyanosis (a dusky or blue color of the skin) caused by a higher arterial blood concentration of reduced hemoglobin. The turbulence produced by blood flow through the septal defect during systole causes a systolic murmur.

References

Armour JA and Randall WC. Structural basis for cardiac function. *Am J Physiol* 218:1517–1523, 1970.

Brecher GA and Galletti PM. Functional anatomy of cardiac pumping. In: *Handbook of Physiology*, Section 2: *Circulation*, edited by WF Hamilton and P Dow. Washington, D.C.: American Physiological Society, 1963, Vol. II, pp. 759–798.

Hurst JW (ed.). *The Heart, Arteries and Veins.* New York: McGraw-Hill, 1982, 5th ed., pp. 22–32.

Leon DF and Shaver JA (eds.). *Physiologic Principles of Heart Sounds and Murmurs*, Monograph No. 46. Dallas: American Heart Association, 1974.

Moskovitz HL, Donoso E, Gelb IJ and Wilder RJ. *An Atlas of Hemodynamics of the Cardiovascular System.* New York: Grune & Stratton, 1963.

Rushmer RF. *Cardiovascular Dynamics.* Philadelphia: W.B. Saunders, 1976, 4th ed.

Sokolow M and McIlroy MB. *Clinical Cardiology.* Los Altos, Calif.: Lange Medical Publications, 1981, 3rd ed.

Streeter DD. Gross morphology and fiber geometry of the heart. In: *Handbook of Physiology*, Section 2: *The Cardiovascular System*, edited by RM Berne, N Sperelakis and SR Geiger. Washington, D.C.: American Physiological Society, 1979, Vol. I, pp. 61–112.

chapter 4

Electrical Properties of the Heart

Just as an auto engine requires a well-tuned electrical system to coordinate its pistons to produce power, so the heart needs a system to coordinate contraction of its chambers; without this it is impossible for the pump to bring about the orderly sequence of atrial and ventricular systole. In this chapter, we will consider (a) how the contraction signal (action potential) is spread through the heart, (b) the different types of action potentials and how they are generated and controlled, (c) how action potentials are detected for medical diagnostic purposes, and (d) a brief description of a few conduction abnormalities and some principles of their treatment.

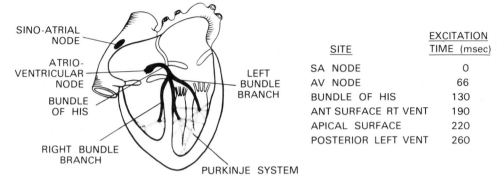

SITE	EXCITATION TIME (msec)
SA NODE	0
AV NODE	66
BUNDLE OF HIS	130
ANT SURFACE RT VENT	190
APICAL SURFACE	220
POSTERIOR LEFT VENT	260

Figure 4.1. The conduction system of the heart. *Left*, the action potential normally originates at the sinoatrial (SA) node, travels over the atrial muscle to the atrioventricular (AV) node and then through the bundle of His, the bundle branches and the Purkinje system to the ventricular muscle. *Right*, the time of arrival of the action potential at different parts of the heart. (Reprinted with permission from A.M. Scher and M.S. Spach, *Handbook of Physiology: Cardiovascular System*, The Heart. Bethesda, Md.: American Physiological Society, 1979, Vol. I.)

Spread of Cardiac Impulse

In order to coordinate the contraction of its different parts, the heart has a specialized conduction system that consists of the sinoatrial (SA) node, atrial bundles, the atrioventricular (AV) node, the bundle of His with its right and left branches and the Purkinje networks (Fig. 4.1). The SA node, the AV node, and the remaining specialized conduction tissue can all discharge spontaneously, *i.e.*, can initiate action potentials (APs) and serve as "pacemakers." However, the SA node ordinarily has the fastest discharge rate and, as a consequence, is the normal cardiac pacesetter or "pacemaker." The impulse is conducted via self-propagating depolarization currents in a fashion similar to the APs in nerve fibers.

The transmission velocity in the SA node is about 0.05 m/sec and in the atrial muscle, bundle of His and ventricular muscle 0.8 to 1.0 m/sec. The conduction velocity in the AV node is 0.03 to 0.05 m/sec, but increases to 5 m/sec in the Purkinje tissue, *i.e.*, to a speed about 100 times greater than in the nodal systems. The transmission times to the various regions are shown in Figure 4.1 (*right*). The AV node is a critical element in the system since it is the only normal avenue over which an impulse can be transmitted from atrium to ventricle. An important characteristic of the AV node is its exceedingly low conduction velocity, making it responsible for the delay between atrial and ventricular activation. The Purkinje fibers, on the other hand, have a high conduction velocity, which facilitates coordinated contraction of the entire ventricular mass.

Action Potentials at Different Sites

Two main types of AP are generated in the heart, *i.e.*, those charac-teristic of nonpacemaker tissues such as atrial muscle, Purkinje fibers and ventricular muscle (Fig. 4.2*B*, *C* and *D*) and those found in pacemaker tissues such as the SA and AV nodes (Fig. 4.2*A*). A typical AP of ventricular muscle, nonpacemaker tissue, (Fig. 4.2*D*) shows a rapid initial depolarization from about −90 mV to about +10 mV (phase 0), a quick partial repolarization (phase 1) and then a "plateau" voltage near zero (phase 2) which is maintained for several hundred milliseconds; this is followed by a rapid repolarization (phase 3) and a return to resting potential (phase 4, Fig. 4.2*D*).

Electrical and Ionic Events of Contraction

Resting Membrane Potentials

The intracellular negative charge of the cardiac cell is substantial, varying from about −60 to −90 mV. This resting transmembrane

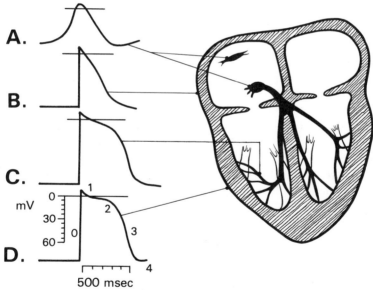

Figure 4.2. Intracellular action potentials (AP) in different regions of the heart. The pacemaker type of potential (sinoatrial or atrioventricular node) is shown in *A*, the atrial AP in *B*, the Purkinje fiber potential in *C* and ventricular cell AP in *D*. Zero voltage shown by horizontal lines. Note the depolarization potential and lack of plateau in the pacemaker tissue (*A*). The different phases of the AP are sometimes identified by numbers as shown in *D*. (Reprinted with permission from A.M. Scher and M.S. Spach, Cardiac depolarization and repolarization and the electrocardiogram. In: *Handbook of Physiology*, Section 2: *The Cardiovascular System*, The Heart, edited by R.M. Berne. American Physiological Society, 1979, Vol. I, pp. 357.)

potential is maintained primarily by three factors, *i.e.*, the chemical concentration gradients across the membrane, the internal and external cellular electrostatic forces and the membrane itself. The excess of intra- over extracellular K^+ ions (*i.e.*, $K^+_i > K^+_e$), and the reverse situation with respect to Na^+ and Ca^{2+} (*i.e.*, $Na^+_e > Na^+_i$ and $Ca^{2+}_e > Ca^{2+}_i$), tend to move the ions down their respective concentration gradients. The negative electrostatic charge tends to retain the positively charged K^+ ions within the cell and draw in the extracellular Na^+ ions. The crucial role, both in maintaining the resting potential and in generating and transmitting the action potential, is played by the membrane through exercise of selective permeability and operation of its pump mechanisms.

In the case of the resting potential, the two key membrane activities are its selective permeability to K^+ ions and the action of its Na^+ pump. The permeability (P) of the cardiac cell membrane to K^+ is much greater than to Na^+ or Ca^{2+} so that the ratio of $P_K^+ : P_{Na}^+$ is about 100:1. Since Ca^{2+} has only a small effect on resting potential, the K^+ ion concentration dominates the ionic balance of the resting cell. This is shown by the fact that estimation with the Nernst equation of cellular electropotential on the basis of K^+ ion balance alone (E_K) yields a negative charge very close to the -90 mV, which actually exists inside the resting ventricular cell. Nonetheless, the net result of the above forces would ordinarily be a steady inward leak of Na^+ ions into the cell, with a resultant lesser negativity and eventual depolarization. This is prevented by the Na^+ pump, which transports Na^+ outward against the chemical and electrical gradient and maintains the negative intracellular charge. The enzyme Na^+, K^+ activated ATPase supplies the energy for the Na^+ pump. Pathologic conditions, such as ischemia, can reduce ATP and prevent the pump from functioning, thereby leading to a loss of the ionic gradients necessary for the AP. Large doses of digitalis may also block the Na-K pump.

The level of resting membrane potential is a critical factor in determining the rate of rise and propagation velocity of the ensuing AP; *e.g.*, the greater (more negative) the resting potential, the steeper the rise and the greater the velocity of the AP.

Action Potentials—Fast and Slow Responses

The initiation of the AP is associated with quick changes in membrane permeability. The rapid depolarization at phase 0 is due almost exclusively to a sudden increase in Na^+ conductance (gNa^+) with a resulting inrush of Na^+ down its concentration gradient into the cell (Fig. 4.3); there is a simultaneous but much smaller decrease in gK^+ which permits the Na^+ ions to enter the cell faster than the K^+ ions can leave. When the ensuing negativity of the resting cell reaches a critical level or

Figure 4.3. Relationship between electrical and ionic events during action potential in a cardiac pacemaker cell. There is a sharp increase in sodium conductance (gNa$^+$) and a decrease in potassium conductance (gK$^+$) during the spike of the AP and a reversal of these tendencies shortly thereafter. Changes in Ca^{2+} conductance (gCa^{2+}) indicate the slow channel current. (Reprinted with permission from D. Noble, *The Initiation of the Heart Beat.* Oxford: Clarendon Press, 1975.)

threshold (which in the case of a ventricular cell is about −65 to −70 mV), an AP results and the membrane potential overshoots to about +10 mV. This initial phase of the AP is known as the "fast response." There now follows a quick reversal of these changes, *i.e.*, a rapid fall in gNa$^+$ and a rise in gK$^+$. In many excitable tissues (*e.g.*, nerve fiber) this rise in K$^+$ permeability restores the resting potential within a few milliseconds, but in cardiac tissue it takes several hundred milliseconds. The relation of these ionic events to cellular potentials is shown in Figure 4.3. The importance of the Na$^+$ transfer in phase 0 is indicated by the fact that the amplitude of the AP at 0 varies linearly with the log of the resting extracellular Na$^+$ concentration (Na^+_e); thus, when Na^+_e is reduced from its normal value of 140 mM to about 10 to 30 mM, the cell is no longer excitable.

During the plateau (phase 2), there is a slow inward current of Ca^{2+} and Na$^+$ ions into the cell through slow channels called the "slow response." The delay in repolarization of the cardiac cell and the resultant prolongation of the action potential is due to this slow inward

Ca^{2+} current which opposes the repolarizing effect of the extrusion of Na^+ from the cell. An additional and physiologically important facet of the inward migration of Ca^{2+} is that these Ca^{2+} ions now become available for excitation-contraction coupling, which is an essential part of the contraction process (Chapter 5). Repolarization (phase 3) involves an increase in gK^+, a decrease of P_{Ca}^{2+} and an inactivation of the slow Ca^{2+} and Na^+ current.

Studies of these ionic phenomena suggest that cardiac cells are of two general physiological types, depending upon whether the fast or slow response predominates. Fast responses (*i.e.*, those in which phase 0 depolarization is prominent) are characteristic of atrial and ventricular muscle cells and Purkinje fibers; the resting membrane potential in these cells is more negative (−80 to −90 mV), the upstroke velocity of the AP is greater (100–500 V/sec), and the conduction velocity is more rapid than in slow cells. In slow response cells, which are located in normal SA and AV nodes, the resting potential is −40 to −70 mV, the upstroke velocity of the AP is 1 to 10 V/sec, and conduction velocity is very slow. While our knowledge of these phenomena is still incomplete, current evidence suggests that the slow inward Ca^{2+} response, which is present in all types of cardiac cells and is responsible for maintaining the plateau phase of the AP in "fast response" cells, is the primary and perhaps only mechanism for producing the AP in "slow response" nodal cells.

The basic cause of these cellular differences in ionic flux in the fast and slow responses is not known. It is currently theorized that Na^+ channels are guarded by "gates" that are probably charged electrical fields in the phospholipid matrix of the membrane. Opening of the "fast gate" during the first phase of the AP in nonpacemaker cells would permit the rapid Na^+ migration responsible for the quick depolarization in the 0 phase. The absence or closure of such a gate would eliminate the Na^+ fast response and permit a slower response characteristic of pacemaker cells.

The "gate" theory has gained credence with the discovery that myocardial anoxia or chemical agents, *e.g.*, tetrodotoxin (a poison derived from the Japanese puffer fish), can so alter a nonpacemaker cell that it will lose its fast response and be converted into a pacemaker type cell in which the slow response (no longer overwhelmed by the fast initial Na^+ current) becomes the dominant mechanism. The conversion from a fast to a slow response is characterized by a shift of resting membrane potential from a more negative value (*e.g.*, −90 mV) to a less negative one (*e.g.*, −60 to −70 mV).

It is also known that certain pharmaceutical agents such as verapamil and nifedipine, a new class of drugs known as calcium antagonists, can partially block the slow response and decrease the firing rate of pace-maker cells, thus tending to prevent arrhythmias (abnormal rhythms of the heart). Catecholamines such as norepinephrine, on the other hand, enhance the slow response and increase the firing rate of pacemaker cells.

The discovery that slow channel Ca^{2+} blockers are highly beneficial in the treatment of arrhythmias and other circulatory disorders has sparked considerable clinical interest in those drugs (Chapter 15).

Automaticity and Pacemaker Potentials

As mentioned above, the SA node, AV node and the remaining specialized conduction tissue are all characterized as potential pace-makers, but the SA node, because of its inherently faster discharge rate, is the normal cardiac pacemaker. It was also pointed out that these pacemaker cells have slow response types of APs; also characteristic of this type of AP is the slow membrane depolarization during diastole. This property permits "spontaneous diastolic depolarization," *i.e.*, au-tomaticity in the pacemaker cell (Fig. 4.2*A*) but not in the atrial or ventricular muscle cell (Fig. 4.2*B* and *D*). The magnitude and slope of these diastolic pacemaker potentials have an important influence on the heart rate.

The rate of the heart may slow through (a) a decrease in the slope of diastolic depolarization (Fig. 4.4, *left*, *a* and *b*), (b) a rise in the threshold potential (TP-1 to TP-2 in Fig. 4.4), or (c) an increase in the magnitude

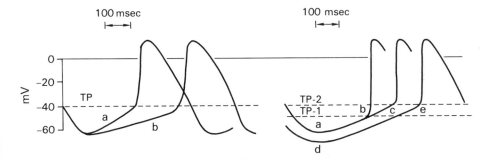

Figure 4.4. Pacemaker potentials in sinoatrial node. Illustrating the effect of diastolic depolarization slopes and potentials on heart rate. The action potential is initiated when the depolarization potential reaches threshold potential (TP). *Left*, slowing of rate of depolarization from *a* to *b* increases the time required to reach TP and lessens heart rate. *Right*, increase of level of TP from 1 to 2 or increased magnitude of resting potential from *a* to *d* also slows the discharge rate and, therefore, the heart rate. (Reprinted with permission from B.F. Hoffman and P.F. Cranefield, *Electrophysiology of the Heart*. New York: McGraw-Hill, 1960.)

of the resting potential (Fig. 4.4, *right, a* and *d*). In case of myocardial ischemia, toxins or other injury, an existing pacemaker may be displaced by a latent pacemaker elsewhere in the heart. There are, in any event, interactions between pacemaker regions of different inherent rhythmicities; when a frequency of excitation greater than that which is inherent to one group of cells is superseded by another group, the rate of firing of the first group is suppressed, a phenomenon known as "overdrive suppression."

Electrical and Mechanical Events of Contraction

A cell is refractory, *i.e.*, is unable to respond to a stimulus, if the stimulus arrives during depolarization or the initial phase of repolarization, *i.e.*, if the voltage of the cell has not become sufficiently negative to initiate the next AP. When the intracellular voltage is greater (less negative) than about -50 mV, there will, during this time, be no inward Na^+ current and no new AP, so that the cell is totally unexcitable. This is called the absolute refractory period (Fig. 4.5). Because the duration of this prolonged refractoriness is of the same order of magnitude as the

Figure 4.5. Relation between electrical and mechanical events of cardiac contraction showing the transmembrane action potential (AP) in isolated papillary muscle (*A*) and the subsequent isometric contraction curve (*B*). There is a considerable delay between the spike of the AP and the peak of the contraction. The graph also shows the refractoriness of the muscle to a subsequent stimulation. ARP, absolute refractory period; RRP, relative refractory period; and SNP, supernormal period. (Adapted from W.R. Milnor, Properties of cardiac tissue. In: *Medical Physiology*, 14th ed., edited by V.B. Mountcastle. St. Louis: C.V. Mosby, 1980.)

duration of contraction, the heart cannot be tetanized. As the voltage of the cell becomes more negative (during the latter part of repolarization) it requires a stronger than normal stimulus to evoke a response; this is the "relative refractory period" (RRP). Immediately following the RRP there is—particularly in the Purkinje fiber—a supernormal phase of increased excitability. The refractory period varies in different parts of the heart, being shortest in the atrium and longest in the Purkinje system and AV node. The long refractory period protects the Purkinje cell against reentry of excitation from adjacent myocardium in a retrograde manner.

Electrocardiography

In 1903, Einthoven developed the first practical device for recording cardiac potentials—a string galvanometer—which subsequently was refined into the electrocardiograph. Since the tissues of the body surrounding the heart are conductors of electricity, a small but constant fraction of the cardiac potentials may be picked up between two surface points (bipolar recording), amplified and recorded. Such a graphic record is termed an *electrocardiogram* (ECG); if the electrodes are placed directly on the heart surface, the resulting trace is called an *electrogram*. A conventional method of electrocardiography is to record from electrodes on three extremities of the body, *i.e.*, left and right arms and left leg, using the right leg electrode as ground. The arrangement of these classical "limb leads" is shown graphically in Figure 4.6 (*left*). These leads were defined by Einthoven so that the major deflections in each lead would be upright (positive) in a normal subject.

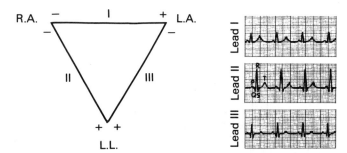

Figure 4.6. *Left*, classical ECG limb leads. *Lead I*, right arm (RA) electronegative with respect to left arm (LA). *Lead II*, RA negative to left leg (LL) and *lead III*, LA negative to LL. *Right*, normal electrocardiogram from limb leads showing P, QRS and T waves. Wide vertical lines, 0.2 second; narrow horizontal lines, 0.1 mV.

The ECG is the algebraic sum of all the myocardial APs as recorded at the surface of the body. Depolarization moving toward an active electrode produces a positive deflection and if moving away, a negative one. By convention, vertical lines are spaced at 0.04-second intervals and a paper speed of 25 mm/sec is usually employed. The vertical voltage scale is calibrated at 10 mm/mV (Fig. 4.6, *right*).

Scalar Electrocardiography—The Normal ECG

Atrial depolarization, represented by the P wave, begins at the SA node and is conducted over the atrial muscle in all directions. There are three specialized, small bundles of atrial muscle (internodal bundles) running toward the AV node which are preferential pathways in which conduction velocity is somewhat greater. The P wave normally does not exceed 0.11 seconds—which is the time for the impulse to travel over the atrium to the AV node.

At the AV node the conduction velocity slows to about 5 cm/sec, then again speeds up to velocities of 1 m/sec in the AV bundles and to about 5 m/sec in the Purkinje system before activating the ventricular muscle to contract. The time for the passage of the AP from the atrium to the ventricular muscle is called the P-R interval (Fig. 4.7). It ordinarily ranges from 0.12 to 0.21 seconds and over half of this period (from the end of the P wave to the Q wave) is taken up in transmission through the AV node. Prolongation of this interval is usually due to abnormal delay in the AV node, to bundle branch disease or to metabolic effects of chronotropic drugs such as digitalis.

Ventricular depolarization begins at the left side of the interventricular septum (Q wave), spreads from the endocardial to epicardial surface of the left ventricle (R wave) and finally to the right ventricle (S wave). The conduction velocity through ventricular muscle is about 0.8 to 1.0 m/sec and the width of the QRS ordinarily does not exceed 0.06 to 0.11 second. The activation times of the different parts of the heart are shown in Figure 4.1 (*right*). Ventricular repolarization proceeds from epicardial to endocardial surface and is represented by the T wave. It normally takes 0.1 to 0.25 second.

The S-T segment is that period between the end of the QRS complex and the beginning of the T wave and represents the interval between completion of depolarization and the time when electrical recovery (repolarization) begins (Fig. 4.7). Its configuration is importantly affected by injury or ischemia of the myocardium as will be further discussed in Chapters 12 and 14. The T-P interval is an isoelectric period of quiescence whose duration varies inversely with the heart rate. The T-P interval sometimes contains a small oscillation called the U wave

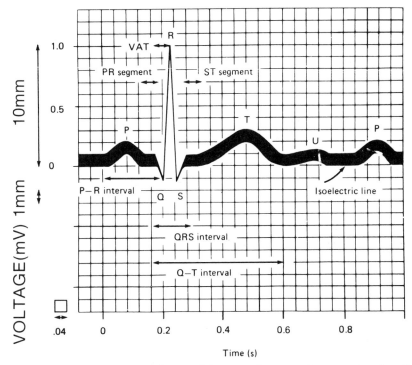

Figure 4.7. Configuration of normal human electrocardiogram showing the primary waves, intervals, segments and ventricular activation time (VAT). The U wave is seen only occasionally and has only minor significance. (Reprinted with permission from M.J. Goldman, *Principles of Clinical Electrocardiography*, 10th ed. Los Altos, Calif.: Lange Medical Publications, 1979.)

which is thought to represent the slow repolarization of papillary muscle; some cardiologists have reported that U wave inversion is suggestive of myocardial ischemia but otherwise the U wave has apparently little physiological or pathological significance.

Vectorcardiography—Electrical Axis of the Heart

While the procedure described above yields a measure of the magnitude of the voltage (scalar electrocardiography) it is possible by summation to determine a resultant vector with both magnitude and direction (vectorcardiography). This is done by recording two leads simultaneously and measuring their respective voltages at the same point using the peak of the R wave. An example of such a determination of a resultant vector is shown in Figure 4.8.

The orientation of the resultant QRS axis in the frontal plane (the

Figure 4.8. Einthoven triangle—calculation of electrical axis of the heart. Perpendiculars from the midpoint of the sides of the equilateral triangle intersect at the center of electrical activity (*a*). RA, right arm; LA, left arm; LL, left leg. If from the midpoint distances equivalent to the wave voltage (in this case the R wave) are laid off parallel to the respective lead, perpendiculars from these end points will intersect at a point designating the magnitude and direction of the resultant R vector (from *a* to *b*).

electrical axis) is usually inferior and to the left at an angle from 0° to +90°; this is in accord with the usual left ventricular predominance. If the angle is more positive, *i.e.*, rotated more to the right, it is suggestive of right ventricular preponderance (right axis deviation). Change in the electrical axis of the heart can be produced by mechanical alteration of the cardiac position and also by a wide variety of cardiac and pulmonary disorders which may change the anatomical position or wall thickness of the heart.

Unipolar Leads

Bipolar leads, as described above, measure potential differences between two points on the surface of the body; however, they cannot record actual potentials at either electrode; thus waves of depolarization and repolarization at different points on the myocardium may neutralize each other and not be accurately recorded.

In 1934, Wilson introduced unipolar lead electrocardiography in which one electrode (the exploring electrode) is placed at different points on the body surface and the other, indifferent electrode, is kept at zero potential by connecting all three limbs to a central terminal through a 5,000-ohm resistance. Unipolar leads are labeled V followed by a letter

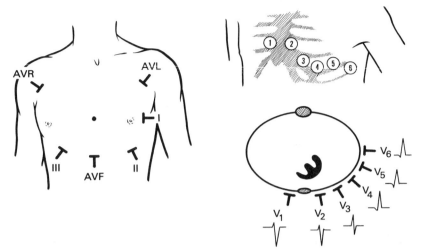

Figure 4.9. Limb leads (*left*) and precordial leads (*right*) in standard 12-lead ECG. Limb leads include leads I, II and III and augmented limb leads with exploring electrodes on right arm (AVR), left arm (AVL) and left foot (AVF). Precordial leads V₁ to V₆ (*right*) record cardiac potentials in a transverse plane. (Reprinted with permission from R.L. DeJoseph, *Introduction to Electrocardiography: The Vectorial Approach.* East Hanover, N.J.: Sandoz, 1977.)

or number which describes the position of the exploring electrode. Because potentials so recorded may be somewhat smaller than desirable, a system of "augmented" leads is commonly used for the unipolar limb leads, *i.e.*, AVR, AVL and AVF (Fig. 4.9, *left*).

The Standard ECG

In the standard 12-lead ECG, six leads are recorded in the frontal plane and six in the transverse plane. The leads in the *frontal* plane are referred to as standard limb leads, *i.e.*, leads I, II and III and the augmented limb leads, AVR, AVL and AVF. These are, in effect, positive poles of a bipolar recording system "looking at" the depolarization vectors from six different positions in the frontal plane (Fig. 4.9, *left*). The other six leads are the precordial chest leads which record the depolarization vectors in the *transverse* plane and are numbered V₁ to V₆. They are placed in positions varying from near midsternum to left midaxillary line, as shown in Figure 4.9, *right*.

In Figure 4.9 (*right*), leads V₁ to V₆ represent summation of electrical activity of both ventricles. The QRS of the left ventricle dominates because of its thicker musculature. As the excitation spreads toward the

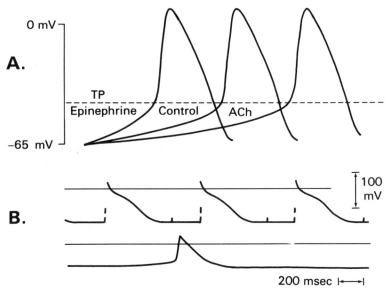

Figure 4.10. Effects of epinephrine (E) or sympathetic stimulation, and acetyl-choline (ACh) or vagal stimulation on heart rate (*A*) and Purkinje fiber action potentials (AP) (*B*). E increases and ACh decreases the slope of diastolic depolarization (*A*). E converts Purkinje fiber APs (*B, upper strip*) to pacemaker type (*B, lower strip*). (Reprinted with permission from E.E. Selkurt, *Physiology*, 4th ed. Boston: Little, Brown, 1976.)

recording electrode, the deflection is positive or upward and as it moves away the deflection will be downward.

Extrinsic Influences on the Heart

The innate automaticity and rhythmicity is independent of neural influences; however, extrinsic factors—neural, thermal, metabolic and ionic—can and do significantly influence cardiac function.

Neural Effects

Vagal stimulation or acetylcholine (ACh) will (a) slow the heart, (b) decrease the strength of atrial contraction, and (c) cause a marked reduction in conduction velocity through the AV node. ACh apparently acts on the heart in two ways: it increases K^+ permeability, thereby shortening the AP, slowing conduction and slowing the pacemakers; and it also decreases the Ca^{2+} current. The reduction of Ca^{2+} current reduces the excitability of the SA and AV nodes and reduces the contractile strength of the myocardium. Strong vagal stimulation will arrest the heart; however, even with continued stimulation the normal heart will, after a short interval, again resume beating (vagal escape).

The endogenous sympathetic transmitter is norepinephrine (NE) but epinephrine (E) has similar effects. Sympathetic stimulation or administration of NE or E will (a) increase the rate and force of cardiac contraction, (b) increase the conduction velocity through the AV node, atria and ventricles, and (c) increase the tendency of Purkinje fibers to exhibit pacemaker activity (Fig. 4.10). The rate effect is due to an increased rate (or slope) of membrane depolarization in the SA node. The mechanism of the sympathetic effect on the heart is most likely twofold, *i.e.*, (a) an increase in the number of Ca^{2+} channels, which lowers the excitability threshold, speeds nodal conduction and increases myocardial contractility, and (b) alteration in the voltage dependence of pacemaker currents, which accelerates firing rate and favors spontaneous depolarization. The myocardial action of catecholamines may also be due, in part, to stimulation of the intracellular enzyme adenylcyclase with a resultant increased concentration of $3'5'$-AMP in the myocardial cell, an increase in Ca^{2+} accumulation and enhanced contractility.

Temperature

Warming the SA node increases its spontaneous activity and its slope of diastolic depolarization, thereby speeding heart rate. There is approximately a 10 beat/min rate increase per 1°C elevation of temperature. Cooling has the reverse effect and severe cooling may arrest the heart.

Inorganic Ions

Electrolyte abnormalities, particularly of K^+ and Ca^{2+} have important and potentially serious effects on cardiac function. Hyperkalemia (elevation of serum K^+) influences depolarization through the direct effect of increased K^+ on lowering the resting potential; the resulting decrease in the fast inward current reduces the rate of rise and amplitude of the AP and slows the conduction velocity. As a result, there is a reduction of P wave amplitude and a widening of the P-R interval and QRS complex, along with a decrease in the rate and force of contraction. The increased K^+ concentration also accelerates repolarization, shortens the plateau phase of the AP and the Q-T interval and produces characteristic tall, peaked T waves. With more severe hyperkalemia, there may be disappearance of the P waves, AV nodal block and possibly ventricular fibrillation and sudden death.

Potassium depletion (hypokalemia) causes first an increase in the magnitude of the resting potential but with further lowering of serum K^+ (*e.g.*, below 3 mM), there will be a decrease in resting potential with slowing of repolarization and prolongation of the AP. The result is usually a flattening of the T waves, prominent U waves, prolongation of the P-R and Q-T intervals, and with severe hypokalemia, a tendency toward AV block and ventricular fibrillation.

Hypercalcemia shortens the duration of the AP, increases the slow inward current and accelerates repolarization. The characteristic ECG changes are a shortened Q-T interval (due to shortening of the AP) and abnormal S-T segments and T waves. Hypocalcemia causes opposite changes, *i.e.*, prolongation and reduced amplitude of the AP and a prolongation of the Q-T interval and S-T segment.

As will be described in Chapter 5, the presence of an adequate extracellular Ca^{2+} concentration is essential for normal cardiac muscle contraction. At low concentrations of intra- and extracellular Ca^{2+}, contraction will not take place. In animal experiments it can be shown that very high levels of extracellular Ca^{2+} concentration will greatly increase the strength of cardiac contraction and if exposure is prolonged, there is less and less relaxation after each contraction until finally the heart stops in sustained calcium rigor.

Arrhythmias

Arrhythmias are disturbances of rate, rhythm or sequence of depolarization which are due either to disorders of impulse formation or impulse conduction. Normal sinus rhythm indicates that the SA node is the pacemaker and that the rate, form and order of excitation is within normal limits. *Sinus arrhythmia,* which is common in normal young adults and children, refers to phasic rate changes with respiration. In sinus bradycardia the rate in the adult is by definition less than 60/min and in sinus tachycardia greater than 100/min but the rhythm, form and succession of the various ECG waves are normal. The causes of arrhythmias are manyfold and include myocardial ischemia, heart failure, blood electrolyte imbalances (especially K^+), high epinephrine levels (*e.g.*, in excitement) and certain drugs such as amphetamines, caffeine and alcohol.

Premature Contractions and Pathological Tachycardias

It is thought that many arrhythmias arise because of an unequal transmission velocity through branches of the conduction system with "reentry" into a proximal conduction site. The reentry theory suggests that because of ischemia or other injury there is a unidirectional block in one fiber bundle (because of partial depolarization) and a delayed or slow retrograde conduction in the previously blocked but now repolarized bundle (Fig. 4.11*B*). The retrograde impulse from the unblocked limb may penetrate the damaged segment, reenter, and cause a premature contraction since, because of the delay, it has reached the original pathway after the refractory period. Bidirectional block will stop the reentrant impulse (Fig. 4.11*D*). The process may become repetitive and result in tachycardia.

In addition to disordered conduction, arrhythmias may also arise because of newly developed centers of impulse formation. All cardiac tissue may, as a result of ischemia, injury or heightened excitability, become a temporary or permanent pacemaker for the heart and thus usurp the normal pacemaker. Such sites are called "ectopic foci" and the anomalous complexes are referred to as premature or extrasystoles. These abnormal impulses may be formed in the atrium outside of the SA node (atrial premature beats), in the AV node (junctional premature beats), in the bundle of His or in the ventricular muscle (ventricular ectopic beats).

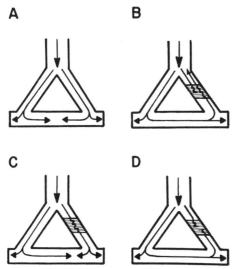

Figure 4.11. Diagram to show "reentry" pathways and possible modifications. *A*, normal velocity of propagation through Purkinje bundle branches. *B*, unidirectional (antegrade) block through a diseased branch with retrograde penetration of the depressed segment and impulse activation through reentry. The extrasystole may be suppressed by improved antegrade conduction (*C*) or development of bidirectional block (*D*). (Reprinted with permission from M.R. Rosen, B.F. Hoffman, and A.L. Wit, *Am Heart J* 89:526, 1975.)

The ectopic beat may also be conducted in a retrograde direction and may depolarize the SA node, atria or AV node; in this case the normal pacemaker cannot generate an impulse until repolarization is complete so that there may be an interval between beats (a compensatory pause). During this pause there may be increased ventricular filling and an increased stroke volume in the succeeding systole. The pause and the increased stroke volume are often sensed by the patient as a "skipped beat."

Atrial premature contractions result from a nonnodal atrial pacemaker and may show an abnormal P wave; usually normal QRS and T complexes occur unless aberrant intraventricular conduction is also present (Fig. 4.12, *left*).

Ventricular extrasystoles are usually caused by an irritable or ectopic focus within the ventricle; the QRS complex may be normal but is usually abnormal (Fig. 4.12, *right*). If the ectopic focus discharges rhythmically and thus has a constant relation to the normal QRS complex, the beat is "coupled"; if it occurs after every normal beat it is called "bigeminy" and if after every second normal beat "trigeminy" etc.

Paroxysmal supraventricular tachycardia occurs if the ectopic focus maintains a very high atrial rate (Fig. 4.13*A*, *top*); the episodes often have a sudden onset and offset. If the rate is 250 to 300/min, the disorder becomes an atrial flutter. Flutter is a serious arrythmia because it often has a rapid ventricular response. Either atrial flutter or fibrillation may be followed by various degrees of heart block. In atrial flutter, the rate is rapid but coordinated contractions can occur; however, in fibrillation, contraction is not coordinated, so the muscle cannot develop sufficient power to propel blood.

APC   VPC

Figure 4.12.   *Left*, in atrial premature contraction the extra systole is due to an atrial premature beat which causes a deformity of the preceding T wave. *Right*, in contrast, the ventricular premature contraction is not preceded by any evidence of atrial activity. In both cases, a wide QRS premature wave follows the sinus beat. [Reprinted with permission from M.D. Alpert, *Cardiac Arrhythmias.* Chicago: Year Book Medical Publishers, 1980 (*left*) and J.J. Gallagher in Cecil's *Textbook of Medicine*, edited by J.B. Wyngarden and L.H. Smith, 16th ed. Philadelphia: W.B. Saunders, 1982, (*right*).]

A. PAT

B. VT
aVF

AF
II

VF
V4

Figure 4.13.   Paroxysmal atrial tachycardia (*A, top*) showing normal complexes; atrial fibrillation (*A, bottom*) with irregular, uncoordinated atrial waves dissociated from QRS waves. Ventricular tachycardia (*B, top*) showing rapid, abnormal QRS complexes. Ventricular fibrillation (*B, bottom*) with very irregular, uncoordinated QRS complexes. (Reprinted with permission from M. Sokolow and M.B. McIlroy. *Clinical Cardiology*, 3rd ed. Los Altos, Calif.: Lange Medical Publications, 1981.)

It has been suggested that atrial fibrillation (Fig. 4.13*A, bottom*) results from alteration of an excitation wave so that it travels around a damaged area in a circle or "circus movement." In animal experiments, the behavior of induced atrial fibrillation is consistent with such a concept. If the ectopic focus is in the ventricle, paroxysmal ventricular tachycardia may occur (Fig. 4.13*B, top*). This is a dangerous arrythmia since it frequently degenerates into ventricular fibrillation (Fig. 4.13*B, bottom*) in which there is complete cessation of effective ventricular contraction. Ventricular fibrillation is a common cause of sudden death.

Conduction Blocks

Blockade of the conduction path may occur anywhere between the SA node and ventricles. One of the more common sites is AV nodal block of which three degrees are usually distinguished. In first degree block all the atrial impulses reach the ventricles but the P-R interval is prolonged, *i.e.*, greater than 0.2 seconds (Fig. 4.14, *top*); this is usually due to AV junctional delay.

Second degree block, in which not all P waves are followed by QRS complexes, may be of two types. In the first type, the P-R interval is relatively fixed and the ratio of transmission may be 2:1, 3:1, 4:1, etc. (Fig. 4.14, *2nd from top*). In partial progressive AV block, the P-R interval progressively increases, culminating in a dropped beat (Wenckebach phenomenon) shown in Figure 4.14, *3rd from top.*

In a third degree, or complete heart block, the impulses are completely interrupted between the atria and ventricles and the QRS complexes are dissociated from the P waves (Fig. 4.14, *bottom*). The ventricular rate is

Figure 4.14. Atrioventricular heart block. *Top:* Incomplete first degree block with prolonged P-R interval but otherwise normal ECG. *Second from top:* Second degree, 2:1 block, ventricle responds only to every other atrial beat. *Third from top:* Wenckebach phenomenon showing progressive AV nodal delay and finally a P wave without a following QRS. *Bottom:* Complete AV heart block; atria are activated by normal impulses from SA node but ventricular rate is slow and independent of atrial rate.

much slowed (usually 35–40/min) so that cardiac output is inadequate. This leads to a sharp fall in arterial pressure, inadequate perfusion of the brain, cerebral ischemia, and fainting (Stokes-Adams syndrome).

Ischemic heart disease, a common cause of arrhythmias, is discussed in Chapter 14.

Treatment of Arrhythmias

While the ECG is a most valuable diagnostic tool, it should be emphasized that it can only assess the electrical aspects of impulse generation and conduction and cannot measure cardiac contractility. A patient may have a normal ECG and yet the myocardial contractile ability may be inadequate; conversely marked ECG abnormalities may be associated with a competent heart. In diagnosis and treatment the contractile, metabolic and electrical aspects of cardiac function must all be considered.

A recent development in the diagnosis of arrhythmias is continuous ECG recording for a period of 12 to 24 hours. With a small tape recorder (Holter monitor) strapped to the patient's waist, an ECG may be obtained while the patient goes about normal activities. By scanning of the playbacks, the actual incidence and severity of the arrhythmias over a prolonged period can be determined.

Some disturbances such as premature beats, AV block and paroxysmal atrial tachycardia may occur without detectable structural disease of the heart. Other disorders such as second or third degree heart block, atrial flutter and fibrillation and ventricular tachycardia are usually associated with organic disorders such as metabolic or electrolyte disturbances or with cardiovascular disease such as ischemic injury or cardiomyopathy.

The treatment of arrhythmias is highly complex and requires considerable skill and judgment; therefore, only a few general principles will be discussed in this section for the purpose of pointing out the pathophysiology involved. Aside from the effort directed toward the primary cause of the disease, therapy usually involves drugs aimed at the specific cardiac disability. Inotropic agents such as digitalis glycosides which enhance the force-velocity relation of the myocardium (Chapter 5) are used to treat heart failure and will slow sinus tachycardia by improving cardiac output. Digitalis slows the heart rate partly through its vagal action and partly through direct effect on the SA node and AV node; in the latter case it slows the supraventricular tachycardia by increasing the block at the AV node. Digitalis overdosage may, however, lead to advanced AV block or tachyarrhythmias.

Antiarrhythmic agents such as quinidine and procainamide are useful in disorders such as atrial fibrillation primarily because they decrease the rate of ectopic pacemaker excitation and prolong the absolute refractory period of the atrium—thus interrupting the "circus movement."

Noninvasive methods of stimulating the vagus nerve will sometimes abort attacks of paroxysmal atrial tachycardia. These methods include carotid sinus massage, the Valsalva maneuver (Chapter 13), lateral pressure on the eyeball or the application of cool water to the face (the face immersion reflex, Chapter 13). Whenever the sinus or AV node is directly involved in the reentry circuit in a condition such as paroxysmal supraventricular tachycardia, the tachycardia may be terminated in this manner; such maneuvers cause increased vagal activity (vagotonia) and act by slowing or blocking conduction within the reentry circuit. However, when these nodes are not directly involved, the vagal maneuver may temporarily decrease the ventricular rate without affecting the atrial rate. Caution must be used during these procedures since strong vagal stimulation may induce asystole, and carotid sinus massage occasionally results in cerebrovascular accident (stroke).

In the last several years in Europe and Japan and very recently in the United States, Ca^{2+} slow channel blocking agents such as verapamil have been used with considerable clinical success in the treatment of arrhythmias and other cardiac disturbances. The effectiveness of these slow Ca^{2+} inhibitors in conditions such as atrial tachycardia, flutter and fibrillation are the result of their direct electrophysiologic action (*i.e.*, the slowing of AV node conduction velocity and the blocking of reentry mechanisms). Lidocaine, which diminishes the automaticity of the His and Purkinje system, raises the threshold for ventricular fibrillation and causes bidirectional block in areas of conduction delay. It is also used in ventricular arrhythmias. Through its β-adrenergic blocking action, propranolol has a primary antiarrhythmic effect. It will reduce heart rate and is used to treat certain ectopic tachycardias and premature ventricular contractions.

In some disorders of ectopic rhythm, such as atrial flutter or fibrillation, cardioversion may succeed in restoring normal rhythm. Cardioversion consists of a direct current shock applied momentarily to the chest early in systole. It temporarily depolarizes the entire heart and interrupts the circus movement of the ectopic disorder thus permitting the sinus node pacemaker to reestablish sinus rhythm.

Artificial pacemakers are often inserted in cases of heart block, Stokes-Adams syndrome and other conditions in which an inadequate heart rate is a threat to the patient. In this procedure a "demand-type," transvenous pacemaker is usually placed *via* the subclavian vein into the right ventricle. The demand, noncompetitive pacemaker releases an electrical signal (1–2 mA) at a rate of about 70/min only when no intrinsic cardiac impulse is sensed by the pacemaker within a preset period. Extensive experience has demonstrated the clinical usefulness of this procedure in maintaining adequate heart rate and preventing fainting attacks.

References

Berne RM and Levy MN. *Cardiovascular Physiology.* St. Louis: C.V. Mosby, 1981, 4th ed., pp. 5–51.
Goldman JJ. *Principles of Clinical Electrocardiography.* Los Altos, Calif.: Lange Medical Publications, 1978, 10th ed.
Harvey WP, Kirkendall WM, Kirklin SW, Nadas AS, Resnekov L, and Sonnenblick EH (eds.). *Yearbook of Cardiology.* Chicago: Year Book Medical Publishers, 1981, pp. 22–52.
Hoffman BF and Cranefield PF. *Electrophysiology of the Heart.* New York: McGraw-Hill, 1960.
Katz AM. *Physiology of the Heart.* New York: Raven Press, 1977.

Scher AM. Electrocardiogram. In: *Physiology and Biophysics*, edited by TC Ruch, HD Patton and AM Scher. Philadelphia: W.B. Saunders, 1974.

Schlant RC and Hurst JW (eds.). *Advances in Electrocardiography.* New York: Grune & Stratton, 1972.

Sokolow M and McIlroy MB. *Clinical Cardiology.* Los Altos, Calif.: Lange Medical Publications, 1981.

Trautwein W. Generation and conduction of impulses in the heart as affected by drugs. *Pharmacol Rev* 15:277, 1963.

Wallace AC. Electrical activity of the heart. In: *The Heart, Arteries and Veins*, edited by JW Hurst. New York: McGraw-Hill, 1982, 5th ed.

chapter 5

Contractile Properties of the Heart

Structural and Functional Characteristics of the Myofibril

The muscle fiber is composed of myofibrils which on microscopic section show longitudinal strands of thick myosin and thin actin filaments. The basic structural unit is the sarcomere, that portion between the Z lines (Fig. 5.1).

Contraction of the myocardial fiber involves a complex series of chemical and physical events which are not well understood. The essential process consists of chemical activation by Ca^{2+} of the proteins of the actin and myosin filaments and of the crossbridges which run between them. It is visualized that as a result of this activation, the repetitive attachment of the thin (actin) filaments to the crossbridges of

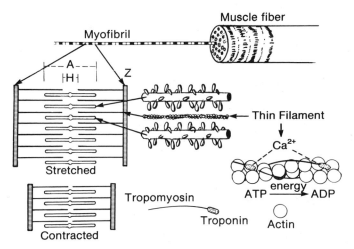

Figure 5.1. Structure of myocardial muscle cell. The myofibrils consist of overlapping thick (myosin) and thin (primarily actin) filaments with crossbridges between them. The actin of the thin filament is closely bound to two additional proteins, *i.e.*, tropomyosin and troponin complex. During the plateau of the action potential, Ca^{2+} ions bind with troponin, which triggers the coupling of actin and myosin and the movement of the crossbridges. Pulled by the crossbridges, the filaments slide across each other pulling the Z lines together and causing contraction. (Adapted from R. Rushmer, *Structure and Function of the Cardiovascular System*, Philadelphia: W.B. Saunders, 1976.)

the thick myosin filaments and their subsequent release causes a "pulling" of the thin actin strands toward the center of the sarcomere with ratchetlike movements. The two types of filaments then slide upon each other (sliding filament hypothesis) pulling the Z lines toward one another, thus shortening and contracting the muscle.

Four major proteins are concerned with the contractile process. Aside from actin and myosin, the thin filaments of the myofibrils contain at least two other proteins, *viz.*, tropomyosin, which has the function of modulating the interaction between actin and myosin, and "troponin complex" which is itself composed of three separate proteins. Troponin (bound to tropomyosin) is distributed at intervals along the actin strand (Fig. 5.1). In the absence of sufficient Ca^{2+}, troponin complex blocks the formation of crossbridges between myosin and actin. As Ca^{2+} in the cell rises, this inhibition is removed and actin-myosin interaction begins. The sequence of "making and breaking" crossbridges in quick succession "pulls" the actin filament along and causes the sarcomere to shorten.

Hydrolysis of the terminal phosphate on ATP by ATPase in the crossbridges supplies the chemical energy required for generation of the mechanical force at each crossbridge attachment.

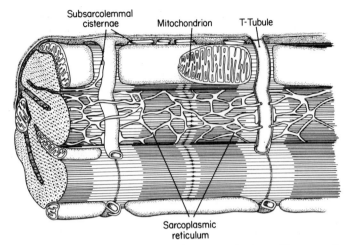

Subsarcolemmal
cisternae   Mitochondrion   T-Tubule

Sarcoplasmic
reticulum

Figure 5.2. Myofibril showing sarcoplasmic reticulum. The muscle fibril is enveloped by a cell membrane which has tubular projections (T or transverse tubules) which are open to the extracellular space. A second completely intracellular membrane system, *i.e.*, the sarcoplasmic reticulum, makes close contact with the T tubules and sarcolemma. (Reprinted with permission from W. Bloom and D.W. Fawcett, *Textbook of Histology.* Philadelphia: W.B. Saunders, 1969.)

Excitation-Contraction Coupling

The combination of Ca^{2+} with the muscle proteins is a key factor in excitation-contraction coupling. Essentially, such coupling involves depolarization of the transverse (T) tubules and release of Ca^{2+} from storage sites within the sarcoplasmic reticulum (Fig. 5.2).

Small saclike expansions of the sarcoplasmic reticulum, called subsarcolemmal cisternae (Fig. 5.2), are located near the Z lines. The three units—the longitudinal superficial sarcoplasmic reticulum, the transverse system (T tubes) and the cisternae—are closely involved in the contraction-relaxation sequence.

The ionic and electrical aspects of the cardiac action potential (AP) were described in Chapter 4. Although the exact relationship between the AP and muscle contraction is not fully understood, the intracellular mobilization of Ca^{2+} in adequate quantities in its so-called "activator" state undoubtedly plays a pivotal role. This is shown by the fact that at low concentrations of extracellular Ca^{2+}, the AP will not elicit a contraction. Furthermore, the contractile process necessitates an influx of Ca^{2+} and the resultant strength of contraction is directly correlated with the extracellular Ca^{2+} concentration.

During the plateau of the AP there is an influx of extracellular Ca^{2+} into the cell which triggers the release of large amounts of previously bound Ca^{2+} from intracellular stores, primarily in the sarcoplasmic reticulum and cisternae. The combination of the "activator" Ca^{2+} with troponin complex results in the removal of an inhibitory effect of tropomyosin, permitting attachment of myosin bridges to sites on the actin filament. The ATP energy conversion results in interdigitation of the filaments with consequent contraction of the muscle fiber. After the plateau phase of the AP and repolarization of the cell membrane, the intracellular Ca^{2+} is again bound to the sarcoplasmic reticulum or extruded from the cell, and the myofibril relaxes.

Thus, the AP, through its regulation of the intracellular concentration of activator Ca^{2+}, not only triggers the contraction but also influences its magnitude and duration. The force of contraction appears to depend on the number of crossbridges formed and this number is related to the intracellular Ca^{2+} concentration. Inotropic agents may act at several possible sites.

Digitalis glycosides have been used for over 200 years in the treatment of heart failure but, until recently, their mode of action has been poorly understood. It is now generally agreed that these glycosides increase the force of myocardial contraction through the action of Ca^{2+} on the excitation-contraction coupling system. Digitalis inhibits the Na^+-K^+ pump in the sarcolemmal membrane which results in a small net increase of Na^+ ions on the intracellular side of the membrane. This excess, in turn, initiates a Na^+-Ca^{2+} exchange system and the increased movement of Ca^{2+} into the cell during the AP is responsible for the heightened contractile force. Digitalis glycosides are capable of increasing myocardial force development by 50 to 60% and can completely reestablish cardiac function in many instances of heart failure. Catecholamines appear to increase contractile force by increasing the intracellular concentration of cyclic AMP and thus of available energy for the crosslinkage.

Elastic Properties of the Myocardium

Heart muscle possesses elastic as well as contractile properties. If a strip of myocardium is passively elongated it will develop tension disproportionate to the applied stretch. It is advantageous for conceptual purposes to separate the contractile and elastic elements of cardiac muscle. Compliance (elasticity) is an important factor in determining the resistance to diastolic inflow into the ventricle and ultimately, therefore, in determining stroke volume.

The elastic components of myocardium have been visualized by some investigators as separate parallel and series elements as shown in Figure 5.3.

The parallel element, PE, (Fig. 5.3) represents the elastic behavior of resting muscle and SE the elastic behavior of contracting muscle. CE

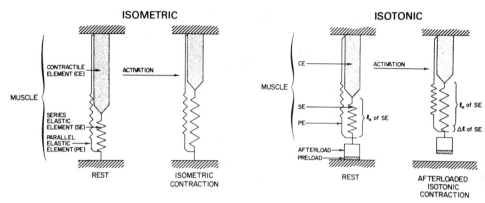

Figure 5.3.   The three-component functional model of the myocardium showing the contractile component (CE), parallel elastic component (PE) and series elastic component (SE). CE and SE are in series with each other and PE is parallel with them. The elastic elements are passive springs and the contractile element is freely extensible. (Reprinted with permission from E.H. Sonnenblick, *Fed Proc* 21:975, 1962.)

represents all the contractile elements. When muscle first contracts, shortening is rapid because the resisting load is small but as shortening develops in isotonic contraction, the SE lengthens and with the tension increase, the velocity of contraction decreases. The force registered at the ends of the muscle will depend, therefore, not only on the contractile properties of CE, but on the elastic properties of SE and the time allowed for interaction between the lengthening of SE and shortening of CE. It should be emphasized that this concept is a theoretical one useful for analytical purposes. No anatomical analogues actually exist as purely contractile or elastic elements.

Myocardial Contractility

How well the heart can propel blood is unquestionably a crucial determinant of circulatory performance. But what factors regulate myocardial contractility and how it can be measured are questions which still provoke frequent debates and sharply dissenting views among investigators. In the following, emphasis will be placed on those aspects which seem most relevant to cardiac function in the intact human.

We will consider cardiac muscle from two standpoints: first, its *intrinsic regulation*, *i.e.*, the basic contractile properties inherent in the muscle itself; and secondly, its *extrinsic regulation*, *i.e.*, its response to conditions imposed from the outside such as neural stimulation, hormones, drugs and disease.

Intrinsic regulation involves an analysis of myocardial response to (a) stretching prior to contraction, *i.e.*, to added *preload stress* such as increased diastolic filling, known as the Starling effect, (b) myocardial response to *heart rate alteration,* and (c) myocardial response to increased load imposed after contraction has begun, *i.e.,* to *afterload stress,* such as a rise in aortic diastolic pressure.

Intrinsic Regulation of the Myocardium

Preload Stresses—Starling's Law of the Heart

This very basic concept, originally described by Frank and Starling, states in effect that within physiological limits, the force or tension generated by the contracting muscle is greater if the muscle is previously stretched. This can be shown *in vitro* by determining the peak tension developed at different precontractile lengths (Fig. 5.4).

As indicated in Figure 5.4, not only the time to peak tension but also the time to relaxation was unchanged when fiber length was altered. This would imply that during diastole a greater influx of blood into the ventricle will cause the ensuing contraction to be more forceful. This may be thought of as a "preload" stimulus since it was applied before contraction began.

Starling, an English physiologist, studied this phenomenon further in an isolated, canine heart-lung preparation in which he controlled the right atrial pressure (and thereby the ventricular diastolic pressure or preload) by raising or lowering an infusion bottle connected to the vena

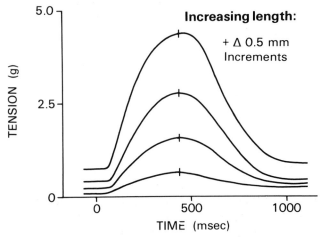

Figure 5.4. Effect of increased stretch of isolated papillary muscle on contractile force showing isometric contractions of the isolated muscle at different precontractile lengths while using stimuli of the same strength. Note that while the generated tension increases progressively, the time to maximal tension is constant. (Reprinted with permission from E.H. Sonnenblick, *Fed Proc* 21:975, 1962.)

Figure 5.5. Starling volume-pressure curve of myocardial function. Classical curve indicating that within physiological limits, increased end-diastolic ventricular volume will result in increased peak ventricular pressure. Beyond the *dotted line* the ventricle is overstretched and the heart will respond to increased filling with less pressure. (Reprinted with permission from S.W. Patterson, H. Pipers, and E.H. Starling, *J Physiol* 48:465, 1914.)

cava; he also controlled the aortic pressure (or afterload) by means of an artificial aortic resistance. From a series of such experiments Starling showed that with increased diastolic volume, the subsequent contraction of the isolated heart did indeed result in a higher peak systolic pressure. His data showed that if the ventricle is stretched beyond the physiological limit, the systolic pressure will then decline, indicating impending failure (Fig. 5.5).

Sarnoff and Mitchell found that similar relationships existed between left ventricular end-diastolic pressure (LVEDP) and LV stroke work; because the length-tension relationship of the two ventricles is usually comparable, graphs depicting *right* ventricular volume and *left* ventricular pressure—as was done originally by Starling—also show similar configurations.

This characteristic of the myocardium—also called "heterometric autoregulation"—is an inherent, intrinsic property of the muscle fiber which is evident in the heart fully isolated from all neural or humoral influences. It has been suggested that this property is due to the apposition—as the muscle is stretched—of more crossbridges between the actin and myosin. It was further theorized that the "failure" part of the curve occurs because sarcomeres are stretched beyond their normal length of about 2.2 μm and that fewer crossbridges are thereby formed between the filaments.

However, in a recent study of heart failure in dogs, investigators did not find increases in sarcomere lengths and expressed the belief that the reduced contractility of the failing myocardium is related to an intrinsic defect of the muscle rather than to its position on the descending limb of the Starling curve. Further evidence is needed on this question.

The Starling effect is an important one, however, since it enables the heart to adapt its pumping capacity to alterations in venous return. The contractile response to altered myocardial length is particularly helpful in matching the output of the two ventricles and thus keeping the pulmonary and systemic systems in balance.

Heart Rate Alteration

Aside from precontractile length, alteration of the heart rate and heart rate interval may, under certain circumstances, also influence the contractile response. This may occur in two ways, *i.e.*, through an *intrinsic increase in stroke power* associated with an increase in rate and through so-called *interval-strength effects*.

Interval-Strength Effects

Heart rate will influence stroke volume through its temporal effect on diastolic filling time, *i.e.*, with greater filling time, there will be increased stroke volume (Chapter 7). But there are additional intrinsic "interval-strength" factors which can produce temporary alterations in myocardial contractility. Interval-strength relationships are complex and only three effects will be considered here. A rapid rate increase will progressively augment cardiac contractility—this is known as the staircase or "treppe" phenomenon (Fig. 5.6, *left*).

Similarly, a longer than normal delay between beats, or a pause after an extrasystole (post-extrasystolic potentiation) will be followed by stronger contractions. These effects, which are clearly intrinsic and not

Figure 5.6. Myocardial contraction: the interval-strength relation. An increase in heart rate, a prolonged beat interval and a delay after an extrasystole all result in stronger subsequent contractions. (Reprinted with permission from E.O. Feigl, *Physiology and Biophysics*, edited by T.C. Ruch and H.D. Patton. Philadelphia: W.B. Saunders, 1974.)

dependent on increased filling, are nonetheless amplified in the intact heart by the added mechanical effect of increased diastolic filling.

In the intact ventricle, as well as in isolated cardiac muscle, a premature depolarization results in a reduced mechanical contraction, the magnitude of which is a function of the degree of prematurity of the extra depolarization. The next contraction then is more forceful than normal, the degree of augmentation being greater the earlier the extra depolarization is introduced. The interval-strength relation, which is of relatively minor importance in the intact human, is probably due to a time-induced alteration in Ca^{2+} availability to the muscle cell.

Intrinsic Increase in Stroke Power

With increase in heart rate, Mitchell et al. demonstrated that in the areflexic, open-chest dog preparation, the left ventricle can produce the same stroke work over a wide range of heart rates, *i.e.*, with no change in end-diastolic volume. Thus, the ventricle, as it beats faster, becomes stronger, *i.e.*, develops more stroke power as its rate increases. The mechanism of this intrinsic response is not known.

It is therefore evident that alteration of heart rate affects ventricular contraction in two ways. A rate alteration will clearly affect the time for diastolic filling so that if other factors are held constant, a slowing of the rate will increase stroke volume through this mechanical effect. The degree to which heart rate affects stroke volume depends on the degree of heart rate change. The effect of heart rate on stroke volume will be discussed further in Chapter 7. However, in addition to this factor, as described above, alteration of heart rate interval has intrinsic effects on myocardial contractility, which become evident in carefully designed, isolated heart preparations. The role of these intrinsic effects in the intact, awake animal or human (with functioning reflexes) is not yet certain.

Afterload Stresses—Force-Velocity Curves

If a cardiac muscle strip is made to lift a load after contraction has begun (afterloading), the muscle gradually develops tension as the series elastic element (Fig. 5.3) is stretched, so that after a brief interval the muscle begins to shorten. At first the velocity of shortening is high but as the elastic tension rises, the velocity gradually diminishes. When the afterload is increased in steps, the degree of shortening, the velocity of shortening and the total time of contraction all decrease (Fig. 5.7, *bottom left*).

The counterpart of this in the intact human is the decreased stroke volume, decreased ejection velocity and shortened ejection time when the aortic pressure rises (Chapter 7); the myocardial fibers need a longer

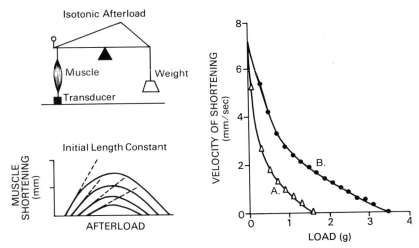

Figure 5.7. Influence of afterload on velocity and degree of shortening of myocardium. When a muscle is permitted to shorten (isotonic contraction) against different afterloads (*top left*), the degree of shortening and initial velocity (*dashed lines*) decrease as afterload is increased (*bottom left*). *Right*, the plot of force (afterload) *vs.* initial velocity of shortening with different afterloads. At 1.6 g (*curve A*) the load is too heavy to lift, the velocity is 0 and the contraction is isometric. A greater preload (*curve B, right*), and therefore a greater initial muscle length, shifts the curve to the right, but the maximum velocity (V_{max}) is unchanged. (Reprinted with permission from E.H. Sonnenblick, *Fed Proc* 21:975, 1962.)

time to develop the tension required to overcome the greater afterload. At the lightest load, the initial velocity of contraction is greatest. If the velocities are plotted against afterload (Fig. 5.7, *right, curve A*), the velocity curve extrapolated to the *y* (velocity) axis would represent the velocity at zero load, *i.e.*, maximum velocity (V_{max}).

In the above experiment, the initial muscle length (preload) was held constant and the afterload varied. If now, the preload is varied, *i.e.*, the muscle stretched to a larger precontractile length and the muscle again subjected to different afterloads, a curve similar to that of Figure 5.7, *right, curve B*, will result.

It will be noted in Figure 5.7 (*right*) that the muscle with the greater preload (and thereby stretched) can overcome a larger afterload, which is in accord with Starling's law; but in addition, it is significant that V_{max} is independent of preload.

Homeometric Autoregulation

As described above, increase in afterload will cause a decrease in strength, velocity and duration of contraction of the isolated heart muscle. Similarly, increase in aortic pressure will cause comparable effects in the intact ventricle (Chapter 7). However, in certain instances, particularly in anesthetized animals after abrupt increase in aortic pressure, there may be an initial decrease followed by a temporary *elevation* of stroke work. This is not a mechanical but rather an intrinsic, inotropic response of the myocardium; it is known as the "Anrep" effect or "homeometric autoregulation" since it occurs without any change in fiber length. Existing evidence suggests that this phenomenon, which may be related to an improved myocardial blood flow, plays only a minor role in myocardial contraction in the intact human circulation.

Extrinsic Regulation of the Myocardium—Inotropic State

Outside factors which affect the inotropic state or contractility of the heart may be of three general types: (a) *neurohormonal effects*, due to influences of the sympathetic or parasympathetic systems or of the catecholamines; (b) *chemical and pharmacological effects, e.g.*, contractile changes due to alterations in blood K^+, Ca^{2+} or pH, or to drugs such as digitalis and sympathetic "blockers"; and (c) *pathological effects, e.g.*, those due to ischemia incident to coronary occlusion or toxic effects resulting from bacteria or chemicals.

As shown in Figure 5.8 (*left*), sympathetic stimulation will produce a positive inotropic effect and move the Starling curve upward and to the left depending on the strength of stimulation. Increased contractility will also result from injection of norepinephrine, digitalis or Ca^{2+} ions. If these same stimuli are applied either to the isolated muscle or to the

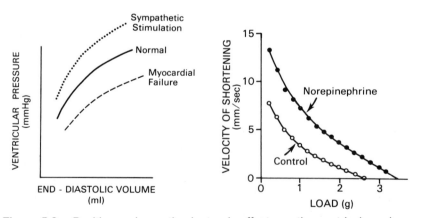

Figure 5.8. Positive and negative inotropic effects on the ventricular volume-pressure (Starling) curve (*left*) and on the myocardial force-velocity curve (*right*). Sympathetic stimulation or administration of norepinephrine or digitalis will move the Starling curve up and to the left and the force-velocity curve up and to the right and will increase V_{max}. Myocardial ischemia, toxic agents or heart failure will have opposite effects.

intact heart, the force-velocity curve is moved upward and to the right and V_{max} is increased (Fig. 5.8, *right*). Therefore, in these cases a stronger myocardial contraction has resulted from an extrinsic influence as evidenced (a) by the shift to a higher Starling curve or (b) by a shift to a higher force-velocity curve with an increased V_{max}. Conversely, myo-cardial ischemia, toxic and anesthetic agents, hypocalcemia, hyperkale-mia or cardiac failure will result in a negative inotropic effect; these are manifested by a lower Starling curve and a lower force-velocity curve with a decreased V_{max}.

As previously described, an increase in the length of the cardiac muscle fiber or augmentation of end-diastolic volume (as occurs within an individual Starling curve) causes an increase in the ability of the contractile machinery to develop force. While this is an exceedingly important characteristic of the heart muscle that enables it to adapt itself to variations in venous return, it does not affect the inotropic state. The change in sarcomere length alters the degree of filament overlap but does not change the number of contractile sites and is not considered an alteration in contractile state. In contrast, a shift of the curves denotes an increase in the rate of activation of contractile sites, an alteration in the velocity of shortening and a change in the basic inotropic state of the muscle.

The alteration of the inotropic state of cardiac muscle is probably related to the rate of Ca^{2+} binding to troponin. The normal serum calcium concentration (about 4.3–5.3 mEq/L) is about 10,000 times that of the myocardial cell; yet a reduction of serum calcium will lessen myocardial contractility.

Assessment of Cardiac Contractility

As described above, in the intact human circulation, the strength of cardiac contraction may be altered in two primary ways: (a) by altering diastolic filling, *i.e.*, by changing precontractile muscle length, an intrin-sic effect; or (b) by altering the inotropic state or contractility, an extrinsic effect, which is usually brought about by neural or hormonal influences. For clinical as well as experimental purposes, the measure-ment of contractile capability of the heart is a highly important objective.

In evaluating cardiac function, a distinction should be made first of all between "performance" and "contractility." Cardiac performance refers to measurements such as stroke volume and cardiac output which depend on contractility but are also influenced by mechanical or other extraneous factors. Contractility is the more important measurement and refers to a careful estimate, under controlled conditions, of the basic ability of the heart muscle to generate power, *i.e.*, its inotropic state. Circulatory performance such as cardiac output may, for example, be adversely affected by decreased blood volume or an incompetent valve while the contractile ability of the myocardium may be entirely normal. This distinction would be an important one for instance after a myocardial infarct, when it would be helpful to have a quantitative measure of the remaining myocardial contractile ability so that an estimate might be made as to whether the patient may be an acceptable risk for myocardial revascularization surgery.

There are four major determinants of myocardial performance, *i.e.*, preload, afterload, heart rate and contractility (inotropic state). As previously noted, preload and inotropic capability are major determinants of myocardial contractile power while afterload and heart rate (to be discussed in Chapter 7) are mainly mechanical factors which affect performance. By maintaining preload, afterload and heart rate constant, one may determine the effect of drugs, catecholamines or other interventions on contractility. Alternatively, one may maintain the heart rate, afterload and extrinsic factors constant and determine the effect of preload. If one could control external factors in this fashion, ideal measures of cardiac contractility would be the determination of ventricular pressure and work at different levels of end-diastolic volume (Starling curve) or the measurement of V_{max}.

While such procedures are possible with cardiac muscle strips or isolated heart preparations, they are difficult to achieve in the intact organism. Many methods have been designed to approximate this ideal and to estimate myocardial contractility in the intact subject but none is as yet fully satisfactory.

In clinical studies, some of the more commonly used measures of cardiac contractility are (a) ejection indices, (b) ventricular dimensions and their rate of change, (c) isovolumic indices and (d) systolic time intervals. Ejection indices, which are based on the effectiveness of left ventricular ejection, include aortic flow velocity, acceleration of blood in the aorta (dV/dt) and ejection fraction (the ratio of stroke volume and end-diastolic volume). Ventricular dimensions and their rate of change can be estimated by ventricular angiography, radionuclide ventriculography and echocardiography; these techniques will be described in Chapter 7.

Isovolumic indices are based on the pressure rise during the isovolumic contraction period (Fig. 3.5) when the ventricle is a closed chamber and is undergoing isometric contraction. One of the more commonly used of these indices is left ventricular dP/dt_{max}.

In this method, sensitive manometers are used to record the ventricular pressure curve; the tangent of the steepest point of the curve (or the peak of a wave recorded by a differentiating circuit) indicates the maximum rate of pressure change. This occurs during the isovolumic phase and is a reasonable index of the initial velocity of myocardial contraction (Fig. 5.9).

Although dP/dt_{max} will vary to some extent with preload and heart rate, it is very responsive to changes in the inotropic state and has been used clinically to characterize the contractile ability of the heart. The left ventricular dP/dt_{max}, which is normally about 1,600 mm Hg/sec, tends to be less than 1,200 mm Hg/sec in patients with disorders of the left ventricular myocardium. One of the problems with this determination is a technical one, *i.e.*, even with high-fidelity, catheter-tip manometers which eliminate much of the distortion of the pressure wave due to fluid transmission through the catheter, recording artifacts are still difficult to avoid. Moreover, insertion of the catheter is an invasive procedure and carries with it some risk to the patient.

Systolic time intervals (STI) have also been proposed as useful measures of cardiac contractility. STIs are based on the relative duration of contraction and relaxation phases of the cardiac cycle and on the generalization that at a fixed heart rate, the more competent ventricle will, if all other factors are held constant, eject a given stroke volume in less time, *i.e.*, have a shorter ejection period. One of the commonly used STIs is PEP/VET, *i.e.*, the quotient of the preejection period (from the

Figure 5.9. Maximum rate of rise of left ventricular pressure (peak dP/dt). Left ventricular pressure curves with the tangent at the steepest part of ascending limb designating maximum dP/dt. *A*, control; *B*, after norepinephrine; and *C*, cardiac failure. (Reprinted with permission from R.M. Berne and M.N. Levy, *Cardiovascular Physiology.* St. Louis: C.V. Mosby, 1981, p. 81.)

onset of the QRS complex to the beginning of the aortic pulse wave) and the ventricular ejection time (from the beginning of the aortic pulse to the incisura). In an extensive comparative analysis of 32 separate indices of cardiac contractility, Abel found that PVP time (time from the beginning of systole to peak ventricular pressure) was more sensitive to myocardial contractility and less sensitive to changes in preload, afterload and heart rate than any of the other parameters measured.

While all of the currently available indices have certain shortcomings, they can, in many instances, provide valuable information if used in carefully defined circumstances and provided that the techniques and their limitations are understood.

Oxygen Consumption and Work of the Heart

The "resting" O_2 consumption of the heart is about 8 ml/100 g/min of which about one-fourth is for basic maintenance and the remainder for its work of contraction. Of the total oxygen consumption, only 35 to 40% is normally due to oxidation of carbohydrates; thus the major cardiac energy (in postabsorptive states) is derived from noncarbohydrate sources, mainly fatty acids. The amino acid contribution is small. As with other tissues, about 95% of the energy is used to form ATP in mitochondria. The main determinants of myocardial oxygen consumption are (a) ventricular wall tension, (b) heart rate, and (c) velocity of myocardial shortening.

The main work of the heart is expended by pumping a volume of fluid against a pressure head. For this reason the external cardiac work (for the left ventricle) is usually estimated as the product of the stroke volume ejected and the mean aortic pressure during systole (stroke work). The "pressure work" may also be approximated as the product of the cardiac output and the mean arterial pressure. Since the mean pulmonary arterial pressure is about one-sixth that of the aorta and the output of the right ventricle the same as the left, the work done per minute by the right ventricle is about one-sixth that of the left.

In addition to the potential energy in the form of pressure-volume work, kinetic energy is also generated by virtue of the velocity imparted to the blood. Although at rest only about 2 to 4% of the useful work of the heart is in the form of kinetic energy, this fraction may increase to 20 or 25% in exercise.

Because cardiac pressure work is more demanding of oxygen than "flow work," Sarnoff and associates suggested that myocardial O_2 consumption ($M\dot{V}O_2$) might be indirectly estimated by the "tension-time index" (TTI) which is the product of the mean systolic pressure, the duration of systole and the heart rate. In a condition such as aortic stenosis (Chapter 3), intraventricular pressure (and thus TTI and cardiac work) will be much elevated; this increased work requirement prevails in the face of a lessened aortic pressure available for coronary perfusion.

Recent exercise studies by Bruce and others in normal subjects and cardiac patients have indicated that certain indices such as the product of systolic pressure and heart rate (pressure-rate or "double product") or the systolic pressure-heart rate-systolic ejection time product ("triple product") are highly correlated with myocardial oxygen consumption ($M\dot{V}O_2$). The double product at maximal exercise can thus provide a reasonable noninvasive estimate of the limit of left ventricular capability. It should be pointed out, however, that TTI and double product estimations of coronary $M\dot{V}O_2$ do not take into account the metabolic effect of increase in wall tension which occurs in dilated hearts (Laplace's law, Chapter 1) or the alteration in contraction velocity which also has a metabolic effect as mentioned above.

Pressure-Volume Loops

The stroke work of the heart may be represented graphically by a pressure-volume diagram (Figure 5.10). Such a diagram or "loop" represents, in a different way, the events of the cardiac cycle previously

Figure 5.10. Pressure-volume loop showing left ventricular volume and pressure changes during a single heart cycle in a normal adult at rest.

discussed in Chapter 3 and shown in Figure 3.5; in addition (since work = pressure × volume) it also represents the external stroke work expended during a single cardiac cycle. Kinetic energy is omitted.

Diastole, or ventricular filling, consists of the first or rapid filling stage followed by the slow filling phase called diastasis with a final contribution from atrial contraction. Note that there is only a small increase in pressure with the increase in ventricular volume. At the end of diastole, the mitral valve closes and the period of isovolumic (isometric) contraction takes place. During ejection, ventricular pressure is greater than aortic pressure and the myocardium shortens isotonically. At the closure of the aortic valve, isometric relaxation of the ventricle takes place. The diagonally marked area represents work done through venous filling of the ventricle. The area within the loop is the work done by the contracting heart. In certain experimental and clinical situations, pressure-volume loops of disordered hearts may be useful for analyzing the energy exchange and efficiency of the heart.

Efficiency of the Heart

Mechanical efficiency is usually estimated as external work done divided by energy consumed. The work may be calculated as described above and the energy by conversion of O_2 consumption (1 ml of O_2 liberates 2.06 kg-m of energy). The efficiency of the myocardium is ordinarily about 5 to 15%, although this may be considerably increased in exercise in which the cardiac output or flow component increases disproportionately to the pressure component. The remaining 85 to 95% of the energy produced is in the form of heat. Because of the metabolism-stimulating and flow-stimulating effects of temperature itself, physical work capacity is importantly influenced by the ability of the body to maintain optimum temperature. The increased blood flow to skin which occurs in order to dissipate the excess heat, adds to cardiac work demands and, therefore, to coronary flow requirements. This may be a limiting factor in the work capacity of cardiac patients.

References

Abel FL and McCutcheon EP. *Cardiovascular Function: Principles and Applications,* Boston: Little, Brown, 1979, pp. 197–216.
Braunwald E and Ross J Jr. Control of cardiac performance. In: *Handbook of Physiology,* Section 2: *The Cardiovascular System,* The Heart, edited by RM Berne, N Sperelakis and SR Geiger. Bethesda, Md: American Physiological Society, 1979, Vol. I, pp. 533–580.
Galosy RA, Mitchell JH, Atkins JM and Reisch J. Sympathetic stimulation, hemodynamic factors and indices of cardiac inotropic state. *Am J Physiol* 234:H562–H566, 1978.
Langer GA. Myocardial force development in health and disease. In: *Pathophysiology of the Heart,* edited by G Ross. New York: Masson Publishers, 1982, pp. 1–39.

Mitchell JH, Wallace AG and Skinner NS. Intrinsic effects of heart rate on left ventricular performance. *Am J Physiol* 205:41–48, 1963.

Randall WC. *Neural Regulation of the Heart.* New York: Oxford University Press, 1977.

Rothe CF. The venous system: the physiology of the capacitance vessels. In: *Handbook of Physiology. Section 2: The Cardiovascular System,* edited by FM Abboud and JT Shepherd. Bethesda, Md.: American Physiological Society, 1982, Vol. III.

Sarnoff SJ. Myocardial contractility as described by ventricular function curves. *Physiol Rev* 35:107, 1955.

Sonnenblick E. Force-velocity relations in mammalian heart muscle. *Am J Physiol* 202:931, 1962.

Starling EH. *The Linacre Lecture on the Law of the Heart.* London: Longmans, Green & Co., 1918.

Weissler AM. *Non-Invasive Cardiology.* New York: Grune & Stratton, 1974.

Winegrad S. Electromechanical coupling in heart muscle. In: *Handbook of Physiology, Section 2: The Cardiovascular System,* The Heart, edited by RM Berne, N Sperelakis and SR Geiger. Bethesda, Md.: American Physiological Society, 1979, Vol. I, pp. 393–428.

chapter 6

Pressure and Flow in the Arterial and Venous Systems

Aortic Pressure and Flow

As indicated in a previous chapter (Fig. 3.5), during the first third of left ventricular emptying, about two-thirds of the stroke volume is ejected into the aorta. Simultaneous aortic recordings with a pressure transducer and a sensitive flowmeter illustrate this rapid emptying as a quick rise in aortic flow in early systole (Fig. 6.1). This rapid ejection is followed by a sharp fall in ejection rate. At the end of systole there is actually a small, transient reverse flow due to (a) an influx of blood into the coronary arteries, (b) a slight regurgitation of blood back into the left ventricle through the aortic valve, and (c) the distension of the valve as the bolus of blood is stopped from reentering the ventricle.

The pressure wave (Fig. 6.1, *top*) is the shock impulse due to the sudden ejection of blood into the aorta. This wave is transmitted through the aortic blood column and aortic wall at a velocity of about 4 to 6 m/sec which is about 20 times greater than the mean velocity imparted to the blood itself (20 to 40 cm/sec). The pressure wave has, therefore, no direct relationship to flow and could occur fully as well if there were no flow at all. Because the transmission velocity of the pulse wave is increased when the arteries become less distensible, the speed of the wave has sometimes been used as an index of arterial distensibility.

Aortic Pressure Wave

Components

Because pressure is technically easier to record than flow and since the aorta stands between the heart and the circulatory beds of the tissues,

Figure 6.1. Simultaneous flow and pressure tracing in the aorta. There is a rapid ejection of blood from the left ventricle into the aorta followed by a rise in the aortic pressure. (Reprinted with permission from H.P. Peiper, *Rev Sci Instrum* 29:965, 1958.)

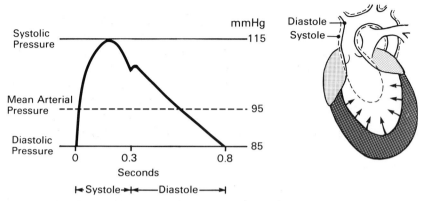

Figure 6.2.   Aortic pressure curve. During systole the ejected volume distends the aorta and aortic pressure rises. The peak pressure is known as the aortic systolic pressure. After the peak ejection, the ventricular pressure falls and when it drops below the aortic pressure, the aortic valve closes, which is marked by the incisura, the end of systole. During diastole, the pressure continues to decline and the aortic wall recoils, pushing the blood toward the periphery. The trough of the pressure wave is the diastolic pressure. The difference between systolic and diastolic pressure is the pulse pressure.

the analysis of the aortic pressure wave can yield valuable information about both central and peripheral circulatory events.

The ascending or anacrotic limb of a typical aortic pressure wave (shown in Fig. 6.2) is the result of the forcible ejection of the left ventricular blood into the aorta with resultant distension of the aortic wall. After it reaches its peak (*i.e.*, the systolic pressure) the ventricular pressure declines to a level below the aortic (the catacrotic limb); at this point the aortic valve closes with a small rebound wave marking the incisura and the end of ventricular systole. At a heart rate of 75 per minute, the cycle length is 0.8 sec or 800 msec, of which about three-eighths or 0.3 sec is taken up by systole.

Diastole, which occupies the rest of the descending limb of the curve is characterized by a long, declining pressure wave during which the aortic wall recoils and propels blood distally to the tissues (the "diastolic runoff"). Meanwhile the ventricle is relaxing and filling for the next stroke. Diastole occupies about five-eighths of the cycle or 0.5 sec. The lowest point of the pressure wave, which occurs at the end of isovolumic ventricular contraction, is called the diastolic pressure.

The difference between systolic and diastolic pressure is the pulse pressure. The mean aortic pressure is the average for the complete period, which is the pressure-time integral for the entire cardiac cycle. The mean pressure can be determined electronically with a polygraph recorder or by determining the area under the curve (the pressure-time product) and dividing by the length of the cycle.

The true mean pressure in an artery is less than the arithmetic average of the systolic and diastolic pressures because the lower half of the curve has a greater area than the upper half. Under ordinary conditions and at normal heart rates, the mean arterial pressure can be roughly estimated as the diastolic pressure plus one-third of the pulse pressure. At high heart rates, it approaches the diastolic plus one-half the pulse pressure. Mean pressure values are essential for certain calculations, *e.g.*, in determining pressure gradients or peripheral resistance.

Transmission

Both the pressure values and the wave configurations are altered during transmission through the peripheral arterial tree (Fig. 6.3). With increasing distance from the heart, the dicrotic notch becomes less sharp (smoothed or filtered) and dicrotic waves appear. In the descending aorta and large arteries, the systolic pressures are higher and diastolic pressures are lower (with a resultant higher pulse pressure) than in the ascending aorta (Fig. 6.3). This is due to (a) the reflection of the pulse waves from the distal vascular bed with subsequent summation at those points, and (b) resonant oscillations of the ejected bolus of blood acting on the elastic arteries.

Figure 6.3. Pressure waves at different sites in arterial tree. With transmission of the pressure wave into the distal aorta and large arteries, the systolic pressure increases and the diastolic pressure decreases, with a resultant heightening of the pulse pressure. However, the mean arterial pressure declines steadily.

It is important to note, however, that the mean pressure—the best single measure of effective driving pressure—is lower in the more distal arteries than at the arch of the aorta as might be expected at a point downstream from the pressure source. However, the pressure loss in the large arteries is small because of their large radius.

With further peripheral transmission and with progressive decrease in size of the arterial radii, the pulse waves are gradually dampened, particularly in the arterioles where the pressure reaches values of 40 to 60 mm Hg. The pulsatile characteristics of the pressure waves are ordinarily extinguished at the capillaries and veins. The venous pressure waves, which reappear in the large veins close to the heart, are similar to the atrial waves (Chapter 3, Fig. 3.4); they are due to backward transmission and reflect events of the right heart and not the left.

Determinants of Aortic Pressure

If the cardiac output (CO) is the ratio of the driving pressure (ΔP) and the total peripheral resistance (TPR) and if we assume the vena caval pressure is approximately zero, then ΔP becomes mean aortic pressure (MAP) and we can, as stated in Chapter 2, formulate the generalization that: MAP = CO × TPR.

If the remaining factor is held constant, an increase or decrease in either cardiac output or total peripheral resistance will result in a corresponding increase or decrease in mean aortic pressure. Cardiac output may, in turn, be altered either by a change in heart rate or stroke volume so that changes in either of these factors may affect MAP depending on the net effect on cardiac output.

An analysis of the factors influencing arterial pressure (systolic, diastolic, pulse and mean) is important (a) because in the cardiovascular system, arterial pressure is the prime regulated variable, and (b) because clinically, disturbances of these different pressure parameters may suggest the specific nature and site of the hemodynamic disorder.

Systolic and Diastolic Pressure

While mean pressure is a valuable measure, it is also possible to obtain useful information from the systolic and diastolic portions of the aortic pressure curve. The primary hemodynamic factors which produce and maintain these components of the pressure curve are shown in Figure 6.4. The relative importance of each factor has been determined mainly from circulatory models.

An increase in stroke volume will cause an increase in systolic pressure, mean pressure and pulse pressure. A decrease in aortic distensibility, *e.g.*, with advancing age, will result in an increase in systolic pressure; the lack of recoil will not sustain the diastolic pressure which

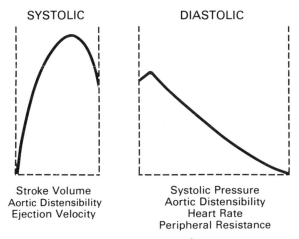

SYSTOLIC   DIASTOLIC

Stroke Volume   Systolic Pressure
Aortic Distensibility   Aortic Distensibility
Ejection Velocity   Heart Rate
                                   Peripheral Resistance

Figure 6.4. Main determinants of aortic systolic and diastolic pressures.

will then fall off more rapidly and as a consequence the pulse pressure will increase substantially. More rapid ejection will cause greater pulse pressure because of inadequate time for the aortic wall to distend in response to the ejected volume. An increased heart rate will interrupt the diastolic decline at a higher point on the curve and raise the diastolic pressure. An increased peripheral resistance will, as previously noted, raise the mean arterial pressure; the diastolic pressure, and eventually the systolic pressure, will also be raised depending on the degree of change in peripheral resistance.

It should be emphasized that the above represent hemodynamic tendencies with a change in one variable. In the intact organism, the situation is often more complex since two or more factors may coexist and the resulting compensatory reflex responses may be superimposed. However, changes in the systolic and diastolic pressure and in the wave configuration can and do provide useful clues to important central and peripheral hemodynamic events.

Arterial Blood Pressure

Pulse Pressure

The pulse pressure is the difference between the systolic and diastolic pressures and would, of course, not exist in a constant flow system. It is due to the force imparted to the arterial blood column by left ventricular contraction which produces a pressure increment over and above the existing diastolic arterial pressure. The pulse wave excursions, when recorded from the body surface (*e.g.*, over the radial artery at the wrist) are damped versions of the arterial pressure wave. The area of the wave will be roughly proportional to the ventricular stroke volume and the character of the wave, *e.g.*, the upstroke, will generally reflect aortic distensibility and ejection velocity, as previously described.

Palpation of the pulse at the carotid or radial artery can give general indications of: (a) *rate and rhythm of the heart*—extrasystoles may be detected if the ejection is forceful enough to transmit the impulse to the periphery; (b) *pulse pressure*—often will be increased in advanced arteriosclerosis or aortic regurgitation; it will be decreased in deep shock in which the rapid, "thready" pulse is characteristic; (c) *approximate level of arterial pressure*—may be gauged by the tension required to obliterate the pulse entirely with one finger while palpating with an adjacent finger.

Normal Values

In the foregoing section, emphasis has been placed on the components of arterial pressure and the central and peripheral hemodynamic factors which may affect arterial pressure in an acute situation. There are other factors which affect arterial pressure on a long term basis. Individuals who are more responsive to stress may show rather wide variations in arterial blood pressure. In such individuals repeated daily measurements after a brief rest period will help to determine the true normal value for that individual.

Age is an important factor; with advancing years there is a progressive tendency toward increase in both systolic and diastolic pressures (Fig. 6.5). Indications of abnormal values should be checked by repeated determinations. The problem of hypertension is discussed in Chapter 15.

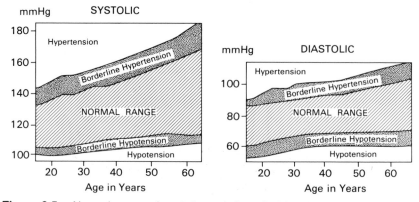

Figure 6.5. Normal range of systolic and diastolic blood pressure in different age groups. (Reprinted with permission from R.F. Rushmer, *Cardiovascular Dynamics*, 4th ed. Philadelphia: W.B. Saunders Co., 1976.)

Venous System: Pressure-Volume-Flow Relations

The study of venous hemodynamics is complicated by: (a) the low intravascular pressure, (b) the intermittent nature of the flow (which varies between high velocity and absolute cessation), (c) the gravity effect, (d) the retrograde pulse transmission, (e) the presence of valves and (f) the collapsible nature of the venous wall. Thus, in many respects, venous flow patterns are more complex than those of the arteries.

As previously shown (Fig. 1.4), the veins constitute the most voluminous portion of the circulatory system. Their compliance, *i.e.*, the unit volume accommodated per unit pressure (dV/dP), is about 25 to 30 times greater than that of the arterial tree. Consequently, when blood or plasma is infused into the vascular system, these fluids, since they seek pressure equilibrium, tend to distribute themselves rather rapidly in the venous and arterial system in the same ratio, *i.e.*, from about 25:1 to 30:1. Similarly, in case of hemorrhage, the decrease in vascular volume is predominantly on the venous side. This can be demonstrated either *in vivo* or in an artificial system containing tubes of similar distensibilities and capacities (Fig. 6.6).

Venous Pressure

Measurement

Venous pressures, either peripheral or central, are ordinarily determined by intravascular catheterization. Because venous pressures are low, they are usually expressed as centimeters of H_2O in a vertical

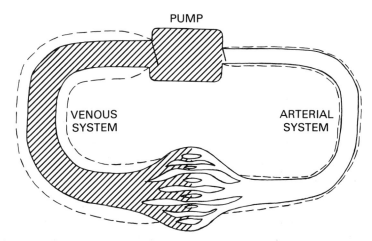

Figure 6.6. Simplified artificial circulation. The "venous" and "arterial" tubes have compliance ratios of about 30:1. Upon overfilling the system, the additional fluid distributes itself in about the same ratio.

manometer using a sensitive pressure transducer. The pulsatile arterial pressure is ordinarily damped out and becomes nonpulsatile at the capillary level. In the venules and large peripheral veins, the pressures remain nonpulsatile, but at the vena cavae level, pulsations again appear, reflecting contractile events on the right side of the heart. These pulsations resemble pressure wave patterns in the right atrium (Chapter 3, Fig. 3.4). Mean pressure values on the venous side normally range from 10 to 15 mm Hg in small venules, from 4 to 8 mm Hg in peripheral veins and from 0 to 2 mm Hg in the vena cavae. Thoracic vena caval pressure is also called "central venous pressure."

Gravity Effect on Venous Pressures

Posture will have marked effects on vascular pressures and volumes in various parts of the body, depending on the vertical distance of the blood column from the heart. Upon quiet standing, the foot veins and arteries in a normal adult are about 120 cm below the heart; this adds a hydrostatic pressure of 120 cm of H_2O, *i.e.*, about 88 mm Hg (Fig. 6.7). It is important to note that although the pressures inside the dependent vessels are increased, the driving pressure, *i.e.*, the impetus forcing blood from the arterial side to the venous side and back toward the heart is unchanged, *i.e.*, it is unaffected by gravity because the increases in pressure on the arterial and venous sides are the same.

Figure 6.7.   Effect of erect position on vascular pressures in the foot and head. Pressures taken in the lower part of the body should be corrected by subtracting the pressure equivalent of the vertical distance below the heart. (Reprinted with permission from A.C. Burton, *Physiology and Biophysics of the Circulation*, 2nd ed. Chicago: Year Book Medical Publishers, 1972.)

The effective driving pressure at any point propelling blood toward the heart will, therefore, be the gauge pressure (that relative to the atmosphere) minus the gravity pressure. All intravascular pressures must be so "corrected" by adding or subtracting the vertical height of the fluid column. If, for example, the pressure in a foot vein of this subject is 102 mm Hg, the effective driving pressure (ΔP) will be 14 mm Hg. On the other hand, this gravity (hydrostatic) pressure will be effective laterally, *i.e.*, across the vessel wall, and, in the upright position, might be expected to increase transmural pressure and capillary transudation of fluid from the capillaries (Chapter 8). This pressure effect is largely offset in normal individuals (as described below) by the skeletal muscle pump, venous valve action and a concomitant gravity effect on interstitial tissue fluid in the legs. In certain cardiac patients, however, the added hydrostatic pressure will increase net capillary transudation of fluid from capillaries causing dependent edema (Chapter 14).

In the upright position, gauge pressures in the arterial tree above the heart will be negative and the true arterial driving pressure is obtained by *adding* the appropriate hydrostatic correction factor. However, venous pressures in the cranium are more complicated and less predictable. In the upright position, the veins inside the skull do not collapse because of their close equilibrium with cerebrospinal fluid, which is at a negative pressure, and because of the anatomical fixation of certain cranial veins (Cerebral Circulation, Chapter 11).

In order to compare venous pressures in different individuals, it is customary to use a common reference point; for this purpose, venous pressures are commonly expressed in terms of vertical height above or below the "phlebostatic level," which passes transversely through the thorax between the anterior and posterior surfaces of the trunk at the level of the fourth intercostal space.

Volume (as well as pressure) changes will also occur in the upright posture because of the height of the vertical blood column. As described in Chapter 1, in the erect position about half of the central blood volume in the chest (about 500 ml) gravitates toward the lower extremities. The veins because of their thinner and more distensible walls will accumulate over 90% of this displaced volume. This migration of blood toward the legs has important hemodynamic effects which will be discussed in Chapter 13 (Postural Effects).

Venous Return to the Heart

The factors influencing the return of blood from the low pressure side of the circulation may be classified as primary and secondary. The primary and by far the dominant factor is the pressure transmitted from the left ventricle through the arteries and veins to the right atrium. Secondary factors are (a) the skeletal muscle pump, (b) the respiratory pump, (c) the venous valves, (d) the "suction" effect of ventricular contraction and relaxation on the atria and (e) venomotor tone, *i.e.*, the state of contraction or relaxation of the smooth muscle of the veins.

Primary Factor Influencing Venous Return

The dominant force which drives blood back to the heart has been called the systemic filling pressure (P_{SF}), *i.e.*, the "mean circulatory pressure" of the systemic circuit. The P_{SF} represents the hemodynamic gradient for the entire systemic circulation, from the root of the aorta to the right atrium; its value is about 7 mm Hg in man. The net driving pressure returning blood to the heart can then be visualized as the difference between the P_{SF} and right atrial pressure. The P_{SF} and its role in venous return is discussed further in Chapter 7.

Secondary Factors Influencing Venous Return

Skeletal Muscle Pump

In certain situations (*e.g.*, in adjustment to the erect posture) skeletal muscles play a significant role. Immediately upon standing, blood gravitates toward the veins of the lower extremity. The venous valves temporarily prevent this retrograde flow but the veins fill rapidly from below. Within a few seconds they are engorged and the pressures in the foot and ankle veins increase to reflect the increased height of the hydrostatic blood column. Shortly thereafter the skeletal muscles of the lower extremity begin rather rhythmical cycles of reflex contraction and relaxation which are responsible for the unconscious swaying action of the body during quiet standing. During the contraction, the blood is squeezed centrally, and during relaxation the veins refill. The valves permit movement of the blood only toward the heart. Without competent venous valves, the muscle pump will be much less efficient. The skeletal muscle pump plays a particularly important role during physical exercise such as running.

This "muscle pump" action serves to lower venous pressure in the dependent parts of the leg, facilitate venous return and relieve venous congestion in the area. Excess blood in the extremities not only creates a deficit in circulating blood volume but in some circumstances also hampers capillary exchange and cellular nutrition of the part. The effectiveness of the muscle pump is illustrated by a marked fall in calf venous pressure with only a single step after quiet standing (Fig. 6.8*A*). With several steps, the muscle action will milk the blood toward the heart and maintain a lower volume and pressure in the dependent veins (Fig. 6.8*B*). As might be expected, the effectiveness of the muscle pump is also dependent on the rate of inflow of blood into the leg, *i.e.*, the rate of venous filling. If the leg is kept cool (25°C), the arterial inflow is

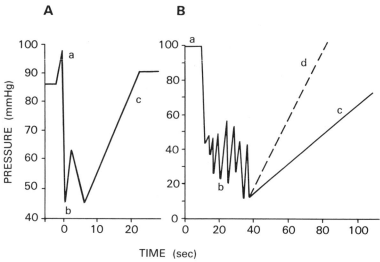

Figure 6.8. Effect of gravity and leg movement on venous pressure in the ankle. *A*, shows at (*a*) a decrease of pressure of 50 mm Hg from quiet standing position to completion of first step and at (*b*) a rapid rise of pressure toward control with resumption of quiet standing at (*c*). *B*, venous pressure at the ankle during quiet standing (*a*) and during walking (*b*). The slope of pressure return during quiet standing is relatively shallow if the skin of the foot is cool (25°C) (*c*). But the rate of rise is doubled at a higher foot temperature (33°C) (*d*). (Adapted from A.A. Pollack and E.H. Wood, *J Appl Physiol* 1:649, 1948–1949; and from J.P. Henry and O. Gauer, *J Clin Invest* 29:855, 1950.)

less and the return to control venous pressure after quiet standing will take about 80 seconds (Fig. 6.8*Bc*). At a higher skin temperature (33°C), arterial inflow to the veins is faster and the return to the higher venous volume and pressure is more rapid (Fig. 6.8*Bd*). At a still warmer skin temperature of 39°C (not shown), the venous pressure returns to the standing level in less than 10 seconds, *i.e.*, the muscle pump during quiet standing is still less efficient in milking blood centralward and in counteracting the increased venous volume and pressure in the lower extremities. This diminished effectiveness of the muscle pump at higher temperatures is instrumental in decreasing the postural tolerance of heart failure patients during hot weather. These patients already have a deficient cardiac pump and generally lessened skeletal muscle tone.

In order for the lower extremity muscles to serve as an effective pump during standing, it is also necessary for the feet to anchor the body so that skeletal muscles may have a counterweight against which to contract. The importance of this factor is underscored by the fact that if the body is suspended in an upright position so that the feet dangle and cannot reach the ground, the unconscious milking action of lower extremity muscles is largely prevented. In this situation most individuals suffer marked reduction of venous return and cardiac output. A 20- to 40-minute suspension in this fashion will produce fainting and a longer exposure may be life threatening. The ancient practice of execution by crucifixion was largely based on the resultant circulatory stress from upright suspension.

Conversely, massive and widespread skeletal muscle contraction such as a grand mal epileptic seizure will cause excessive venous return with increased cardiac output and heightened arterial pressure. A similar increase in venous pressure and venous return will result from widespread sympathetic stimulation of the vascular system (Chapter 7).

Respiratory Pump

This refers to the assistance given to venous return by the mechanical movements of respiration. The intrathoracic pressure is usually slightly subatmospheric and varies during quiet breathing from about −2 to −4 mm Hg during expiration to about −5 to −7 mm Hg during inspiration. As the intrathoracic pressure falls during inspiration, the intraabdominal pressure rises due to the descent of the diaphragm. These changes in pressure gradient facilitate venous return from extrathoracic veins during inspiration and diminish it during expiration.

In this regard, Honig has pointed out that during inspiration, there is about a 250-ml increase in thoracic blood volume due to the decreased (more negative) pressure in the pulmonary vessels; during expiration, there is a comparable expulsion of intrathoracic blood due to the more positive pressure. The increased flow and volume in the vena cavae during inspiration aid right ventricular filling and increase right ventricular stroke volume by about 20 ml. However, the simultaneously increased capacity of the pulmonary vessels (during inspiration) temporarily decreases left ventricular filling and stroke volume. This process is reversed during expiration so that during a full respiratory cycle the left ventricular output shows only a 5 to 7% variation.

The above tendencies are exaggerated with heightening of the respiratory movements and the consequent increases in respiratory pressure increments. However, the effect is limited because of the likelihood of venous collapse at the point of entrance of the veins into the thorax if intravenous pressure becomes negative at that level (Chapter 7).

Venous Valves

Venous valves are very thin, transparent, cusplike structures in the veins of the extremities which insure unidirectional flow. They are placed at about 2- to 4-cm intervals in deep and superficial veins of the extremities, skeletal muscles and skin but are absent in the splanchnic circulation. The walls of veins surrounding valves are usually expanded into a sinus which allows the cusps to separate fully without contraction of the walls, permitting rapid valve closure. As mentioned above, valves are essential for effective muscle pump action.

"Suction" Effect of Ventricular Contraction and Relaxation on the Atria

While the P_{SF} (systemic filling pressure) is the main force driving blood toward the heart, the ventricles also contribute to venous return. During ventricular systole, when the AV valves are closed, the AV ring is drawn downward by the ventricles, enlarging the atria, thereby lowering their relative internal pressures and thus increasing flow from the vena cavae and pulmonary veins. Current evidence further suggests that during diastole, the ventricles also exert a negative pressure by virtue of the "diastolic recoil" of their walls, particularly in hypotensive states such as circulatory shock.

Venomotor Tone

The state of contraction of venous smooth muscle is a significant factor in venous return but the effect of this muscle contraction depends on the intravascular pressure. At low pressures (0–5 mm Hg), veins take on an eliptical shape and contraction of the vascular muscle has little effect on volume; thus the venous wall movement is mainly passive. However, when venous pressures exceed 5 to 10 mm Hg, veins assume a more circular cross section and muscle fibers have increasing length and tension; in this case, venomotor activity is much more effective and a small increase in tone or contractile state, *e.g.*, through venoconstriction, can shift a large amount of blood toward the heart (Chapter 1, Fig. 1.6).

The efferent neural control of venous smooth muscle is exclusively sympathetic and has important functional distributions, *e.g.*, to the splanchnic and cutaneous tissues. The constriction of splanchnic veins in certain stresses (*e.g.*, hemorrhage and shock) shifts the important reservoir of splanchnic blood into the general circulation and thus substantially aids venous return and cardiac output. Superficial veins of the extremities—especially of the skin—show sympathetic venoconstrictor responses during a deep inspiration or hyperventilation and may show contractile responses to a variety of emotional and physical stresses such as pain, fear, anger and hemorrhage. Cutaneous vessels, including veins, play an important role in temperature regulation by constricting in cold and dilating in heat (Chapter 11). While superficial veins of the extremities respond strongly to sympathetic stimulation, deep veins of the calf and forearm respond very little and veins of skeletal muscle not at all to neural stimuli.

Disturbances of Venous Pressure and Flow

Varicose veins refer to vessels which have become distended and tortuous because of incompetent valves and/or prolonged obstruction due to pregnancy, abdominal tumor or prolonged weight bearing. Venous valves usually become incompetent because of congenital defects or previous attacks of thrombophlebitis (inflammation of the vein). The essential defect is a chronic venous hypertension in the lower extremities due to valvular insufficiency in the superficial veins, usually the greater saphenous, the deep veins, or the communicating veins. Resting venous pressures are not abnormally high in varicose veins but the pressure fall during walking is much less and the return to the higher pressures upon quiet standing is much faster. Varicose veins are more common in the female at a ratio of about 5:1.

In the dependent position, limbs with varicose veins contain more blood than normal because of their greater diameter, length and distensibility. In view of this, one might anticipate an exaggerated physiologic response to the head-up position. However, this does not ordinarily occur. The lack of fainting or other reaction to the head-up position may be due to an increase in total blood volume that is often found in varicose vein patients and which may exert a partially compensating effect. The Brodie-Trendelenberg test for varicose veins involves placing a tourniquet on the upper thigh (below the sapheno-femoral venous junction) and noting, after the patient stands, the rate and degree of venous filling before and after release of the tourniquet. Although not a serious circulatory disorder, per se, varicose veins, if widespread and chronic, may lead to dependent edema and persistent ulcers. Elastic stockings (to prevent progression) or surgical removal are common forms of treatment. The most serious complication of a varicosity is a thrombosis (clot) in the vein with subsequent breaking off of a clot segment and central embolization (blood stream conduction) via the vena cavae and impaction into a branch of the pulmonary artery in the lungs. Small emboli are generally absorbed without difficulty but massive widespread embolization with occlusion of more than 50% of the pulmonary vascular bed may produce hypoxemia, pulmonary hypertension, shock and death.

Blood Flow Measurement: Methods

Because the interpretation of blood flow and blood pressure data is closely linked with how the data are obtained, a brief review will be made of the more common methods in current use. Flow methods applicable to cardiac output, *i.e.*, central blood flow, will be discussed in Chapter 7. Following is a brief description of the principles involved in sensing peripheral flow.

Electromagnetic Flowmeter. This invasive method is widely used in experimental studies to determine pulsatile flow in individual arteries (Fig. 6.9). A collar or probe which has two small electrodes positioned on opposite sides of the artery is placed around the blood vessel. Two small magnets in the probe produce a magnetic field across the blood vessel. When a conductor such as blood moves through this field, the electric potential developed at the electrodes is proportional to the velocity of the stream. Knowing the cross-sectional area of the vessel, the volume flow per minute can be calculated. This is an excellent method for accurate flow measurement in an isolated vessel and is particularly applicable to animal studies.

Ultrasonic Flowmeter. There has been increasing interest in the use of ultrasound for a variety of biological measurements including the detection of arterial and venous flow. High frequency sound waves are directed across the vessel and reflected back from the moving erythrocytes to a sensor. There is a shift in frequency of the sound, depending on the velocity of flow, known as the Doppler effect. By detecting the relative velocities of these sound transmissions, the volume flow in the blood vessel can be estimated knowing the cross-sectional area of the vessel. One advantage of the ultrasonic method is that the detector can be positioned on the surface of the body so that blood flow may be determined in a noninvasive manner.

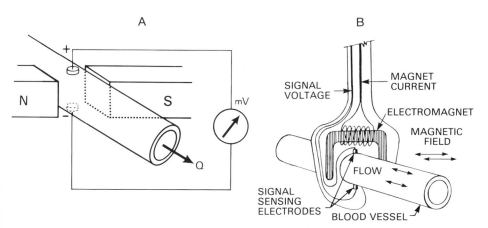

Figure 6.9. *A*, principle of the electromagnetic flowmeter. When a conducting fluid containing ions flows through a magnetic field, an electromagnetic force will be generated perpendicular to the field and proportional to the velocity of the fluid. (Reprinted with permission from T.C. Ruch and H.D. Patton, *Physiology and Biophysics.* Philadelphia: W.B. Saunders, 1974.) *B*, schematic showing incorporation of the elements into a flowmeter probe.

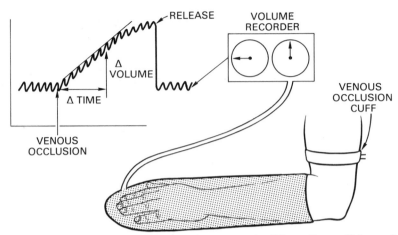

Figure 6.10. Venous occlusion plethysmograph. When the cuff is rapidly inflated to 50 mm Hg, venous outflow is prevented and for the next few seconds, the volume increase in the plethysmograph will reflect the arterial inflow. The initial slope of increased volume per unit time on the calibrated volume recorder will indicate the blood flow to the forearm in milliliters per minute.

Impedance Flowmeter. If band electrodes are placed about a limb, *e.g.*, the calf, and the electrodes excited by a high frequency (100 kHz) sinusoidal current, the observed voltage and impedance changes are dependent on the blood volume changes. From the impedance wave forms, the volume flow through the limb may be calculated. The low amplitude, high frequency current has no injurious effect on the tissues; the impedance method is also adaptable for noninvasive determination of cardiac output (Chapter 7, Impedance Cardiography).

Venous Occlusion Plethysmography. This method is particularly suitable for blood flow determination in an intact limb (Fig. 6.10). By enclosing the extremity in an airtight container and sealing the skin junction, sudden temporary occlusion of the venous return with an occlusion cuff will permit the registration of the volume change of the limb per unit of time on a recorder. Since a temporary venous occlusion will not affect arterial flow, this limb volume change will, for the first 6 to 8 seconds, faithfully record the arterial inflow to the limb. The determination can be repeated after relatively short intervals. By means of an arterial tourniquet at the wrist or ankle, the hand or foot blood flow, which is primarily skin flow, can be excluded; this will permit flow measurements on the forearm or calf alone, which consist primarily of skeletal muscle tissue. This is a convenient and useful noninvasive method in which flows to different tissues of a limb can be determined, for example, in patients with peripheral vascular disease.

Blood Pressure Measurement: Methods

Direct Method of Measuring Arterial Blood Pressure

This involves the placement of a needle or catheter directly into the artery. Pressure and flow studies in a pulsatile system have helped to clarify the requirements for such direct arterial pressure recording; in order to adequately register pressure fluctuations at a given heart rate, a manometer system must accurately respond to frequencies of pulsation at least seven times the frequency of the heart rate.

The strain gauge pressure transducer, which is commonly employed for such arterial pressure sensing, consists of a stiff diaphragm to which are bonded several strain gauges capable of responding rapidly to the transient pressure changes. The hydraulic system which couples the transducer to the artery by means of a catheter is an important element. To retain maximum frequency response, it should be of maximum bore and of minimum length in order to avoid excessive damping of the pressure wave.

The direct method provides the most accurate pressure data; however, it is invasive and, since it involves the placement of a catheter in the vessel, requires that the procedure be performed under sterile conditions.

Figure 6.11.   Illustration of the auscultatory and palpatory techniques for the indirect method of measuring arterial blood pressure. The appearance and disappearance of the ausculatory sounds are illustrated. (Reprinted with permission from R.F. Rushmer. *Cardiovascular Dynamics*. Philadelphia: W.B. Saunders, 1976.)

Figure 6.12. Korotkoff sounds characteristic of the auscultatory phases during measurement of blood pressure in the human. (Reprinted with permission from L.A. Geddes, *The Direct and Indirect Measurement of Blood Pressure.* Chicago: Year Book Medical Publishers, 1970.)

Indirect Blood Pressure Methods

These are most commonly used because of their practicability and ease of repetition. The method depends either (a) on the production of Korotkoff sounds, which are mainly the result of turbulence in the stream, or (b) on the appearance and disappearance of the palpated arterial pulse (Fig. 6.11).

The instrument used is a sphygmomanometer which consists of an inelastic cuff which encloses a rubber bag. Inflation of the cuff to a level above systolic pressure will occlude all blood flow to and from the arm. Gradual reduction of the cuff pressure will permit a return of arterial flow as detected by the appearance of an audible tapping sound at the brachial artery below the cuff, marking the systolic pressure. Progressive decrease of the pressure will produce characteristic sound fluctuations (Fig. 6.12) until final muffling and disappearance of the sound. Muffling is the best index of diastolic pressure in children. Disappearance of the sounds is regarded as the best index of diastolic blood pressure in adults. In some individuals (especially in hypertensive patients), during the lowering of the cuff pressure, the sounds may temporarily disappear and then reappear, a possible source of error in the determination (auscultatory gap, Fig. 6.12). To avoid errors in reading, the cuff must be the correct width for the patient's arm. If it is too narrow, the pressure reading will be erroneously high; if it is too wide, the reading may be erroneously low. The width of the inflatable bladder should be 40% of the circumference of the midpoint of the limb (or 20% wider than the diameter) on which it is to be used. For the average adult arm, a bladder 12 to 14 cm wide has been found to be satisfactory.

Although the indirect method does not provide a continuous recording and is not as accurate as the direct, it is rapid and convenient. If carefully performed, this method serves adequately in most clinical circumstances.

References

Abel FL and McCutcheon EP. *Cardiovascular Function: Principles and Applications.* Boston: Little, Brown, 1979.

Alexander RS. The peripheral venous system. In: *Handbook of Physiology,* Section 2: *Circulation,* edited by WF Hamilton and P Dow. Washington, D.C.: American Physiological Society, 1963, Vol. II, p. 1075.

Geddes, LA. *Direct and Indirect Measurement of Blood Pressure.* Chicago: Year Book Medical Publishers, 1970.

Geddes LA and Baker LE. *Principles of Applied Biomedical Instrumentation.* New York: John Wiley & Sons, 1975, 2nd ed.

Honig CR. *Modern Cardiovascular Physiology.* Boston: Little, Brown, 1981, pp. 127–131.

Kirkendall WM, Feinleib M, Freis ED, and Mark AL. *Recommendations for Human Blood Pressure Determination by Sphygmomanometers.* Dallas: American Heart Association, 1980.

Milnor WR. *Hemodynamics.* Baltimore: Williams & Wilkins, 1982.

Rothe CF. The venous system: The physiology of the capacitance vessels. In: *Handbook of Physiology,* Section 2: *The Cardiovascular System,* edited by FM Abboud and JT Shepherd. Bethesda, Md.: American Physiological Society, 1982, Vol. III.

Shepherd JT and VanHoutte PM. *Veins and Their Control.* Philadelphia: W.B. Saunders, 1975.

Strandness DE and Sumner DS. *Hemodynamics for Surgeons,* New York: Grune & Stratton, 1975, pp. 21–30.

Whitney RJ. The measurement of volume changes in human limbs. *J Physiol (Lond)* 121:1, 1953.

chapter 7

Venous Return and Cardiac Output

Undoubtedly one of the most basic cardiovascular measurements is the output of the heart. It is usually defined as the volume of blood ejected by either ventricle per minute and since the two ventricles, except in unusual circumstances, are in balance, the two outputs are essentially equal. In the resting human adult, mean flow to the entire body is about 80 ml/kg/min so that total flow or cardiac output in an average sized subject (70 kg) is about 5.6 L/min. The two prime determinants of tissue blood flow are its mass and metabolic rate. Cardiac output is correlated with both body mass and body surface area. The latter is in more common clinical use and on this basis, the average value, called the *cardiac index*, is about 3.2 L/min/m² body surface.

Regulation of Cardiac Output—General

In a closed, artificial, hydraulic system consisting of a pump and pipes, the output depends on the characteristics of the pump, of the system and of the fluid. To obtain the required flow, the usual procedure is to determine the resistance, and then set the pump speed at the level necessary to overcome that resistance and thus achieve the desired output.

In the human circulation, however, the situation is quite different; both the pipe system and the fluid are able to change characteristics from time to time and thereby impose varying demands on the pump. On the other hand, the pump has, in its own right, a wide latitude in altering its own characteristics in order to meet these demands.

As will be discussed in Chapter 9, the overriding determinant of total flow in any organism of fixed mass is the metabolic rate; as a consequence, flow requirements will rise markedly in fever or exercise and decrease in conditions such as sleep or hypothyroidism. But these changes in output are induced by metabolic requirements of the body and not by switching the pump to a different setting; in other words it is the body which sets the pace and not the pump.

Thus from a flow standpoint, the heart plays a "permissive" role and does not regulate its own output. So in the human circulation, the heart functions as a "demand" pump and will eject only the minimum volume demanded of it. The healthy, normal heart does, however, have impressive resources at its own disposal and is well able to meet a large range of ordinary demands; nevertheless, when diseased, the heart becomes the limiting factor in controlling the output and when it cannot cope, signs and symptoms of failure appear (Chapter 14).

For these reasons it is necessary to consider the regulation of cardiac output from two different standpoints: (a) *the role of systemic factors* in determining cardiac output (*i.e.*, what influences the return flow of blood to the heart) and (b) *the role of cardiac factors* in determining cardiac output (*i.e.*, what influences the ability of the heart to pump out the blood returned to it).

Systemic Factors Determining Cardiac Output—Venous Return Curves

In a discussion of venous flow in Chapter 6, it was pointed out that the primary factor influencing the return of blood to the heart was the force transmitted by left ventricular ejection through the arteries to the veins. This pressure gradient is sometimes called the *vis a tergo* ("force from behind").

Guyton has analyzed the forces responsible for venous return to the heart from a somewhat different perspective. He has suggested the concept of a "mean circulatory filling pressure" which is the average of the pressures in all segments of the vascular system when each of these pressures is weighted in proportion to the compliance of its respective segment. This average pressure would be a single, integrated, hydrostatic measure of the degree of filling of the circulation and would represent the force tending to propel blood toward the right atrium. He pointed out that without such a filling pressure and return force, the cardiac output would be zero no matter how actively the heart would pump.

Guyton found that this single mean circulatory filling pressure of the systemic circuit could be measured in animals by suddenly arresting the heart and rapidly pumping blood from the aorta to the vena cavae until the pressures equalized. The pressure measurements must be made quickly (within about 7 seconds), *i.e.*, before any autonomic reflexes become effective.

Determined in this manner, the mean circulatory filling pressure for the systemic system, called the *systemic filling pressure* (P_{SF}), is about 7 mm Hg in the dog and is believed to be very similar to this in man. The *mean pulmonary filling pressure* (P_{PF}), *i.e.*, the comparable figure for the pulmonary circuit, is about 2 mm Hg.

Viewed in this perspective, the beating heart in the living animal has the essential function of transporting blood from the low pressure-high compliance venous system to the high pressure-low compliance arterial system. This rearrangement of volumes and pressures enables the arterial system to provide the necessary pressure head for perfusion of all the peripheral tissues. In a normal, unstressed circulation, the mean circulatory pressures would be similar to those determined in the arrested heart.

Under circumstances in which nervous and other controls are not operative, the venous return to the right atrium may be theoretically determined as the balance between the "systemic filling pressure" (P_{SF}), *i.e.*, the force tending to return blood to the right atrium, and the right atrial pressure (P_{RA}), *i.e.*, the opposing force. The resulting venous return at different levels of P_{SF} and P_{RA} are shown in the form of venous return curves in Figure 7.1.

Figure 7.1. On the normal venous return curve (*solid line*), the venous return is about 5.5 L/min when the systemic filling pressure (P_{SF}) is 7 mm and the right atrial pressure (P_{RA}) about 0. If on the normal curve, the P_{RA} is increased to about 2 mm Hg or the P_{SF} decreased to 5.2 mm Hg, the venous return would decrease to about 4 L/min. (Reprinted with permission from A.C. Guyton, *Circulatory Physiology*: *Cardiac Output and Its Regulation*. Philadelphia: W.B. Saunders, 1973.)

In the schema of Figure 7.1, the estimated venous return can be read off the y axis at the intersecting point of the P_{RA} and P_{SF} curve. At normal values of 7 mm Hg P_{SF} and about zero for P_{RA}, the 7 mm gradient will induce a venous flow of about 5.5 L/min. In case of decreased blood volume (*e.g.*, hemorrhage) or loss of sympathetic tone, which would decrease both arterial and venous pressure, the P_{SF} will also decrease; if the P_{SF} decreases to 5.2 and P_{RA} remains at zero, the net pressure gradient would be reduced to 5.2 and venous return will decrease to about 4 L/min. If the P_{SF} is 7 and P_{RA} is increased to 2 mm Hg, the gradient for venous return will be reduced to 5 mm Hg and the output will also be reduced to about 4 L/min. Increased venous return curves, *e.g.*, the above-normal P_{SF} curve of 10.5 mm Hg in Figure 7.1 might occur with increased blood volume, increased sympathetic stimulation or a massive contraction of skeletal muscle with excessive skeletal muscle pump action and heightened peripheral venous pressure.

It will be noted that the P_{SF} curves become flat at right atrial pressures below the zero level. This plateau is due to the collapse of veins entering the chest whenever the transmural pressure is less than zero. This stops effective flow no matter what the right atrial-P_{SF} gradient may be.

While the venous return curves involve certain abstractions and include parameters which are difficult to measure, Guyton's analytic approach has been of considerable theoretical and practical assistance in understanding the basic factors concerned with venous return. This concept also permits, *e.g.*, a combination of venous return and cardiac output curves into a single graph (Fig. 7.2). In Figure 7.2*A* are shown normal venous return and cardiac output values in which these two variables are both related to right atrial pressure. The two curves intersect at a value of 5 L/min (point *a*). If the blood volume is increased by transfusion, the P_{SF} will be considerably increased as will the venous return and cardiac output (point *b*).

Sympathetic stimulation has two effects: (a) contraction of the peripheral vasculature, particularly of the venous bed, will increase the P_{SF} and therefore the pressure gradient for venous return, and (b) increase in cardiac contractile strength will move the ventricular function curve to the left (Fig. 5.8). As shown in Figure 7.2*B*, the venous return and cardiac output would both increase and their junction point would move from point *a* to *c*. Decreased sympathetic activity will have the reverse effect and move the cardiac output from point *a* to *b*.

It should be emphasized that the responses to stresses such as increased blood volume, hemorrhage and sympathetic stimulation are ordinarily damped by autonomic circulatory reflexes (Chapter 10) with a gradual

RIGHT ATRIAL PRESSURE (mmHg)

Figure 7.2.   Combined venous return and cardiac output curves. *A*, a large blood transfusion increases the systemic filling pressure (P_{SF}) from 7 to 16 mm Hg and the right atrial pressure from 0 to 8 mm Hg. As a result, the venous return and cardiac output are considerably increased, *i.e.*, from point *a* to point *b*. *B*, sympathetic stimulation increases P_{SF} through contraction of peripheral vessels (particularly veins) and so moves the venous return curve from the *solid line* to the *upper dashed line*; simultaneously it increases ventricular contractility and shifts the atrial pressure-cardic output curve to the left. The cardiac output is, therefore, moved from point *a* to point *c*. Conversely, with sympathetic inhibition, the cardiac output might be reduced from point *a* to point *b*. (Reprinted with permission from A.C. Guyton, *Circulatory Physiology: Cardiac Output and Its Regulation*. Philadelphia: W.B. Saunders, 1973.)

Figure 7.3.   Reserve stroke volume. Schematic representation showing ventricular volume and stroke volume (SV). Upon standing, heart rate is increased and stroke volume decreased; with exercise in the erect position, SV is increased through encroachment on both diastolic and systolic reserve. (Adapted from R.F. Rushmer, *Cardiovascular Dynamics*. Philadelphia: W.B. Saunders, 1976.)

return to the normal state. However, an understanding of the initial tendencies is important because they may persist for appreciable periods of time and in the diseased state may even progress.

Cardiac Factors Determining Cardiac Output

Since the heart is a demand pump, it must be able to make moment by moment adjustments in order to cope (a) with shifting preload requirements as manifested by alterations in venous return, and (b) with sudden circulatory demands which may arise as a result of stress and which require rapid changes in output. Since cardiac output is the product of stroke volume (SV) and heart rate (HR), such adjustments may be made by alteration in either or both of these two parameters.

At a HR of 70/min the SV of a normal resting adult will be approximately 80 ml. The mean end-diastolic volume (EDV) at rest is variable but will normally range from about 110 to 130 ml. The ejection fraction (EF), *i.e.*, the ratio of SV/EDV, is normally about 67% in man but somewhat lower (45 to 65%) in the faster-beating canine heart; the blood remaining after ejection is called the end-systolic volume (ESV). As shown in Figure 7.3, there is usually a diastolic and systolic reserve volume.

In the supine position, central blood volume, atrial filling pressure and EDV are all relatively high; with exercise in this position, CO is increased mainly through a HR increase and only secondarily by greater ventricular emptying and a decrease in ESV. In the quiet, erect position, atrial filling pressure, SV and EDV are all decreased (Fig. 7.3*B*) and HR is increased. Upon exercise in the erect position, HR is further increased and SV is increased by both a greater diastolic filling with increased EDV, and a more complete systolic emptying and decreased ESV (Fig. 7.3*C*).

Regulation of Stroke Volume

The four primary factors described in Chapter 5 as determinants of myocardial performance are also the main determinants of stroke volume; these factors are *diastolic filling* (*preload*), *inotropic state* (*contractility*), *aortic pressure* (*afterload*) and the *heart rate*. The first two of these factors importantly affect myocardial contraction; the last two exert mainly mechanical effects on cardiac output.

Diastolic Filling (*Preload*). As described in Chapter 5, the heart has an important intrinsic capability enabling it to make adjustments to changes in EDV (heterometric autoregulation). With increased venous return and increased filling, there is increased strength of the subsequent contraction and increased stroke volume; with decreased filling the reverse occurs.

Inotropic State. This important extrinsic factor enables the heart to contract more strongly at an equivalent diastolic volume. In the normal circulation, a positive inotropic effect is commonly mediated through sympathoadrenal discharge which will improve cardiac performance in several ways, *viz.*, ventricular contraction is more rapid (increased V_{max} and dP/dt) and is stronger. As a result the ventricles empty more completely, *i.e.*, there is a decreased ESV and increased SV, which will produce higher systolic pressures in the ventricle and aorta. Diastolic compliance, however, is not affected. If the cause of the increased inotropic state is sympathetic stimulation, there will be an associated increase in heart rate; as discussed below, the degree of stroke volume increase may be limited by the shortening of ventricular filling time incident to the rate increase. However, with sympathetic stimulation, the net result is usually an increased cardiac output. A negative inotropic effect, by vagal stimulation, will decrease heart rate and impulse conduction and diminish atrial contractility.

Aortic Pressure (*Afterload*). Alteration of aortic pressure will produce important effects on cardiac function because of the mechanical resistance it imposes on left ventricular emptying. Sudden aortic pressure changes will result in inverse changes in strength, velocity and duration of left ventricular ejection and therefore of stroke volume. These effects were discussed in Chapter 5 and shown in isolated cardiac muscle in Figure 5.7 and in a denervated animal preparation in Figure 7.4. In the intact animal, there is, at the same atrial pressure, an inverse relation between aortic pressure and stroke volume when the arterial pressure is high. However, at normal mean arterial pressures (up to about 100 mm Hg), the cardiac output is relatively independent of arterial blood pressure. Even though the left ventricular stroke volume may be temporarily reduced by a moderate increase in systemic arterial pressure, the right ventricle continues to pump, which maintains the left ventricular filling pressure and end-diastolic volume. This factor, as well as

Figure 7.4. Relationship of left ventricular output and aortic pressure in a denervated animal preparation. As aortic pressure is increased, the left ventricular output decreases at the same left atrial pressures. The heart rate was constant so that the afterload effect was on the stroke volume. (Reprinted with permission from K. Sagawa, *Physical Bases of Circulatory Transport*: *Regulation and Exchange*. Philadelphia: W.B. Saunders, 1967.)

homeometric autoregulation (Chapter 5), combine to help restore the left ventricular output at these arterial pressure levels.

Effect of Heart Rate on Stroke Volume. At a constant left atrial filling pressure, an increase in heart rate will decrease the diastolic filling time, and consequently, through heterometric autoregulation, decrease stroke volume; however, most of ventricular filling occurs during the rapid filling phase. A modest increase in heart rate will encroach first on diastasis (the slowest filling phase) so the effect on diastolic filling is minimized and cardiac output will increase. If other factors are held constant, the net effect of heart rate on cardiac output will depend mainly on the extent of rate increase, on atrial filling pressure and on the contractile or inotropic state of the ventricle.

If, while at rest, atrial filling pressures remain normal and the heart rate is progressively increased by using a pacemaker, cardiac output will rise at first, then level off, and at rates of 120 to 130/min will begin to decline. However, during sympathoadrenal stimulation or exercise, cardiac output will only begin to decline at rates of about 180/min; this improved cardiac performance is due to a combination of increased venous return with increased atrial filling pressure and the inotropic effects mentioned above, *i.e.*, increased strength of ventricular contraction and a shortening of ventricular systole (with a relative lengthening of diastole). This better performance, however, is contingent on the maintenance of adequate atrial filling pressure and volume. During exercise the increased metabolic rate, the decreased peripheral resistance (especially in the exercising muscle) and the venoconstriction all contribute to the increased atrial filling. As a result, the increase in heart rate will be associated with an increase in cardiac output in the young adult up to rates of about 180/min. With increasing age, this maximum rate will gradually decrease (Chapter 12).

Regulation of Heart Rate

While heart rate does affect stroke volume, it is a separately controlled variable which has other effects on cardiac performance. The chronotropic activity of the heart is normally determined by the rate of impulse generation in the SA node (Chapter 4). This, in turn, is influenced primarily by: (a) the autonomic balance between the sympathetic and vagal impulses to the node—sympathetic stimulation will increase heart rate and vagal stimulation will decrease it; (b) temperature and metabolic activity of the pacemaker tissue—increased temperature and metabolism will increase heart rate, reduced temperature and metabolism will have the reverse effect; and (c) the effect of ionic and pH changes on the heart. The latter effects are less important from a heart rate standpoint.

The autonomic balance—an important factor in cardiac control—is affected by several reflexes which influence heart rate, *e.g.*, distension of the right atrium by increased venous return may increase heart rate (the Bainbridge reflex). The role of these reflexes will be further discussed in Chapter 10.

Integration of Stroke Volume and Heart Rate

As previously mentioned, an increase in thoracic vena caval and right atrial blood volume, *i.e.*, in "central" blood volume and pressure, will cause an increase in the force of ventricular contraction (Starling effect) as well as an increase in heart rate (Bainbridge reflex). But which of these mechanisms will predominate or will both be activated? A recent reinvestigation of this question indicated that there are considerable species differences in such hemodynamic responses and that the results are strongly influenced by the state of the animal or subject.

Two generalizations have emerged from these analyses, *viz.* (a) in normal human subjects, heart rate is much more important in producing major temporary adjustments in cardiac output than is stroke volume, and (b) the response which will ultimately be employed depends mainly on the latitude remaining to that particular response mechanism.

The latter principle is exemplified by the effect of posture on the exercise response. In the supine position, central venous pressure and end-diastolic volume are high and heart rate is relatively low; during exercise in this position, the increase in cardiac output involves a large increase in heart rate, but a lesser increase in stroke volume. Experiments on normal, conscious dogs have yielded similar results, *i.e.*, the reclining animals have a high resting stroke volume and low heart rate; elevation of preload in these dogs induced mainly an increase in heart rate. However, in the same animals, a reduction of cardiac output by volume depletion was mediated almost entirely through a reduction of stroke volume. In other experiments, it was shown that after trauma, hemorrhage, anesthesia or other stress, the heart rate is usually elevated but stroke volume is low; an infusion of blood or plasma at this stage will increase cardiac output mainly through elevation of stroke volume with little change in heart rate.

Thus, it is evident that the cardiac response to altered venous return is an integrated one which depends mainly on the existing heart rate and stroke volume and to a lesser extent on the autonomic balance at the time. In pathological situations, such as myocardial disease, ventricular compliance may also influence the hemodynamic response to increased central venous pressure. In the conditions described thus far, the ventricular wall is assumed to have normal compliance; Figure 5.5 (Chapter 5) showed, *e.g.*, that during normal diastolic filling, left ventricular pressure increases very little, *i.e.*, the chamber walls offer little resistance to filling. However, in congestive heart failure or cardiac hypertrophy, the ventricular wall may become much less compliant and ventricular pressure will rise inordinately during diastole thereby seriously impeding ventricular filling and cardiac output. These special cases will be discussed further in Chapter 14.

Alterations in Cardiac Output

Physiological Alterations

Exercise. The greatest change in cardiac output in normal individuals occurs during intensive exercise with an increase in both rate and stroke volume. During exercise, the cardiac output varies linearly with oxygen consumption and may be increased 4- to 6-fold (Chapter 12).

Postural Changes. On rising from a recumbent to an upright position the cardiac output decreases about 20% because of venous pooling in the lower extremities and a decrease in effective circulating blood volume (Chapter 13).

Pregnancy. Cardiac output is increased about 10% partly because of increased body mass and partly because the blood vessels to the placenta and uterus may act as arteriovenous shunts to lower peripheral resistance; in the latter case cardiac output is then increased to maintain the blood pressure.

Pathological Alterations

Blood Volume Changes. In anemia, cardiac output is increased as a compensatory response to the circulatory hypoxia and to the decreased resistance to flow. Beriberi, a rare nutritional disease, is also characterized by anemia, a decreased peripheral resistance and an elevated cardiac output with an increased heart rate as well as stroke volume. In hemorrhagic and traumatic shock there is a pronounced decrease in cardiac output because of decreased blood volume and lessened venous return.

Metabolic Changes. Since the metabolic rate of an organ or organism is the most important determinant of the blood flow, there are, as might be expected, marked changes in cardiac output with metabolic alterations. During fever and in hyperthyroidism, the increased output is due to the circulatory hypoxia induced by the increased oxygen demand. Studies have also shown that in normal subjects exposed to room temperatures of 30 to 33°C (87–92°F) at high relative humidities, cardiac output may increase as much as 40%.

Peripheral Resistance Changes. Opening of a large systemic arteriovenous fistula, *e.g.*, in the aorta or iliac artery (peripheral shunt) or in cor pulmonale (central shunt), will result in a sudden decrease in peripheral resistance, an increase in blood volume, and a rise in cardiac output.

Cardiovascular Disease. In early hypertension the elevated blood pressure is frequently associated with an increased cardiac output; later in the disease the cardiac output decreases toward normal levels and the peripheral vascular resistance rises (Chapter 15). In congestive heart failure, in which a decreased cardiac contractility exists, the cardiac output is reduced and an inability to increase the output at ordinary work levels leads to shortness of breath and easy fatigability (Chapter 14).

Measurement of Cardiac Output

In experimental animals, cardiac output can be measured by placing an electromagnetic or ultrasonic flowmeter on the aorta or pulmonary artery for direct recording. In the human subject, the two most commonly used methods are the Fick and indicator-dilution methods. Both of these are "invasive" in the sense that they require cardiac catheterization for placement of a catheter into vessels close to the heart.

$$FICK = \frac{QUANTITY\ CONSUMED}{A\text{-}V\ DIFF} = \frac{10/min}{2/ml} = 5\ ml/min$$

Figure 7.5.   Illustration of the Fick principle for calculation of blood flow through an organ or organism. The flow equals the quantity added per unit time (beads/min) ÷ A-V difference (beads out − beads in). (Reprinted with permission from F. L. Abel and E. P. McCutcheon. *Cardiovascular Function: Principles and Applications*. Boston: Little, Brown, 1979.)

The Fick Method

The Fick principle may be used to measure blood flow through an organ or organism (cardiac output). The principle (illustrated in Fig. 7.5) is based on the measurement of the concentration of a substance entering and leaving an organ, and on the total amount of the substance consumed, produced or added. Since the total amount consumed or added will determine the concentration of the substance leaving the organ, flow may be calculated as the amount added per unit time divided by the concentration difference (Fig. 7.5).

To determine the cardiac output in the living organism, the total O_2 consumption is measured over a period of time (usually several minutes) with a respirometer, and a simultaneous determination is made of O_2 concentration in mixed venous blood (from the pulmonary artery) and in the arterial blood. The cardiac output can then be calculated as the quotient of the oxygen consumption (ml/min) and the A-Vo_2 difference (ml/L). If, *e.g.*, an adult resting subject with a heart rate of 80 beats/min had an O_2 consumption of 250 ml/min and simultaneous blood samples from the femoral artery and pulmonary artery (mixed venous blood) were 19.0 and 15.0 ml/O_2/100 ml respectively, the A-Vo_2 difference would be 40 ml/L and the cardiac output would be 250 ml/min ÷ 40 ml/L or 6.25 L/min. The average stroke volume would then be 6,250 ml/min ÷ 80 beats/min or 78 ml.

The Indicator-Dilution Methods

These methods require the injection of a known amount of dye or other indicator substance into the circulation and the measurement of the dilution of this material during a known period of time. The

Figure 7.6. Cardiac output determination by indicator dilution. Plot of time *vs.* the logarithm of indicator dye concentration in the aorta after injection of 5 mg of indicator (*left*). The indicator disappearance time without recirculation is obtained by extrapolation. The area of the curve is represented by the product of $C \times T$ and the cardiac output is the quotient of the amount injected divided by the area of the curve.

indicator must be well mixed into the blood as it is injected, should not be lost from the circulation and must not be toxic or itself affect cardiac output.

Indocyanine green (Cardiogreen), a dye commonly used, satisfies these requirements. In practice a known amount of the dye is injected into the right heart via a cardiac catheter. A few seconds later the dye concentration is detected in arterial blood by withdrawing small samples of blood continuously from an arterial catheter and measuring the dye concentration with a photosensitive device called a densitometer.

The dye concentration gradually increases until it reaches a maximum and then it begins to decline until a second rise in concentration occurs as a result of recirculation (Fig. 7.6). The downslope of the recirculation approximates an exponential decay so that replotting the curve with the logarithm of dye concentration as the ordinate and time as the abscissa permits the time-concentration curve for the dye on its first circulation past the point of sampling to be defined by extrapolating the downslope. Summing the concentration of each sample and dividing by the number of samples will give the average concentration of dye (C). The product of the average dye concentration (C) and the time of this first passage (T) represents the area of the curve. The volume of dye-containing blood (V or CO) that must have passed the sampling site per unit time (V/T) in order to produce the curve can then be calculated by dividing the amount of dye injected (I) by the area of the curve (CT). The larger the area under the curve, the smaller the cardiac output.

A further application of this principle, called "thermodilution," is based on the injection into the right atrium of a bolus of ice-cold dextrose solution; a second catheter in the pulmonary artery with a thermistor tip provides a continuous temperature record. The degree of temperature dilution depends on the flow and, in a manner similar to dye dilution, a temperature-time curve is inscribed which permits estimation of the cardiac output.

Noninvasive Methods for Estimation of Cardiac Output and Performance

In Chapter 3, a brief description was presented of cardiac catheterization and contrast angiography, invasive methods which are at present standard diagnostic procedures in cardiovascular medicine. There have been, in the last 10 years, increasingly intensive efforts to develop noninvasive methods for estimating cardiac output. Such efforts have been made not only because of the higher cost and added risk of invasive techniques, but also because the emotional stress, which even minor invasive procedures sometimes evoke, produces its own physiological effects which may complicate the diagnostic procedure. Following are brief descriptions of three such noninvasive techniques which hold considerable promise as diagnostic aids, *viz.*, (a) echocardiography, (b) radionuclide imaging and (c) impedance cardiography.

Echocardiography. One of the newest and potentially one of the more important noninvasive techniques for cardiovascular diagnosis is the detection of high frequency sound waves (above 20,000 cycles/sec) created by actuating a transducer with alternating electrical current. The sound is emitted from the transducer and directed through the body. The depth and position of the echoes (reflected sonic waves) returned from the body can be detected and recorded. The movement of cardiac structures such as valves, heart wall and pericardium can be tracked and pathological changes can be readily followed with M (for motion) mode echocardiography. The general principle of a M mode echocardiographic scan is shown in Figure 7.7.

A major development in this field has been the introduction of real time, cross-sectional, two-dimensional (2D) echocardiography which provides spatial anatomic information about cardiac structures. More recently a further refinement, using pulsed Doppler echocardiography, permits the recording of actual pattern and velocity of blood flow within the heart and great vessels.

Radionuclide Imaging. Another relatively noninvasive method which has come into increasing use is the visualization of the cardiac chambers with radioisotopes. The intravenous injection of a small bolus of a gamma emitter such as ^{99m}Tc pertechnetate permits rapid sequential visualization of the heart, great vessels and pulmonary vasculature by use of an Anger scintillation camera; the image is usually recorded and stored on tape.

One of the more commonly used radionuclide techniques, "gated

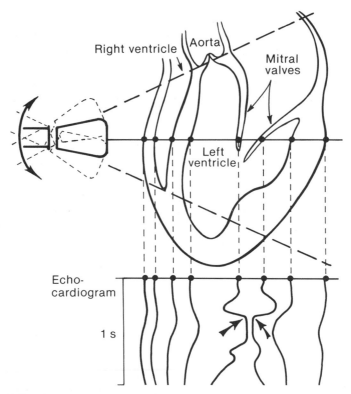

Figure 7.7.   Schematic diagram of principle of echocardiography. The ultrasonic beam is swept in an arc between apex and base. The transducer acts as both sender and receiver in rapid alternation. The distances and movements of the reflecting surfaces are recorded as a function of time. The closing of the mitral valve at the beginning of systole, for example, can be visualized. (Reprinted with permission from *Physiologie des Menschen*, edited by R.F. Schmidt and G. Thews. Berlin: Springer-Verlag, 1980.)

equilibrium radionuclide angiography," consists of injection of a ^{99m}Tc pertechnetate labeled sample of the patients own red blood cells to achieve an intravascular equilibrium concentration of the radioisotope in the blood stream. This label has a biologic half-life of about 4 hours. At a specific signal—usually triggered by the R wave of the ECG—precordial ventricular radioisotope density for one cardiac cycle is divided (gated) into about 20 to 28 sequential subdivisions and automatically counted by computer. The resulting left ventricular time-activity curve yields a ventricular volume record of filling and emptying which permits estimation of left ventricular end diastolic, end systolic and stroke volumes, ejection fraction and wall motion abnormalities.

An important application of this method is the determination of ejection fraction at rest and during exercise. With a healthy myocardium, the ejection fraction is usually increased during physical exercise; in case of a weakened myocardium, *e.g.*, after a myocardial infarct, the ejection fraction may be unchanged or decreased during exercise (Chapter 14).

Impedance Cardiography. This method involves the transmission of a high frequency current across the chest. The ejection of blood into the aorta produces a characteristic impedance wave which permits calculation of cardiac output. Four thin band electrodes are usually placed about the neck and lower chest. The outer two electrodes are excited by a 100-kHz sinusoidal current and the resulting voltage monitored from the inner two electrodes (Fig. 7.8). The method is based upon the principle that if a rapid sinusoidal current is transmitted across a distensible cylindrical fluid system, the ejection of a given fluid volume into the cylinder will cause a negative impedance wave whose area will be directly proportional to the increased cylinder volume. The stroke volume (SV) ejected into the aorta can be estimated with the formula:

$$SV = r \cdot \frac{L^2}{Z_0^2} \cdot T \cdot [dZ/dt_{min}]$$

r is the electrical resistivity of the blood; L is the linear distance between the inner (recording) electrodes; Z_0 is the baseline impedance across the chest; T is the ventricular ejection time and dZ/dt_{min} is the minimum value of the first derivative of the primary (largest) impedance wave. In addition to cardiac output, some investigators have also reported the use of impedance cardiography for estimation of relative changes in regional blood volume and as a clinical index of myocardial contractility.

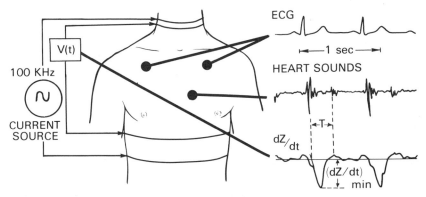

Figure 7.8. Transthoracic impedance cardiography. *Left*, rapid sinusoidal current is transmitted through the two outer electrodes and sensed by the inner ones. *Right*, the minimum value of the first derivative of the main impedance wave (dZ/dt_{min}) and the ventricular ejection time (T) are used to calculate the stroke volume.

A highly sophisticated quantitative imaging method for cardiovascular diagnosis—still in its early developmental stage—is the *dynamic spatial reconstructor* (DSR). This very large and elaborate apparatus performs three-dimensional ray imaging and operates on the principle of computed tomography. This method involves the gathering of anatomical information through cross-sectional (tomographic) roentgenography and computerized synchronous volumetric reconstruction of the photographs. Timed images of the heart and entire circulatory system permit estimation of regional blood flow to all organs of the body. While the applicability of this unique device to routine human studies is still in the future, DSR-based evaluation of cardiac and peripheral circulatory disorders should be possible with greater accuracy and less invasion than with current methods.

References

Feigenbaum H. *Echocardiography*. Philadelphia: Lea & Febiger, 1980, 3rd ed.

Guyton AC. *Circulatory Physiology: Cardiac Output and Its Regulation*. Philadelphia: W.B. Saunders, 1973.

Herndon CW and Sagawa K. Combined effects of aortic and right atrial pressure on aortic flow. *Am J Physiol* 217:65, 1969.

Kubicek WG, Kottke FJ, Ramos MU, Patterson RP, Wittsoe DA, Labree JW, Remole W, Layman TE, Schoening H, and Garamella JT. The Minnesota impedance cardiograph—theory and application. *Biomed Eng* 9:410–416, 1974.

Po Sit S and Vatner SF. Integrated circulatory response to volume expansion. In: *Cardiovascular Physiology IV*, International Review of Physiology, edited by AC Guyton and JE Hall. Baltimore: University Park Press, 1982, Vol. 26, pp. 323–354.

Ritman EL, Kinsey JH, Robb RA, Gilbert BK, Harris LD, and Wood EH. Three dimensional imaging of heart, lungs and circulation. *Science* 210:273–280, 1980.

Rothe CF. The venous system: the physiology of the capacitance vessels. In: *Handbook of Physiology*, Section 2: *The Cardiovascular System*, edited by FM Abboud and JT Shepherd. Bethesda: American Physiological Society, 1982, Vol. III.

Scher A. Control of cardiac output. In: *Physiology and Biophysics*, edited by RC Ruch and HD Patton. Philadelphia: W.B. Saunders, 1974.

Smith JJ, Bush JE, Wiedmeier VT, and Tristani FE. Application of impedance cardiography to study of postural stress. *J Appl Physiol* 29:133–137, 1970.

Vatner SF and Boettcher DH. Regulation of cardiac output by stroke volume and heart rate in conscious dogs. *Circ Res* 42:557–561, 1978.

Zaret BL and Berger HJ. Techniques of nuclear cardiology. In: *The Heart, Arteries and Veins*, edited by JW Hurst. New York: McGraw-Hill, 1982, 5th ed., pp. 1803–1843.

Zelis R, Flaim SF, Liedtke AJ, and Nellis SH. Cardiocirculatory dynamics in the normal and failing heart. *Annu Rev Physiol* 43:455–476, 1981.

chapter 8

The Microcirculation and the Lymphatic System

Anatomy of the Microcirculation

That portion of the systemic and pulmonary circulation especially adapted for exchange of water, gases, nutrients and waste material is known as the microcirculation. It is, in a sense, the most important part of the cardiovascular system since it is here that its ultimate objective, *i.e.*, the exchange with tissue cells, is realized. While the microcirculation is considered a closed system, its walls are much more permeable than those of any other part of the circulation.

As shown in Figure 8.1, microcirculatory vessels have an irregular course and configuration; because of their great cross-sectional area, the flow velocity is least at this point. This slowing of the stream and dispersal over a maximum surface makes the microcirculation particu-

127

Figure 8.1. Schematic drawing of microcirculatory bed showing arterioles, metarterioles, capillaries and venules. Note precapillary sphincters at points where capillaries branch off from the metarterioles. (Reprinted with permission from B.W. Zweifach, *Conference on High Blood Pressure.* New York: Macy Foundation, 1950.)

larly suitable for exchange. It has been estimated that because of the enormous number and wide distribution of capillaries, individual cells are seldom more than 40 to 80 μm from a capillary surface. Arterioles are highly muscular vessels but metarterioles, which generally come off the arterioles at right angles, have only a single discontinuous smooth muscle layer in their walls.

The metarterioles serve to some extent as through-channels to the venules, which are much larger and have a greater capacity than the arterioles. At the point where capillaries branch off the metarterioles, a thin band of muscle, *i.e.*, the precapillary sphincter, encircles the capillary; these sphincters serve as the main control over capillary flow.

Capillaries

Capillaries of different tissues vary considerably, both anatomically and functionally. These differences are usually related to the special role of the respective tissue or organ and will be discussed further in Chapter 11 (Circulation to Special Regions). In the skin, for example, particularly of the toes, fingers and ears, there are arteriovenous anastomoses (AVAs) which are wide-bore, direct channels between the arterioles and venules. Unlike capillaries of other organs, the AVAs are under neurogenic control; their shunting capabilities enable them to reduce heat loss through the skin during cold exposure.

The true capillaries are the most important functional units of the microcirculation. They are short, narrow tubes, about 7 to 10 μm in diameter with a wall consisting of a single layer of endothelial cells and a basement membrane; they have no smooth muscle (Fig. 8.2). Between adjacent endothelial cells are slitlike pores or clefts which range from about 50 to 90 Å in width but which are frequently constricted at one point to about 40 Å.

The cytoplasm of the endothelial cells usually contains pinocytotic vesicles which are believed to play a role in transport processes across the cell. Although there are a wide variety of capillary structures among the different tissues, three main types have been distinguished by electron microscopy on the basis of the continuity of their filtration barriers; these have been labelled continuous, fenestrated and discontinuous types.

Continuous Capillaries

These are capillaries with no recognizable intercellular openings; one subgroup with a "low" or flattened cellular type is seen mainly in muscle, nerve and adipose tissue; a second subgroup with a "high" or

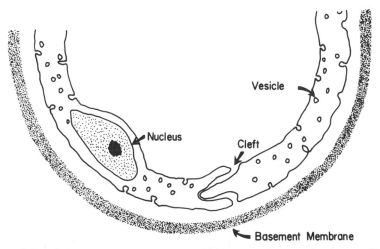

Figure 8.2. Schematic representation of electron micrograph of a capillary. Note the slit-pore (cleft) between the endothelial cells. (Reprinted with permission from C.A. Wiederhielm, in *Physiology and Biophysics*, edited by T.C. Ruch and H.D. Patton, Philadelphia: W.B. Saunders, 1974.)

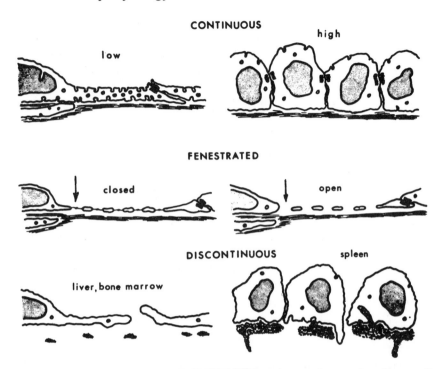

Figure 8.3. Continuous, fenestrated and discontinuous types of capillary wall as shown by schematics of electron micrographs. The classification is based on the completeness of the endothelial layer and in general parallels the extent of the physical barrier to filtration. (Reprinted with permission from G. Majno, in *Handbook of Physiology*, Section 2: *Circulation*, edited by W.F. Hamilton and P. Dow. Washington, D.C.: American Physiological Society, 1965, Vol. III.)

cuboidal epithelial structure is more common in lymph nodes and the thymus gland (Fig. 8.3, *top*).

Fenestrated Capillaries

This type of capillary (Fig. 8.3, *center*) has small gaps which are either "closed" as in endocrine glands and intestinal villi or "open" as in renal glomeruli. These gaps usually range from 800 to 1,000 Å and are, therefore, about 15 to 20 times wider than those of the continuous capillaries.

Discontinuous Capillaries

This type of membrane (Fig. 8.3, *bottom*) has an endothelium with large intercellular gaps; these vessels are usually referred to as sinusoids and are typical of liver, bone marrow and spleen. It should be pointed out that the so-called "tight" junctions of the continuous capillaries are sufficiently wide to permit rapid diffusion of small molecular substances. There is no barrier to diffusion of gases. The other two types of capillaries with larger gaps have much greater permeability, so that in the sinusoids, large proteins and even cells can pass. Thus, to a large extent the transfer of substances between the capillaries and interstitial fluid can be correlated with these anatomical differences in capillary structure.

Regulation of the Microcirculation

As mentioned in Chapter 1, the mean intravascular pressures in the capillary range from about 25 to 30 mm Hg at the arteriolar end to about 8 to 10 mm Hg at the venular end. Flow through the arterioles and metarterioles is controlled mainly by the sympathetic vasoconstrictors on the basis of circulatory reflexes as will be described in Chapters 9 and 10. Flow through the capillaries, however, is not under neural control; rather it is regulated by the precapillary sphincters which are, in turn, influenced by the local metabolic state of the tissue—a process called autoregulation (Chapter 9).

Thus, flow through individual capillary areas can be adjusted to meet both the local demands of the tissues and the overall control of the circulation. Rate of flow through individual capillary beds can vary considerably. In skeletal muscle, for example, only about 5 to 10% of the capillaries are open at rest; however, with increased metabolic activity, the precapillary sphincters open widely. As flow is restored and O_2 needs are satisfied, the sphincters again close.

Transcapillary Exchange

Movement across the capillary wall is influenced by several factors; (a) the shape and molecular size of the substance being transported, (b) the balance of hydrostatic and colloid osmotic forces across the membrane, (c) the capillary surface available for exchange, and (d) the physical characteristics of the capillary membrane.

The continuous type of capillary is often found in muscle, connective tissue, the pulmonary circulation and brain. Consequently the filtration coefficient (*i.e.*, the rate of filtration per unit pressure difference) is relatively low in these tissues. In the renal glomerulus and intestinal mucosa, which have fenestrated capillaries, the filtration rate is moderate to high. In the hepatic sinusoids and spleen with discontinuous or practically "open" capillaries, molecules of all sizes pass readily; these tissues "leak" the greatest amounts of protein and have the highest interstitial plasma protein concentrations.

There are two general methods—*viz.* diffusion and filtration—by which substances pass through capillary walls, depending mainly on their lipid solubility. These are discussed in the following sections.

Diffusion

This is the most important transcapillary exchange mechanism and may take place through the intercellular slitlike pores or through the cell wall itself. Lipid-soluble materials such as oxygen, carbon dioxide and certain anesthetic agents diffuse rapidly with little hindrance through the lipoprotein membrane of the endothelial cell wall. Water-soluble substances on the other hand are limited to diffusion through the intercellular slit-pores in which case the molecular movement is aided by the physical process of filtration.

Filtration-Absorption

Starling described the exchange of fluid across the capillary wall on the basis of the hydrostatic and osmotic pressures on each side of the membrane (law of the capillary). Later, Landis provided specific pressure measurements to verify this concept; Landis found hydrostatic pressures of about 32 and 15 mm Hg in the arteriolar and venular end of a capillary respectively and plasma osmotic pressures due to plasma proteins (oncotic pressures) of about 25 mm Hg. According to the Starling-Landis concept, the resultant pressure gradient along the capillary governs transport across the capillary wall (Fig. 8.4).

At the arterial end, there is an excess of hydrostatic over osmotic pressure tending to promote filtration (movement into the tissue) and at the venous end an excess of osmotic over hydrostatic pressure tending to promote reabsorption. In the intermediate region there is a gradual decline in filtration and a beginning of reabsorption. It should be noted that the areas under the triangles are approximately equal, indicating that filtration and absorption are also balanced and about equal. Further studies have indicated that the total amount of water filtered through the capillaries of the body is about 20 liters per day; of this amount, about 16 to 18 liters are reabsorbed into the capillaries; the remaining 2 to 4 liters per day are removed by the lymphatic system and returned to the circulation.

Although Figure 8.4 refers only to capillary hydrostatic (P_c) and plasma oncotic (π_p) pressures, the interstitial hydrostatic (P_i) and interstitial osmotic pressures (π_i) must also be considered. While P_i and π_i are both quite low compared to the respective P_c and π_p values, the interstitial pressures may, in pathological circumstances, increase and become significant factors in transcapillary fluid exchange as described later in this chapter. Therefore, a more accurate definition of transcapillary forces would be the balance between the net transmural hydrostatic pressure ($P_c - P_i$) and the net transmural oncotic pressure ($\pi_p - \pi_i$).

Two-thirds or more of the oncotic effect of the 7 g/dl of plasma proteins is due to albumin. Because of their large molecular size only a

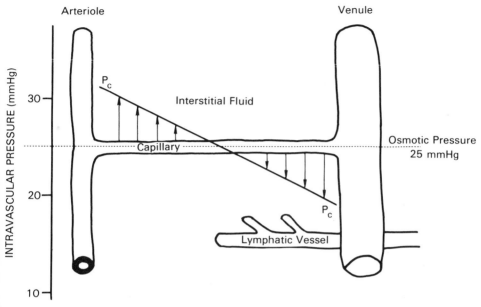

Figure 8.4. Schematic diagram showing filtration and reabsorption along an average capillary. P_c is the capillary hydrostatic presssure, which decreases progressively from the arteriolar to the venular side. The relation of P_c to capillary osmotic pressure causes filtration on the arteriolar side and reabsorption on the venular side. (Adapted from E.M. Landis and J.R. Pappenheimer, in *Handbook of Physiology*, Section 2: *Circulation*, edited by W.F. Hamilton and P. Dow. Washington, D.C.: American Physiological Society, 1963, Vol. III.)

small percentage of plasma protein diffuses across the capillary wall in most tissues. However, as previously mentioned, in the sinusoids, the plasma proteins move more easily into the interstitial fluid so that π_i begins to approach π_p.

Capillary Permeability

As previously stated, the transport of material across the capillary wall depends not only on diffusion and on the balance of pressures across the capillary but also on the structure and porosity of the wall and the nature of the material being transported. For water-soluble substances which are transported primarily via the slit-pores, a single mathematical expression can be used to describe the movement across the capillary wall, *i.e.*:

$$F = (P)(S)[(P_c - P_i) - (\pi_p - \pi_i)]$$

in which F is the net movement of fluid, P is the specific permeability of the capillary and S is the capillary surface area perfused. S depends mainly on the number of capillaries open to flow. P_c and P_i are the hydrostatic pressures in the capillary and interstitial fluid, and π_p and π_i are the osmotic pressure values in the plasma and interstitial fluid respectively. The right side of the equation is a restatement of the balance of hydrostatic and osmotic forces previously described; as will be noted; if F is positive there will be an outward transport of fluid from the capillary and if negative an inward one.

In Table 8.1 are listed the specific permeabilities of a few common substances as well as their molecular weights and sizes. As will be noted in the continuous or tight capillary which prevails in muscle, the permeability ranges from high values for the smaller molecules to practical impermeability for the larger protein molecules; this is consistent with the concept that the movement of these substances across the capillary barrier is essentially a passive one, primarily dependent upon physical forces. The permeability factor may be affected by hypoxia, drugs and certain pathological conditions.

Lymphatic System

The lymphatics comprise a type of secondary interstitial drainage system supplementing venular drainage. Lymphatics are porous, thin-walled vessels resembling capillaries. From closed, blind ends lying in the interstitial space, lymph channels drain centrally and are occasionally interrupted by lymph nodes. Inside the nodes the vessels break up into numerous sinuses, lined by lymphoid cells, which reunite into

Table 8.1.
Permeability of Mammalian Muscle Capillaries to Some Water-Soluble Molecules

Substance	Molecular Weight	Approximate Molecular Radius (Å)	Specific Permeability*
H_2O	18	1.5	28
NaCl	58	2.3	15
Urea	60	2.6	14
Glucose	180	3.7	6
Sucrose	342	4.8	4
Inulin	5,500	12–15	0.3
Myoglobin	17,000	19	0.1
Serum albumin	67,000	36	0.001

* Expressed as $mol/sec/cm^2$ of membrane per mol/concentration difference $\times 10^5$. (From E.M. Landis and J.R. Pappenheimer, in *Handbook of Physiology*, Section 2; *Circulation*, edited by W.F. Hamilton and P. Dow, Washington, D.C.: American Physiological Society, 1963, Vol. II.)

efferent lymph channels. Ultimately, all the lymphatic vessels empty into two main trunks, the thoracic duct (on the left) and the right lymphatic duct; these drain into the junctions of the subclavian and internal jugular veins on their respective sides. The primary function of the lymphatic system is to clear the interstitial spaces of excess fluid, protein, lipids and foreign materials.

Lymph resembles interstitial tissue fluid with which it is in close equilibrium. Its composition is similar to plasma except that its average protein concentration is lower, *i.e.*, about 2 g/dl. The highest protein concentration is that of hepatic lymph which has a range of about 5 to 6 g/dl. Pressure in the lymphatics is similar to that of interstitial fluid and fluctuates from about −3 mm Hg to +5 mm Hg. Guyton and his colleagues have reported that interstitial pressure normally is about −6 mm Hg; these investigators believe that this negative pressure is important to maintain the tissue spaces relatively dry so that diffusion distances between capillaries and cells are optimally short.

Lymph flow is relatively sluggish and total flow in man is about 2 to 4 L/day. This flow is increased by muscular activity or massage, increased venous pressure, hyperemia or inflammation. Lymphatic vessels are highly permeable and are capable of picking up large particles, *e.g.*, dying blood cells, carbon, bacteria, and foreign particles. Intestinal lymphatics (lacteals) pick up large lipid globules, *i.e.*, chylomicra after a fat meal.

Edema

Edema is the accumulation of excess fluid in the interstitial spaces of the body. Clinical edema usually develops in dependent areas such as the feet and becomes more evident in tissues in which expansion is limited, *e.g.*, around the eyes. Edema may be produced in several ways as described in the following.

General Increase in Venous Pressure

As is shown in Figure 8.4 and also in Figure 8.5*A*, when there is a normal balance of filtration and reabsorption forces, there will be no accumulation of interstital fluid. However, if the pressure is consistently increased in the veins, it will also rise in the venules and eventually in the arterial end of the capillary; this will result in an increase in filtration and in the accumulation of interstitial fluid illustrated by the net force tending to move fluid out of the capillary (Fig. 8.5*B*). This condition occurs most commonly in congestive heart failure with elevation of right ventricular end-diastolic pressure, venous congestion and a resultant dependent edema (discussed further in Chapter 14).

Figure 8.5. Effect of variations in hydrostatic and colloid osmotic pressures on fluid filtration-reabsorption balance. *A,* normal balance of capillary hydrostatic and plasma oncotic pressures; *B,* elevation of venular and capillary pressures with excessive filtration and increased interstitial fluid; *C,* decreased plasma protein and plasma oncotic pressure, with excessive capillary filtration and tendency toward edema.

Hypoproteinemia

If the plasma protein decreases to a low level, the plasma oncotic pressure will also fall so that the capillary hydrostatic pressure overbalances the oncotic pressure with a resultant tendency for fluid accumulation in the tissue spaces. The loss of plasma protein—primarily albumin—occurs most commonly in nephrosis, in which large amounts of albumin are continuously lost in the urine, in nutritional edema in which there is inadequate protein in the diet and with severe burns in which the capillaries are damaged.

Lymphatic Obstruction

If the small amount of protein that continually "leaks" through the capillary walls and is normally returned via the lymph cannot be reabsorbed, it will accumulate in the tissue until it reaches a significant concentration and prevents the return of fluid into the venular end of the capillary. This occurs rarely but when seen is usually due to a tropical parasitic disease called "filariasis"; the larvae (microfilaria) gradually obstruct the lymphatic vessels. The edema may become so excessive that a leg may swell to two or three times its normal size— hence the clinical term "elephantiasis" for this type of massive edema.

Local Edema

Localized edema may occur in an organ or region if there is extensive venous obstruction with elevation of venous and capillary pressures, *e.g.*, a widespread venous thrombosis.

References

Bundgaard M. Transport pathways in capillaries in search of pores. *Annu Rev Physiol* 42:325–336, 1980.
Gore RW and McDonagh PF. Fluid exchange across single capillaries. *Annu Rev Physiol* 42:337–357, 1980.
Guyton AC, Granger HJ, and Taylor AE. Interstitial fluid pressure. *Physiol Rev* 51:527, 1971.
Haddy FJ, Scott JB, and Grega GJ. Peripheral circulation: fluid transfer across the microvascular membrane. In: *Cardiovascular Physiology II*, International Review of Physiology, edited by AC Guyton. Baltimore: University Park Press, 1976, Vol. 9.
Intaglietta M and Johnson PC. *Principles of Capillary Exchange in Peripheral Circulation*, edited by PC Johnson. New York: John Wiley & Sons, 1978.
Landis EM and Pappenheimer JR. Exchange of substances through the capillary walls. In: *Handbook of Physiology*, Section 2: *Circulation*, edited by WF Hamilton and P Dow. Washington, D.C.: American Physiological Society, 1963, Vol. II.
Majno G. Ultrastructure of vascular membrane. In: *Handbook of Physiology*, Section 2: *Circulation*, edited by WF Hamilton and P Dow. Washington, D.C.: American Physiological Society, 1965, Vol. III.
Renkin EM. Multiple pathways of capillary permeability. *Circ Res* 41:735–742, 1977.
Wiederhielm CA. Dynamics of transcapillary fluid exchange. *J Gen Physiol* 52:29–63, 1968.

chapter 9

The Peripheral Circulation and Its Regulation

Normal Distribution of Blood Flow

How blood flow is distributed to the various organs is obviously of considerable importance; total flow is limited and it must be disposed only in amounts needed when and where it is needed. If, in a 70-kg adult, a cardiac output of 5,400 ml/min were partitioned evenly on a weight basis, the mean flow would be about 7.7 ml/min/100 g of tissue. However, the actual flow distribution is quite uneven. Figure 9.1 shows average values for tissue blood flow and oxygen consumption in the normal adult human at rest.

As the top bar graph shows, three tissues, liver (hepatosplanchnic region), kidney and skeletal muscle receive about two-thirds of the total flow. If the organ flows are divided by the respective organ weights, the

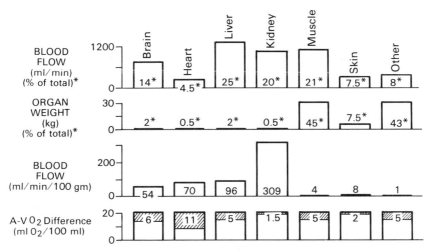

Figure 9.1. Blood flow, organ weight, vascularity (blood flow per unit weight) and A-V oxygen extraction of main organs in normal adult at rest. Body weight, 70 kg; cardiac output, 5,400 ml/min; mean vascularity, 7.7 ml/min/100 g; mean A-V$_{O_2}$ difference, 5 ml O_2 per dl. (Liver flow includes that of the intestinal and other organs draining into the portal vein and therefore actually refers to hepatosplanchnic flow.)

blood flow per unit weight or "vascularity" (Fig. 9.1, 3rd graph) is obtained. As described in Chapter 2, when comparing relative flow or peripheral resistance values, it is necessary to consider the weight and surface area of the respective organ or organism.

Four organs, *viz.*, kidney, liver, heart and brain, all have a high flow/ unit weight because of a relatively low vascular resistance/unit weight; in contrast *resting* skeletal muscle and the relatively avascular tissues such as skin, bone, cartilage, fat and connective tissue etc., which are grouped under "other," have a low blood flow/unit weight because of their relatively high vascular resistance.

Just as the flow distribution to the different organs is uneven, so is the flow distribution *within* organs, *e.g.*, in the heart, kidneys, brain, etc., as will be discussed in Chapter 11. Since these intraorgan flow characteristics have functional significance, regional blood flow determinations have become increasingly important.

The kidneys, being primarily clearance organs, obviously need a very large flow to carry out their function; their close proximity through short arterial vessels to the high aortic pressure and their innate vascularity contribute to the high resting flow. The renal clearance function is associated with only a modest oxygen demand so that the flow is mainly "nonnutritional." As a consequence, the renal A-V oxygen difference is small, *i.e.*, 1.5 ml of O_2/100 ml of blood. Therefore, in spite of the very large flow, the estimated oxygen consumption of the kidneys, *i.e.*, about 4.6 ml/min/100 g (3.09 × 1.5), is less than that of the liver (4.8) or heart (7.7) (Fig. 9.1).

That fraction of the arterial O_2 content taken up in the tissues is usually termed the O_2 extraction ratio. If the arterial O_2 content were 20 ml/dl, the O_2 extraction for resting skeletal muscle (Fig. 9.1) would be 0.25 and for myocardium 0.55. The remaining fraction of unextracted oxygen represents an important reserve.

In certain stress situations, both the total flow and flow distribution shown in Figure 9.1 (*top graph*) would be considerably altered. For example, during severe exercise, cardiac output can increase 4 to 6 times; furthermore, the percentage of total flow received by skeletal muscle would increase to about 90% because of a marked decrease in vascular resistance in the dilated muscle vessels (Chapter 12). Since, in addition to the increased fractional flow to muscle, there will also be an increase in the O_2 extraction ratio, the total O_2 consumption of skeletal muscle can, in severe exercise, increase 15 to 20 times over the resting level.

Range of Flow Responses in Different Organs

Changes in vessel caliber may occur passively in response to transmural pressure changes or through active contraction (vasoconstriction) or relaxation (vasodilation) of its circular smooth muscle; such activity will, in the small arteries and arterioles, mainly influence peripheral

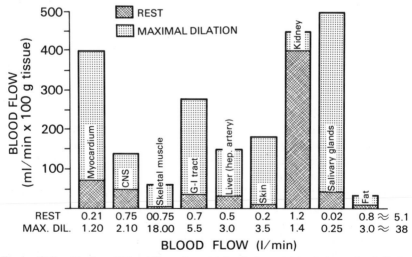

Figure 9.2. Regional blood flow at rest (*shaded areas*) and at maximal dilation (*stippled areas*) per organ and per 100 g tissue. (Reprinted with permission from S. Mellander and B. Johansson, *Pharmacol Rev* 20:117, 1968.)

resistance, but in the small veins and venules, the primary effect is on the capacitance of the peripheral bed.

Vessel caliber may change over a wide range; vasoconstriction of small arterial vessels may be so intense that flow practically ceases; on the other hand if all constrictor nerves are cut and the vessels maximally dilated by pharmacological agents, flow may increase 2- or 3-fold in the brain and liver, 5-fold in the myocardium and over 20-fold in skeletal muscle (Fig. 9.2). In contrast to this, renal vessels can only increase their flow about 16%. Such large flow alterations in certain tissues are possible because of the fourth power effect of the radius on flow (Chapter 2).

Principles of Flow Regulation

Given its inherent vascular architecture, altered flow demands might be met either by a change in the arterial perfusion pressure or by adjustment of vessel caliber. From an organism standpoint, it is most efficient to maintain arterial pressure relatively constant in order to insure adequate coronary and cerebral flow and to meet the peripheral demands through adjustment of individual resistances. In effect this is what normally occurs; the primary objective of this chapter is to consider how this is brought about. The adjustment of vessel caliber is accomplished by two general mechanisms, *i.e.*, through central regulation and local regulation.

Central Regulation of Flow. This may be either *neural control*, which is carried out almost entirely by the autonomic nervous system, primarily via sympathetic nerves, or *humoral control, i.e.*, through bloodborne agents that may be (a) organic substances such as 5-hydroxytryptamine, angiotensin, etc., (b) blood gases, *e.g.*, O_2 or CO_2, or (c) ions such as Ca^{2+} or K^+. All of these control mechanisms are "central," *i.e.*, they originate from a source remote from the tissue affected. However, as discussed below, certain organic factors and inorganic agents may also act locally on the tissues where they are formed.

Local Regulation of Flow. This is carried out either through biological agents, *i.e.*, so-called "local hormones" such as prostaglandins, bradykinin, histamine, etc., or through inorganic agents such as O_2 or CO_2 or H^+, which are derived in the individual tissues and act directly on nearby vascular beds. The flow alterations are due mainly to effects on the precapillary or postcapillary vessels.

In considering the regulation of blood flow to an organ or organism, an important distinction must be made between short- and long-term circulatory adjustments, *i.e.*, those made rapidly over minutes or hours in contrast to those which occur over days and weeks. The mechanisms involved in these two processes are quite different. In the following sections, the short-term adaptations will be considered first and in greater detail.

In the final section of the chapter, long-term regulation of flow will be discussed in general. In succeeding chapters vascular luminal adjustments of greater duration which apply to specific situations will be described at some length. These will include circulatory changes which develop during physical training and those incident to aging (Chapter 12) and circulatory adjustments which occur in pathological circumstances such as ischemic heart disease and congestive failure (Chapter 14) as well as in hypertension and shock (Chapter 15).

Central Regulation of Flow

Neural Control of Flow

Autonomic Transmitters and Receptors

The autonomic nervous system (ANS), which includes the thoracolumbar (sympathetic) outflow and the craniosacral (parasympathetic) outflow, is responsible for integrating and modulating the functions of all the autonomous organs of the body, including the cardiovascular system. Neural transmission along the ANS is done in the usual fashion, *i.e.*, by means of self-propagating action potentials; transmission across synapses and across junctions with other tissues is via rather unique and specific chemical agents known as neurohumoral transmitters. These transmitters combine with receptors on the effector cells to activate the end-organ.

There are two primary transmitters involved in the ANS: (a) acetylcholine (ACh), released at all autonomic ganglia, at parasympathetic nerve endings and at voluntary neuromuscular junctions, and (b) norepinephrine (NE), released at most sympathetic nerve endings. Exceptions to this generalization are the sympathetic cholinergic endings, *e.g.*, at sweat glands, and the cholinergic vasodilators in skeletal muscle. At these endings ACh is released. Epinephrine (E) is liberated (along with a small fraction of NE) by the adrenal medulla into the blood.

Endogenously active sympathomimetic amines (NE, E, dopamine) are known as catecholamines; an outline of the synthesis of these compounds is given in a simplified diagram in Figure 9.3. NE, derived in a series of steps from tyrosine, is for the most part synthesized locally by the adrenergic nerve terminal. About 80% of the NE released by the nerve action potential is removed via an active reuptake process into the neuron for reuse. The remainder either diffuses into the surrounding tissue or blood or is metabolically degraded. The importance of the uptake process lies in the consequent availability (or not) of the NE for continued combination with the effector cell and so is a determinant of the strength and duration of the NE effect. Since this transmitter orginates within the body, it is termed endogenous. The NE secreted by

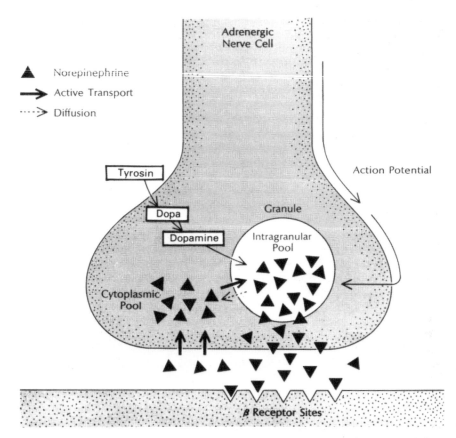

Figure 9.3.   Schema showing local synthesis and release of norepinephrine (NE) in the heart. Ninety per cent of the cardiac NE is synthesized locally. The NE is stored, either in the granules or in the cytoplasm, and is released by the action potential. It then leaves the nerve cell, attaches to the myocardial β-receptor site and stimulates myocardial contraction. (Reprinted with permission from E. Braunwald, *The Myocardium: Failure and Infarction*. New York: HP Publishing Co., 1974.)

the nerve cell remains active for only a few seconds but the E secreted by the adrenal medulla can remain active for several minutes.

If the transmitter (*e.g.*, NE or ACh) is injected (exogenous source) so that it reaches the receptors via the blood stream, the effect will be similar to that of neurally released NE or ACh, so that a "sympathomimetic" or "parasympathomimetic" effect will be produced. But whether generated by neural or humoral means, autonomic effects on the various end-organs are diverse and complex. A significant (and initially baffling) discovery was that specific chemicals could prevent or competitively "block" certain autonomic effects (but not others) and thus render the transmitter temporarily ineffective at these effector sites.

In 1948, Ahlquist proposed that divergent sympathetic responses were due to the existence of two different types of "receptors" at the various anatomical sites, which responded differently to the transmitters. These he called "α" and "β" receptors. Because exogenously administered NE or neurally released NE produces a strong vasoconstriction of the blood vessels of skin, kidney, splanchnic area and skeletal muscle (*i.e.*, a "pure" vasoconstriction), he assumed that such receptors were abundant at these sites. At other sites, *e.g.*, in vessels of the brain and heart, NE produces limited or no constriction since at these locations such receptors are scarce. These were called α-receptors and the action an α-constrictor action. Although NE is the primary endogenous agonist (activator) of α-receptors in the human and most mammals, E also has strong α-stimulating effects.

Specific agents such as phenoxybenzamine (Dibenzyline) or phentolamine (Regitine) will antagonize or block α (but not β) receptors and thus, depending on the dose, will minimize or prevent the α-vasoconstriction. The rapid and effective increase in peripheral vascular resistance produced by reflex sympathetic α-constriction is an important defense mechanism against a blood pressure fall, *e.g.*, during hemorrhage. An animal previously injected with a strong α-blocking dose of phenoxybenzamine will have a much lower resistance to hemorrhage than a control animal.

β-Receptors are most prevalent in the heart, in blood vessels of skeletal muscles and in bronchiolar smooth muscle. They are activated by epinephrine at low doses or by one of its synthetic analogues, isoproterenol (Isuprel). When occupied by the transmitter, β-receptors initiate (a) increased heart rate and contractile strength of the myocardium and (b) vasodilation of skeletal muscle blood vessels. β-Receptors (but not α) can be blocked by propranolol (Inderal). Propranolol is used in the treatment of certain types of hypertension and can assist in controlling blood pressure by reducing the inotropic activity of the ventricle.

As mentioned above, there are postganglionic sympathetic cholinergic nerve endings located in vessels of skeletal muscle. These endings, rather paradoxically, release ACh, which binds "cholinergic" (or more specifically "muscarinic") receptors and causes vasodilation. This effect, which can be blocked by the primary muscarinic blocking agent, atropine, is thought to be involved in certain emotional responses such as fright or rage.

Some investigators have also reported the existence of "dopaminergic" receptors. Dopamine, which is only one of the intermediate compounds in the synthetic pathway of NE, has a vasodilator effect on renal, splanchnic, and coronary vascular beds, an action which can be blocked by specific antagonists, *e.g.*, haloperidol.

It has been shown that in congestive heart failure, there is a depletion of myocardial catecholamines, with consequent reduction of inotropic capability. The depletion is probably due to the marked reduction of tyrosine hydroxylase, the rate-limiting enzyme in the conversion of tyrosine to DOPA.

As is evident from the above, certain tissues, by virtue of having different kinds of receptors, are capable of different types of vascular response if the proper stimuli are provided. This is particularly true of skeletal muscle. Figure 9.4 illustrates the effects of successive blockade of different receptors on skeletal muscle blood flow. Skeletal muscle, because it comprises about 45% of the body bulk and has unusual constrictor and dilator capabilities, represents an enormous pool of vascular resistance.

Parasympathetic control of blood flow (to be discussed later in this chapter) is much more limited than that of the sympathetic system.

Autonomic neurotransmitters and receptors are currently the focus of intensive investigation, and recent studies have revealed that there are many substances and complex interrelationships involved at neuroeffector junctions. There are, *e.g.*, two subtypes of β-receptors—β_1 and β_2; these vary not only in their sensitivity to NE and E but also in the chronotropic and inotropic responses they invoke in different species. In addition, two types of α-receptors have been proposed, *i.e.*, α_1 and α_2. α_1-Receptors are found primarily postsynaptically in vascular smooth muscle; they apparently mediate vasoconstrictor responses to NE. α_2-Receptors are mainly located presynaptically and can inhibit the release of NE from the sympathetic nerve terminals. Thus, NE can inhibit its own release. α_2-Receptors are abundant in the CNS and may be important in the central control of blood pressure. Recent studies have further shown that in addition to NE itself, certain agents such as ATP, prostaglandins and histamine can also act presynaptically to inhibit NE release at the nerve terminal. In contrast, other agents such as angiotensin II can facilitate NE release.

The physiological significance of these complex interactions is not yet clear. The expectation that such developments will eventually lead to progressively greater ability to control regional vasculature with specific autonomic agents has spurred unprecedented efforts to develop more specific and effective agents for the treatment of cardiac and peripheral circulatory disorders.

Sympathetic System—Circulatory Effects

Descending fibers from the cardiac and vasomotor centers of the medulla synapse with cells of the intermediolateral cell column of the spinal cord; preganglionic fibers from the cord travel via the anterior

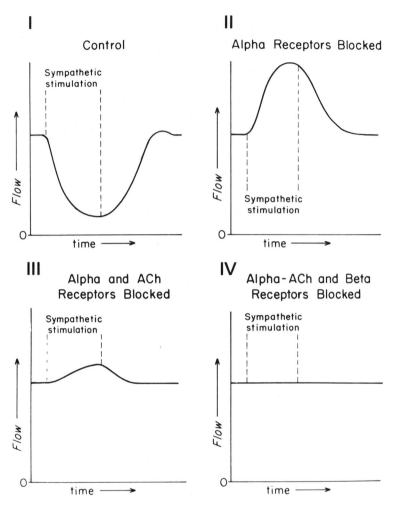

Figure 9.4. Results of stimulation of sympathetic nerves on blood flow in skeletal muscle. *I*, a strong vasoconstriction is present due to α-receptor action; *II*, after α-blockade, a sympathetic vasodilator effect is unmasked; *III*, after atropine the main vasodilator action in *II* is shown to be due to sympathetic cholinergic action. In *IV* the smaller, residual vasodilator action (β-effect) is abolished with a β-blocker. (Reprinted with permission from T.C. Ruch and H.D. Patton, *Physiology and Biophysics*. Philadelphia: W.B. Saunders, 1974.)

spinal roots to the thoracolumbar sympathetic chain (Fig. 9.5). Descending impulses from the cerebral cortex and hypothalamus may also, by way of these spinal pathways, induce sympathetic vascular responses.

The postganglionic sympathetic fibers from the cervical and upper

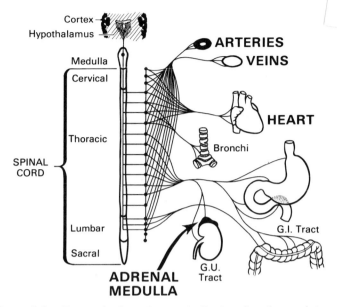

Figure 9.5. Sympathetic pathways to the heart and vasculature.

four thoracic sympathetic ganglia supply the heart and the entire peripheral circulation. The cardiac sympathetics are widely distributed to the SA and AV nodes and to the myocardium. Stimulation of these fibers activates β-adrenergic receptors and causes increases in rate and conduction velocity in the heart and increased myocardial contractility. The effects of sympathetic stimulation on the electrical and contractile events of the heart are discussed in Chapters 4 and 5, respectively. The remainder of this chapter will be concerned primarily with sympathetic effects on the peripheral circulation.

Other sympathetic postganglionic fibers join the somatic and other autonomic nerves to reach practically all arteries and veins of the body. Upon stimulation, these fibers activate α-adrenergic receptors to produce a general vasoconstriction, particularly marked in the skin, skeletal muscle, splanchnic and renal vascular beds. Reports have indicated that sympathetic stimulation may also activate peripheral β-adrenergic receptors which will tend to produce vasodilation, particularly in skeletal muscle. The importance of this response, however, is in dispute. In any event, the β-adrenergic dilator tendency in muscle is overshadowed by the much stronger α-constrictor action.

Preganglionic sympathetic fibers supply the adrenal medulla where they control the release of E and NE into the bloodstream.

Sympathetic stimulation will produce other important, noncirculatory effects, *e.g.*, relaxation of smooth muscle of the respiratory bronchioles, gastrointestinal tract and urinary tract and lessened secretion of sweat and lacrimal glands. Sympathetic stimulation also increases hepatic and muscle glycogenolysis and induces hyperglycemia; these metabolic effects assist in energy maintenance during prolonged stress such as physical exercise.

Parasympathetic System—Circulatory Effects

Preganglionic fibers of the craniosacral division of the ANS arise either in motor nuclei of the brain stem, and exit with the cranial nerves, or in the sacral division of the spinal cord (Fig. 9.6).

The vagus (tenth) cranial nerve supplies the heart. These fibers are distributed to the cardiac pacemakers, conducting tissue and to the myocardium, particularly that of the atrium. Vagal innervation to the SA node and AV junctional region is particularly important; vagal stimulation activates cholinergic (muscarinic) receptors in the heart which exert strong inhibitory effects by slowing heart rate and AV conduction velocity (Chapter 4) and by decreasing cardiac contractility, primarily of the atria (Chapter 5). As described later in this chapter, parasympathetic vasodilator fibers have been reported in vascular beds of the brain, myocardium, salivary glands, sex organs, and possibly intestine.

Preganglionic fibers of this division run to—or almost to—the innervated organs before synapsing so that parasympathetic effects tend to be more discrete and specific than sympathetic effects. Aside from its cardiovascular action, parasympathetic stimulation also induces contraction of nonvascular smooth muscle of bronchioles, gut and bladder,

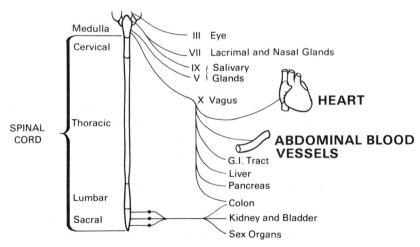

Figure 9.6. Parasympathetic pathways to the heart and vasculature.

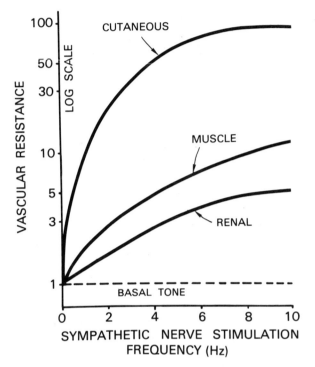

Figure 9.7. Relative responsiveness of skin, muscle and kidney vessels to vasoconstriction. Skin vessels show a greater increase in vascular resistance at equivalent stimulation frequencies. (Reprinted with permission from T.C. Ruch and H.D. Patton, *Physiology and Biophysics*. Philadelphia: W.B. Saunders, 1974.)

contraction of the pupil of the eye (miosis) and increased secretion of certain exocrine glands.

Vasoconstriction

Sympathetic vasoconstrictor impulses arise in the vasomotor center of the medulla as a result of either (a) intrinsic or extrinsic reflexes from various parts of the body, or (b) as descending impulses from the higher centers of the brain. The origin and nature of these two pathways will be discussed in Chapter 10. But however activated, sympathetic impulses will—as described above—promptly and almost simultaneously cause general constriction of the small arteries and veins.

However, all regions are not equally sensitive to constrictor impulses. Skin and muscle arteries show greater constriction at equivalent stimulation frequencies than do renal arteries (Fig. 9.7). The sensitivity of the vascular muscle is also influenced by metabolites so that during physical exercise, sympathetic stimulation will produce a much lesser degree of constriction in skeletal muscle vessels than it will at rest.

In addition to the action of arterial vasoconstriction on peripheral flow, there is an important effect on the transcapillary pressure gradient and therefore on plasma volume. Hydrostatic pressure distal to the point of arterial constriction will be reduced; as a consequence there will be less filtration from and more reabsorption of tissue fluid into the capillaries (Chapter 8). In circulatory shock, for example, the increased vasoconstriction will notably increase the circulating plasma volume.

Fluid replacement is, however, a somewhat slower process than the vasomotor action itself; although vasoconstriction is well advanced within 2 to 3 minutes after the onset of hypotension, the influx of fluid into the capillaries only begins after several minutes but continues for some hours afterward.

An important part of the sympathetic vascular response is *venoconstriction* which can significantly decrease venous capacitance and shift blood toward the heart, thus aiding venous return. At low impulse frequencies in the sympathetic vasoconstrictor nerves, *e.g.*, to skeletal muscle, the venoconstrictors (the capacitance vessels) respond more fully to decrease venous capacitance and move blood toward the heart. However, the decrease in lumen size and the consequent increase in vascular resistance is significantly greater in the precapillary (resistance) vessels than in the capacitance vessels. It is the greater increase in precapillary resistance, *i.e.*, a greater ratio of precapillary to postcapillary resistance increase, which brings about the fall in mean capillary hydrostatic pressure and the reabsorption of tissue fluid into the capillary in response to sympathetic vasoconstriction.

Vascular beds differ in their relative contribution to the resistance/capacitance balance. As mentioned previously, skeletal muscle, because of its bulk, is a large contributor to peripheral resistance; on the other hand, constriction of the splanchnic bed results in a substantial reduction of splanchnic venous capacitance and thus can be a significant factor in assisting venous return.

In summary, it should be noted that generalized vasoconstriction will usually have three vascular effects: (a) arteriolar constriction, which will increase vascular resistance, heighten the central arterial pressure and decrease flow to the constricted beds; (b) a reduction of capillary hydrostatic pressure with a resultant net increase in plasma volume; and (c) venoconstriction which will reduce the caliber of the capacitance vessels and assist venous return.

Vasodilation

While vasoconstriction results primarily from sympathetic stimulation of α-receptors, vasodilation is more complex and may be induced in several different ways.

Inhibition of the Vasoconstrictor Center of the Medulla. This type of vasodilation may be the most common pathway and some investigators have questioned the existence of a true medullary vasodilator center.

Sympathetic Cholinergic (Muscarinic) Vasodilators. As previously mentioned, small arterial vessels in skeletal muscle are unique because they are innervated by sympathetic cholinergic vasodilator fibers which can be blocked by atropine. These receptors are activated only in unusual circumstances such as the "defense reaction" (Chapter 10).

β-Sympathetic Vasodilators. These receptors seem to be present primarily in skeletal muscle; when unmasked by α-blockade, they respond with a mild, relatively transitory, vasodilation.

Parasympathetic Vasodilators. The activation of glossopharyngeal fibers to submaxillary salivary glands can evoke glandular secretions that ultimately result in the release of a neurohormone, bradykinin, which has a strong local vasodilator effect. In addition, sacral vasodilators to genital erectile tissue are important in reproduction; however, the arterioles of most other organs do not have parasympathetic innervation.

Vascular Tone and the Abolition of Tone

Basal tone is the low level, continuous, active tension which exists in the vascular smooth muscle when it is at rest or under "basal" conditions. Even when deprived of all extrinsic neural or humoral influences, a measure of basal tone remains, due to the inherent action of the smooth muscle cells themselves, *i.e.*, the myogenic component of tone.

If the sympathetic constrictor fibers are intact, a somewhat higher level of continuous contractile activity is present due to low-frequency efferent impulses from the vasoconstrictor center of the medulla. Vasoconstrictor tone is not equal in the different tissues; it is highest in skeletal muscle, skin and in splanchnic vessels and least in vessels of the brain, myocardium and kidney. The degree of basal tone of neurogenic origin can be determined in experimental animals by severing of the vasoconstrictor fibers and measuring the change in blood flow and peripheral resistance.

Vascular tone is important in the continuous maintenance of arterial pressure. In case of severance of the spinal cord there will be a flaccid paralysis of all somatic motor elements below the transection (paraplegia); in addition, the sympathetic preganglionic vasoconstrictors will be interrupted and vasoconstrictor vascular tone to the entire body mass below the lesion will be lost. This usually results in a drastic fall in arterial pressure to levels of 60 to 80 mm Hg (spinal shock) due to (a) the abrupt reduction of peripheral resistance, (b) the loss of venoconstriction, and (c) loss of skeletal muscle pump action. A similar, though

temporary and less severe fall in blood pressure, results upon administration of an α-adrenergic blocking agent such as phenoxybenzamine.

The higher the cord lesion, the more serious is the vascular disability.
If the section is above the sixth thoracic segment, a condition of
orthostatic hypotension usually exists; this means that if the patient is
tilted to any type of head-up position, he will be unable to compensate
for the gravity effect on the circulation by invoking the usual baroceptor
reflexes (Chapter 13). The relatively inadequate orthostatic response of
a patient with a cervical cord lesion compared to a patient with a lower
thoracic cord lesion is illustrated in Figure 9.8.

Several days after spinal transection, vascular constriction begins a
slow recovery, perhaps because of heightening of myogenic tone or the
gradual establishment of spinal vascular reflexes. There also begins
within a few days a denervation sensitivity of the vasculature involved.
The vessels become abnormally sensitive to circulating or injected
catecholamines so that local ischemia may develop. This phenomenon
is usually more severe if the postganglionic (rather than preganglionic)
fibers are interrupted. This effect is probably due to an increase in the
number of receptors because of loss of tonic impulses to the smooth
muscle.

Humoral Control of Flow

Probably the most important humoral agents influencing flow are the
circulating catecholamines; these may be (a) endogenous, *i.e.*, derived

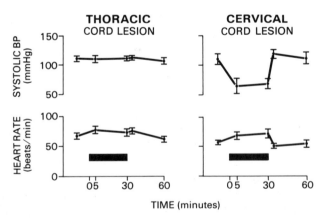

Figure 9.8.   Effect of paraplegia on vascular responses to a posture change.
Black bars indicate change from supine to sitting position. Patient with cervical
cord lesion shows orthostatic fall in arterial pressure compared to patient with
lower thoracic section. (Reprinted with permission from R.H. Johnson and J.M.K.
Spalding, *Disorders of the Autonomic Nervous System*. Philadelphia: F.A. Davis,
1974.)

from the adrenal medulla or from excess catecholamines released at neural endings; or (b) exogenous, *e.g.*, administered intravascularly. In either case, the cardiovascular effects will be similar to those of sympathetic neural action. In severe exercise, circulatory shock or other forms of stress, the plasma concentration of catecholamines (epinephrine and norepinephrine) will increase markedly and reinforce the circulatory effects of sympathetic stimulation. However, the humoral catecholamines normally have only minor cardiovascular effects compared to those resulting from neural stimulation. Norepinephrine, the primary catecholamine, has a pure vasoconstrictor action in most beds. Epinephrine at low doses causes vasodilation through β-receptor stimulation but at high doses, its α-constrictor effect overshadows the β-dilator action, particularly in skeletal muscle. The metabolic effects of sympathetic stimulation are due primarily to epinephrine.

Other humoral vasoactive substances circulating in the bloodstream include angiotensin II, the most potent vasoconstrictor in the body, vasopressin, serotonin (5-hydroxytryptamine) and several prostaglandins. Except for the effect of prostaglandins on the renal circulation (discussed in Chapter 11), the physiological role of these substances in normal cardiovascular regulation is not yet certain.

Local Regulation of Flow

Active Hyperemia

When tissues become metabolically more active, *e.g.*, during exercise or if their temperature is raised, the microcirculatory vessels dilate and flow increases, a process known as active hyperemia. The mechanism of this effect is not certain but is thought to be a vasodilator action of accumulated metabolites such as CO_2 or lactic acid on the precapillary sphincters. The "metabolic" theory is strengthened by the fact that during severe exercise when skeletal muscle metabolism is at its peak and metabolic products such as CO_2, lactic acid, etc., accumulate in the tissues, blood flow is very high.

Other metabolites such as K^+ and H^+ as well as decreased P_{O_2} and increased osmolality have also been proposed as primary dilator agents. There is increasing evidence that the responsible metabolites may vary with the tissue involved; in the hypoxic myocardium, *e.g.*, adenosine and some of its related compounds have been implicated as the active agents. In the salivary gland, bradykinin and in the kidney, prostaglandins are known to have strong local vascular effects. However, some of the evidence is conflicting and further investigation is needed in this important field.

Reactive Hyperemia

If blood flow to a tissue is arrested by arterial occlusion for a period of a few seconds to several minutes, the flow upon release will exceed the control flow for a short period before returning to preocclusion levels. This excess afterflow is known as "reactive hyperemia" and as indicated in Figure 9.9, the resulting degree and duration of the overshoot are roughly proportional to the duration of the occlusion, *i.e.*, to the metabolic debt incurred.

Tissues differ in their reactive hyperemic response; heart and brain show large responses, skeletal muscle intermediate and liver, lung and skin the least. The cause of the increased flow is not clear but the relation between the length of occlusion and degree of hyperemia suggests that either oxygen lack in the tissues or the accumulation of metabolites is responsible. Reactive hyperemia will result after ischemia (partial or full occlusion of arterial supply) or hypoxia (reduced Po_2 in the tissue).

Autoregulation

If individual organs are perfused with blood at different pressures so that flow-pressure relations can be studied, the initial response in almost all cases resembles *curve A*, Figure 9.10. In some tissues, particularly kidney, brain and heart, the flow will change within 30 to 60 seconds to an "autoregulatory" adaptation such as *curve B* (Fig. 9.10), in which there is a tendency to maintain the local blood flow relatively constant in the face of a changing perfusion pressure. Some tissues such as skin and lung show minimal autoregulation.

Curve A is a passive type of curve and its exponential nature is due mainly to the constantly increasing diameter which occurs in a flexible

Figure 9.9.   Reactive hyperemia. *A*, temporary increase in blood flow to forearm after 30-second occlusion. After 60-second occlusion, *B*, the reactive flow is of greater magnitude and duration.

Figure 9.10.   Autoregulation of kidney. Initial pressure-flow response curve (*A*) changes to a plateau-type curve (*B*) within 30 to 60 seconds.

tube when subjected to increasing transmural pressure (Chapter 2). During autoregulation (*curve B*), the higher flows are achieved at low pressure by relaxation of the vascular muscle, and the lower flows at higher pressures by constriction. The net result—the maintenance of a relatively consistent flow—is particularly advantageous to vital organs such as brain and heart; in case of hypotension or failing circulation, local flow will increase. In case of higher pressure, excess flow will be reduced.

Those organs with the smallest neurogenic tone, *i.e.*, brain, heart and kidney, show the highest autoregulatory ability; conversely tissues with the highest resting vascular tone, *e.g.*, skin, have the least autoregulatory ability. Although the ability to autoregulate is affected to some extent by neural and humoral influences such as vasoconstrictor tone and pH of the blood, the autoregulatory response is largely intrinsic and occurs when tissues are fully denervated and isolated; it is, therefore, essentially a local phenomenon.

Different explanations have been advanced for autoregulation; one of these, the myogenic theory, suggests that increased perfusion pressure increases the muscle tension in the vessel wall, stimulating it to contract and thus reduce flow; with reduction in perfusion pressure, there is relaxation of the smooth muscle of the wall and an increase in vessel caliber. This theory proposes, therefore, that distension or relaxation of the muscle is the self-regulating mediator.

Other investigators believe that autoregulation is associated with the

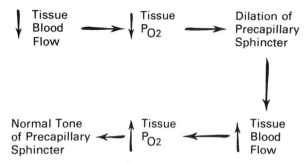

Figure 9.11. Possible mechanism for autoregulation of tissue blood flow involving effect of altered P_{O_2} on precapillary sphincter tone.

state of oxygenation of the tissue; a decrease in flow will produce a decrease in local tissue P_{O_2} and an increase in tissue P_{CO_2}; the decreased P_{O_2} would theoretically relax the precapillary sphincter and the flow would again rise. With restored flow, the P_{O_2} and P_{CO_2} levels are returned toward normal as shown in Figure 9.11. Regardless of the validity of any specific theory, it seems very likely that tissue flow is regulated in some manner similar to the negative feedback mechanism shown in Figure 9.11.

Long-Term Regulation of Flow

The previous portions of this chapter relate to rapid adjustments of the circulation. But what are the responses if demands for additional flow are built up more gradually? If, for example, the main arterial supply to a part of the body such as skin or muscle is gradually occluded, the pressure and flow in the distal vessel will be reduced. What is the response of the tissue to such a situation? In tissues with adequate collateral circulation, *e.g.*, skeletal muscle, collateral vessels will dilate over the ensuing days and weeks so that total arterial flow to the part will gradually be restored to near normal. Thus the local circulatory demand has in some way instigated an increased blood supply. This type of adaptation is, however, severely restricted in tissues such as brain or kidney in which collateral vessels are minimal or absent; in such cases an infarct (area of necrosis) is likely as a result of vascular occlusion with degeneration, loss of function and replacement fibrosis occurring in at least a portion of the involved area. The question of myocardial infarct is discussed in Chapter 14.

On the other hand, if arterial pressure and flow to a part is excessive, *e.g.*, in arteries above the level at which partial occlusion of the abdominal aorta has been produced in an experimental animal, the flow to tissues above the occlusion level will at first be excessive because of the hypertension in this portion of the arterial tree. Gradually, however, the flow to the involved regions will return to normal by virtue of gradually increased constriction of the arteries and arterioles in the area. Thus, if blood flow is artificially increased or decreased, it will, if left alone, tend to gradually return to previous control levels. Similar circulatory responses occur with alterations of oxygen supply. Prolonged hypoxia will stimulate increased flow and in embryonic or fetal tissue will promote the generation of new blood vessels.

It appears, therefore, that the relation of flow to tissue metabolism is the dominant factor in the long-term regulation of blood flow. It seems likely that the mechanism of this effect is either via oxygen demand or through an oxygen-linked metabolite. But how oxygen lack actually brings about increased flow or vascular architectural expansion is not known. The increased physical stretch and tension of vasodilation on growth potential of vascular cells may be a factor; regardless of the actual cause, however, it is known that the vascular cells of younger tissue are more responsive to growth stimuli of hypoxia and ischemia than are those of older tissue.

References

Goodman LS. Neurohumoral transmission and the autonomic nervous system. In: *The Pharmacological Basis of Therapeutics*, edited by AG Gilman, SE Mayer and A Gilman. New York: 1980, 6th ed., pp. 56–70.
Hoffman BB and Lefkowitz RJ. Adrenergic receptors in the heart. *Annu Rev Physiol* 44:475–484, 1982.
Johansson B. Vascular reactivity in hypertension. Symposium. *Fed Proc* 33:121–149, 1974.
Johnson PC. Principles of peripheral circulatory control. In: *Peripheral Circulation*, edited by PC Johnson. New York: John Wiley & Sons, 1978.
Johnson RH and Spalding JMK. *Disorders of the Autonomic Nervous System*. Philadelphia: F.A. Davis, 1974.
Mellander S and Johansson B. Control of resistance, exchange and capacitance functions in the peripheral circulation. *Pharmacol Rev* 20:117–196, 1968.
Randall WC (ed.). *Neural Regulation of the Heart*. New York: Oxford University Press, 1977.
Shepherd JT. *Physiology of the Circulation in Human Limbs in Health and Disease*. Philadelphia: W.B. Saunders, 1963.
Sleight P. Drugs acting on the heart. In: *Circulation of the Blood*, edited by DG James. Baltimore: University Park Press, 1978.
Westfall TC. Neuroeffector mechanisms. *Annu Rev Physiol* 42:383–397, 1980.

chapter 10

Regulation of Arterial Blood Pressure

Arterial Pressure Regulation—General Principles

The two prime objectives for overall circulatory regulation are: (a) the maintenance of an adequate and relatively constant arterial pressure; and (b) a sufficient control of blood flow through local tissues to maintain adequate metabolism, capillary exchange and temperature balance. Blood flow was discussed in Chapter 9. The important topic of arterial pressure control is considered in this chapter.

The method by which arterial pressure is regulated depends upon whether short-term or long-term adaptation is required. Short-term adjustments (over minutes and hours) are intended to correct temporary

158

imbalances of pressure such as those caused by postural change, exercise, hemorrhage or other stress. But whatever the cause of the circulatory imbalance, the reaction is usually a series of rapid autonomic responses intended to return the pressure toward normal.

Long-term arterial pressure adjustments (weeks or months) are usually concerned with the balance between extracellular fluid and blood volume on the one hand and renal mechanisms controlling urinary output on the other. The latter particularly involve pituitary-adrenal cortical mechanisms, which control water and sodium excretion by the kidney; disturbances of this process may result in a gradual increase in arterial pressure and, if continued, in enduring hypertension.

Arterial blood pressure is probably the most important controlled variable in the circulatory system. We know from the general hemodynamic equation discussed in Chapter 2 that blood pressure is, in effect, the mathematical product of cardiac output and peripheral resistance. The cardiovascular centers of the medulla regulate the arterial pressure through adjustment of these two variables. However, these centers are themselves governed by impulses from higher neural centers and from

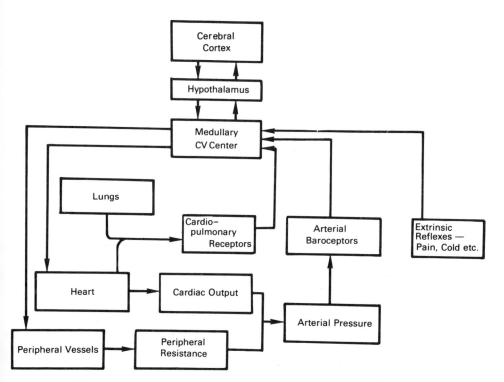

Figure 10.1. Simplified schema showing primary pathways for short-term regulation of arterial blood pressure.

multiple sensors throughout the body. Some of these sensors are in the vascular system. Thus, the arterial pressure, acting through classical feedback mechanisms, is both the controlled and controlling variable (Fig. 10.1).

Cardiovascular Centers of the Medulla

The main nervous control of the circulation resides in several functionally diverse areas or "centers" in the dorsal reticular matter of the medulla and lower pons. These are collectively known as cardiovascular (CV) centers and together with the respiratory center, with which they have close neural connection, constitute the "vital nervous centers" whose integrity is absolutely essential for survival of the organism. There are two major divisions of the cardiovascular control area, *i.e.*, cardiac and vasomotor, which are concerned with the neural control of the heart and peripheral blood vessels, respectively. These two areas are not well defined so that there is both anatomical and functional overlap between them. Careful animal experiments involving surgical transection as well as microelectrode stimulation and functional mapping have indicated that both the cardiac and vasomotor areas have, in turn, further subdivisions with specialized functions.

One of the clearest entities in the cardiac area is a "cardioinhibitory center" located in the nucleus ambiguus and dorsal nucleus of the vagus nerve. Vagal efferents from these sites carry impulses which act primarily to decrease heart rate and to a lesser degree the contractility of the atria. The existence of a corollary sympathetic "cardiostimulatory center" in the lateral medulla has been reported but its identity as a discrete center is less certain.

The "vasomotor center" of the medulla consists, in most species, of a lateral "vasoconstrictor area" whose neurons descend in the spinal cord and synapse with cells of the intermediolateral cell column. Their preganglionic fibers are responsible for the widespread sympathetic vasoconstriction described in Chapter 9. The "vasodilator area" is more questionable and it is probable that vasodilation is mainly due to inhibition of the vasoconstrictor center.

The close proximity of these centers to each other and their tendency to function in a coordinated fashion in the interests of arterial pressure control have led to the characterization of the lateral and superior portions of the CV center area as the "pressor area," and the more medial as the "depressor area" (Fig. 10.2). In most species, stimulation of the pressor area will induce both an increase in cardiac rate and contractility and a generalized increase in peripheral resistance while depressor area stimulation usually elicits the reverse. The "vasoconstrictor," "cardiostimulatory," and "cardioinhibitory" areas are tonically

Figure 10.2. Location of pressor (*crosshatched*) and depressor (*horizontally lined*) areas in the brain stem of the cat. (Reprinted with permission from J. Alexander, *Neurophysiology* 9:205, 1946.)

active, *i.e.*, they emit, even at rest, a constant low level of efferent impulses so that cutting of these efferent fibers will eliminate vasoconstrictor, cardiac stimulatory and cardioinhibitory effects on the respective target organs.

The various CV centers usually function reciprocally, *i.e.*, when vagal slowing is initiated by the cardioinhibitory center, there is simultaneously reduced activity of the cardiostimulatory center.

Intrinsic Reflexes of the Cardiovascular System

"Intrinsic" reflexes, that is those which arise from within the circulatory system itself, are usually distinguished from "extrinsic" or those originating in other systems or organs. The intrinsic reflexes, by far the more important in the short-term regulation of blood pressure, are for the most part activated by special receptors; these receptors are usually sensitive to pressure or to special chemical stimuli. Those sensitive to pressure are termed stretch receptors, baroceptors or mechanoreceptors. The "chemoreceptors" of the vascular system are primarily concerned with respiratory regulation but may in certain circumstances play a secondary role in circulatory control.

A large number of cardiovascular reflexes have been described and through animal experimentation their pathways have been at least partly traced; however, in some cases their role in the intact human circulation is difficult to determine. Our present knowledge, while admittedly incomplete, does, however, permit a few generalizations regarding reflex control of the circulation. These are: (a) the high-pressure, arterial baroceptors of the carotid sinus and aortic arch are by far the key reflexes in short-term regulation of the circulation; (b) the cardiopulmonary baroceptors (all low pressure except those of the left ventricle), while not yet as well defined as the arterial baroceptors, have a significant role in cardiovascular regulation; they elicit circulatory responses which generally supplement and modulate the arterial baroceptor reflexes, the common objective being the stability of arterial blood pressure; (c) the baroceptors also serve as "volume" receptors whose purpose is to maintain the blood volume; and (d) the extrinsic reflexes play a minor role in the normal, healthy subject but may be important in circulatory disease.

Arterial Baroceptors

Afferent fibers from specialized pressure-sensitive endings in the walls of the aortic arch and internal carotid arteries travel via the aortic and carotid sinus nerves, join the vagus and glossopharyngeal nerves respectively, and make connections with the CV centers of the medulla. Impulses from the carotid and aortic chemoreceptors, which are near their respective baroceptor endings, travel over the same afferent nerves (Fig. 10.3).

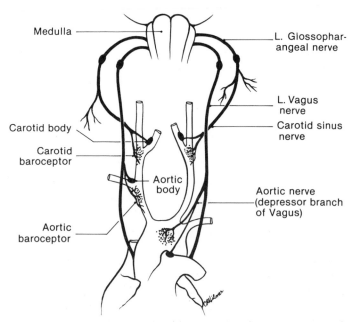

Figure 10.3. Diagrammatic sketch showing the central connections of the aortic and carotid sinus baroceptors.

Figure 10.4.   Hemodynamic response to arterial baroceptor stimulation.

Stretching of these baroceptor endings generates action potentials in the afferent nerves (Fig. 10.3) whose frequency is approximately proportional to the pressure change in the artery. This means that *increased* arterial pressure at the baroceptor site will increase the frequency of afferent impulses in the aortic and carotid sinus nerves. This stimulus results in greater activity in the medullary depressor area and inhibition of the pressor area so that heart rate and myocardial contractility are *decreased* and vasoconstrictor and venoconstrictor tone are *lessened* (Fig. 10.4). Increased blood pressure, therefore, leads to reflex action aimed at reducing the pressure back toward normal (depressor reflex); if baroceptor stretch is decreased, the afferent impulse frequency is decreased and the reverse response occurs (pressor reflex). Thus, in common with most reflexes that stabilize a controlled variable, arterial baroceptors (ABs) involve negative feedback.

The AB vasoconstrictor control is particularly marked in renal, mesenteric and skeletal muscle arteries, and venoconstrictor control in the splanchnic bed. Recent evidence also indicates that during the pressor response, there is an increased release of renin in the kidney, a greater tubular reabsorption of Na^+ and a tendency toward expansion of the plasma volume.

The high-pressure baroceptors respond to absolute stretch, *i.e.*, to changes in both mean arterial transmural pressure and to changes in pulse pressure, but even more strongly to the rate of change of pressure, *i.e.*, dP/dt. The baroceptor response is greatest in the physiological range of blood pressure (80–150 mm Hg) and there is evidence that the carotid baroceptors are somewhat more sensitive than the aortic (Fig. 10.5).

The ABs are particularly important in maintaining adequate pressure and, therefore, flow to the brain and heart during circulatory stresses such as hemorrhage, postural change or any stimulus that will alter arterial pressure. Without AB reflexes, *e.g.*, standing erect would result in a rapid, sharp fall in venous return and cardiac output. But aside from neutralizing abnormal arterial pressure alterations, the ABs tend to damp out the numerous pressure fluctuations that occur during ordinary activity. Studies have shown that even during resting and basal

Figure 10.5. Baroceptor sensitivity at different arterial pressure levels in the dog. At equivalent pressures the carotid baroceptors were more sensitive than the aortic receptors. (Reprinted with permission from D. E. Donald and A. J. Edis, *J Physiol* 215:521, 1971.)

states, dogs with denervated arterial baroceptors tended to show very wide swings in arterial pressure and a striking inability to maintain a constant pressure level. Undoubtedly, this stabilization of arterial pressure lessens flow fluctuations to important organs such as the brain and heart. As indicated in Figure 10.5, at higher arterial pressure levels, the ABs are less sensitive to any given pressure increment, probably because of the lesser compliance of the arterial wall at higher degrees of stretch. There is also some evidence to indicate that arterial baroceptors normally respond more actively to a decrease in pressure than to an increase, *i.e.*, they are more effective in combatting acute hypotension than acute hypertension.

An important property of arterial baroceptors is their ability to adapt to permanent or semipermanent alterations in arterial pressure. Even in acute hypertension (6 hours or less), and in exercise, the ABs continue to function but are "reset" at a higher level, which then becomes the baseline for further baroceptor response. Reports indicate that the baroceptors will also reset to a lower level in case of hypotension. These "resets" are reversible if the baseline pressure changes.

Methods have recently been developed for measuring the sensitivity of the arterial baroceptor response by (a) inducing a mild temporary hypertension with a vasoconstrictor drug, or (b) applying positive or negative pressure to the area of the neck over the carotid sinus receptors. The rapidity and degree of the heart rate response to the transmural pressure change is a measure of the sensitivity of the reflex. Such experiments have shown a decreased responsiveness of ABs with advancing age, hypertension, and coronary artery disease. It has been suggested that arteriosclerotic changes and decreased compliance of the arterial walls are responsible for the decreased sensitivity of the receptors in these conditions.

In general the strength of the baroceptor reflex decrees that in most short-term situations, there is a reciprocal relationship between arterial blood pressure and heart rate. However, this does not universally hold. For example, during static (isometric) exercise, systolic and diastolic blood pressures and heart rate all increase progressively (Chapter 12). In the diving (face immersion) reflex, there is a sharp decrease in both arterial pressure and heart rate (Chapter 13) and during the "defense reaction" (described later in this chapter) there is a pronounced increase in arterial pressure as well as heart rate. It is likely that supramedullary centers, which are involved in all three of these instances, are responsible for the temporary inhibition of the baroreflexes.

Cardiopulmonary Reflexes

Cardiopulmonary receptors are intrathoracic sensors, most of which are located at low pressure sites in the walls of the heart, great vessels and lungs. These receptors are usually classified on the basis of location, *i.e.*, (a) atrial and vena caval, (b) ventricular, and (c) pulmonary (Fig. 10.6).

Atrial and Vena Caval Receptors

These are low-pressure mechanoreceptors whose impulses travel mainly via large, myelinated (fast-conducting) and small, unmyelinated

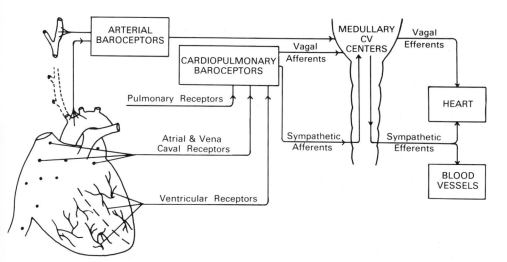

Figure 10.6.   Arterial and cardiopulmonary baroceptors and their central connections.

(slow-conducting) vagal afferent fibers. Three different varieties of these atrial receptors have been recognized: type A, which fire only during atrial systole; type B, which fire only during atrial filling; and an intermediate group, which fire during both atrial systole and filling.

Cardiac reflexes—particularly those arising from atrial and vena caval receptors—are currently a very active focus of research. Our basic understanding of reflexes is mainly derived from animal studies involving the dissection of nerves to their receptor origins, balloon distensions of heart chambers at graded volumes and pressures and electrical stimulation of afferent nerves at different frequencies and intensities. The physiological consequences of such manipulations are noted both in the presence and absence of competing influences (*e.g.*, the arterial baroceptor reflexes). The results of such basic experiments are then compared with studies in human subjects and patients in which cardiopulmonary receptor stimulation is altered, *e.g.*, by changes in central blood volume. While there are some differences of opinion on the scope and function of these reflexes, following is a brief outline of views advanced by most investigators on the probable role of cardiopulmonary (CP) receptors.

Heart Rate Effects. The most widely known of these effects is the *Bainbridge reflex*, which refers to the tachycardia that is sometimes produced by increased filling of the atrium or atriocaval region, *e.g.*, by large intravenous infusions of blood or saline. The afferent pathway is via large myelinated fibers of the vagus nerve, and the efferents are primarily in the sympathetic fibers to the SA node. Although this effect has long been observed in a number of species, the heart rate response to atrial filling in the human, as discussed in Chapter 7 (Integration of Stroke Volume and Heart Rate), seems to depend mainly on the existing heart rate at the time of application of the stress, *i.e.*, the lower the existing rate, the greater the increase, and *v.v.* The variable results reported by different investigators suggest that this reflex probably plays a secondary role in cardiovascular regulation.

Blood Pressure and Renal Effects. There is now considerable evidence that stimulation of other CP mechanoreceptors, whose afferents travel mainly via unmyelinated vagal fibers, trigger a widespread complex of circulatory effects which alter arterial pressure, heart rate and renal function. Recent studies suggest that these CP impulses originate not only in the atria but also in the ventricles and lungs.

Shepherd, Donald and other investigators noted that an increase in central blood volume and pressure (*e.g.*, through large intravenous fluid infusions, prolonged bed rest or the zero gravity state) will increase the firing of these CP receptors. This, in turn, will result in a decrease in sympathetic vasoconstriction of skeletal muscle, renal and mesenteric arterioles, an increase in splanchnic venous capacitance, a diminution in heart rate, *i.e.*, a depressor response. This decrease in sympathetic activity is accompanied by a lesser release of renin by the kidneys, a decreased Na^+ reabsorption from the renal tubules, and a diuresis with a resultant tendency toward a diminution in plasma volume.

Corollary studies have shown that a decrease in central blood volume (*e.g.*, in head-up tilt or hemorrhage), or the cutting of afferent vagal fibers from CP receptors in an experimental animal, result in a sympathetic vasoconstriction of skeletal muscle, renal and mesenteric arterioles, a decrease in splanchnic venous capacitance and an increase in heart rate—a pressor response. This sympathetic hyperactivity is accompanied by increased release of renin by the kidneys, greater Na^+ reabsorption from the tubules, antidiuresis and a tendency toward an increase in plasma volume.

In other words, these CP receptors under normal resting conditions appear to exert a tonic inhibitory effect on sympathetic vasoconstriction and cardioacceleration. A lessening of this receptor stimulation through a decrease in central blood volume, or through cutting of these afferent nerves, "unloads" the receptors and thereby decreases their firing rate. This invokes a sympathetic pressor effect via the vasomotor and cardiac centers of the medulla as well as an antidiuretic effect. It should be noted that the heart rate changes accompanying the reflex induced by these receptors are directionally opposite to those resulting from the Bainbridge reflex.

CP receptors are capable of adapting to a continued increase in atrial pressure by resetting. It has been shown, *e.g.*, that in experimental congestive heart failure in dogs, in which the atria are distended, the atrial receptors gradually adapt and the diuretic reflex is attenuated. This adaptation is reversed if the heart failure is relieved.

From the preceding, it will be noted that the characteristics, effects and general functions of this CP receptor response are similar to those of the arterial baroceptor reflex. It is evident (a) that the low- and high-pressure mechanoreceptors act in concert in an effort to buffer arterial pressure changes, (b) that both have cardiovascular and renal manifestations, and (c) that both can adapt to a sustained alteration in baroceptor stretch by resetting.

However, there are also certain differences between those reflexes: (a) the CP reflexes react to lesser pressure changes—non-hypotensive hemorrhage, *e.g.*, will induce prompt CP responses since these receptors act at low-pressure atrial sites that are affected earlier by the hypotension; (b) CP receptors (at least in man) have stronger reflex vasoconstrictor effects on skeletal muscle arteries while ABs induce stronger splanchnic vasoconstriction and apparently greater effects on heart rate; and (c) the plasma volume effects of CP receptors are more pronounced and the role of CP endings as "volume receptors" appears to be a very significant one.

The mechanism of the renal effects is at present not fully understood. Plasma volume regulation involves complex interrelationships between circulatory reflexes, CNS osmoreceptors and several endocrine systems. Current evidence indicates (a) that the atrial CP mechanoreceptors mediate their plasma volume effects primarily through two mechanisms, *i.e.*, the renin-angiotensin-aldosterone (RAA) system and the antidiuretic hormone (ADH) system, and (b) that the main effector sites are the renal collecting tubules. These mechanisms are further discussed in Chapter 11 (Renal Circulation). The role of these reflexes in hypotensive stresses is discussed in Chapter 13 (Response to Hemorrhage) and in Chapter 14 (Congestive Heart Failure).

Investigators have reported that mechanoreceptors may be stimulated by either stretch or contraction of the muscle with which they are in contact, depending on the orientation of the receptors. It is believed, *e.g.*, that increased atrial muscle contraction is the mechanism for the diuresis seen in certain clinical and experimental pathological conditions, such as paroxysmal atrial tachycardia or atrial fibrillation, in which there is unusual contractile activity of the atrial wall. This effect does not occur in ordinary sinus tachycardia since there is no undue stimulation of the receptors in this case.

Ventricular Receptors

When stimulated by increased stretch or by strong ventricular contraction, afferent impulses from ventricular receptors (traveling mainly via unmyelinated or slow-conducting vagal fibers) reach the medulla and elicit a bradycardia and vasodilation, *i.e.*, a *depressor* response.

A peculiar characteristic of these receptors is that a very similar, hypotensive response is produced by injection into the heart or coronary circulation of a specific chemical agent, called veratrine (an alkaloid extract from lilacs). This unusual chemoreceptor response is known as the *Bezold-Jarisch reflex*. This reflex may also be triggered by intracoronary injections of other chemicals such as nicotine, bradykinin, histamine, or digitalis. A similar response can be elicited by the injection of a contrast medium during coronary angiography and by the accumulation of metabolites under certain pathological conditions. The hypotensive reaction in cardiogenic shock produced by coronary occlusion may be partly due to activation of these ventricular receptors (Chapter 14).

Fox has suggested that under physiological conditions, the decreased peripheral resistance response to strong ventricular contraction may buffer the increased left ventricular ejection and thus minimize the heightened arterial pressure rise, *e.g.*, in severe exercise. Since veratrine also has a positive inotropic action, the Bezold-Jarish effect may also be a special manifestation of the buffering effect of this mechanoceptor reflex.

The above-described responses to stimulation of ventricular receptors are the result of afferent impulses which travel via the vagus nerves. Ventricular distension in experimental animals will also stimulate sympathetic afferent endings in the ventricle which will invoke strong arterial *pressor* responses as well as alterations in respiration. The significance of these sympathetic ventricular CP reflexes is not clear at present.

Pulmonary Receptors

A variety of reflexes arising from the lung are known to be important in the control of respiration but their circulatory significance in man is still uncertain. However, pulmonary congestion, which occurs during severe exercise or increased pulmonary venous pressure, may activate juxtapulmonary receptors (so-called J receptors) and induce reflex tachycardia and dyspnea (difficulty in breathing).

It should be pointed out that most of our information on CP reflexes has been derived from animal experiments. While these have contributed immeasurably to our knowledge, species differences in these types of reflexes are often significant. Thus, the full role of these reflexes in the human is still not known.

Arterial Chemoreceptors

These special endings, located in the carotid and aortic bodies (near the carotid sinus and aortic arch receptors) respond to a reduction in arterial P_{O_2}, an increase in P_{CO_2} or an increase in arterial H^+ concentration, with hyperventilation, sympathetic vasoconstriction (mainly in skeletal muscle) and bradycardia (vagal). While the main purpose of the arterial chemoreceptor reflex is to stimulate respiratory minute volume, its secondary circulatory effects appear to be aimed at increasing oxygen delivery to the brain and heart through general peripheral vasoconstriction and increased arterial pressure. The chemoreceptor reflex becomes a protective factor in certain pathophysiological situations such as the hypoxia of altitude (low arterial P_{O_2}) and circulatory shock (peripheral ischemia). The special role of the chemoreceptors in the diving (face immersion) response is discussed in Chapter 13.

Extrinsic Reflexes of the Cardiovascular System

Certain stimuli originating outside the circulation may invoke cardiovascular responses via somatic afferent pathways. The central connections are not known and the responses are usually less consistent than in the case of the intrinsic reflexes described above. The following are among the more common of these extrinsic reflexes.

Pain

Pain produces a somewhat variable hemodynamic response. Mild to moderate pain usually elicits increased arterial pressure and tachycardia. Severe pain, as might be experienced by undue stretching of the gall bladder, intestine or ureter, or deep trauma to a bone or joint, may induce bradycardia, hypotension and sometimes circulatory collapse and fainting. Overly rapid evacuation of a markedly distended hollow organ may also cause reflex hypotension and sometimes circulatory collapse. This reflex is responsible for the clinical admonition that if pressure in overdistended organs such as the stomach or urinary bladder is relieved by intubation or catheterization, the decompression should be done slowly. Pain accompanying myocardial ischemia is discussed in Chapter 15.

Cold

Somatic afferent fibers from cutaneous thermosensitive endings travel to the hypothalamus and reflexly induce cutaneous vasoconstriction and piloerection (erection of hair). Intense local cold, *e.g.*, by immersion of one hand to the wrist in ice water for 1 minute (the "*cold pressor*" *test*) will result in an increase in arterial pressure through stimulation of pain as well as cold receptors.

It has been reported that in some patients with coronary heart disease, the cold pressor test increases coronary artery resistance, decreases coronary blood flow and sometimes precipitates angina (chest pain) of cardiac origin; these changes did not occur in normal subjects (Fig. 10.7). The cause of angina is not certain but may be due either to reflex coronary vasoconstriction or a relative myocardial ischemia due to the increased aortic afterload.

Special Somatic Reflexes

Strong somatic afferent stimulation may cause circulatory responses, particularly of the depressor type. *Rapid angular acceleration* (rotation or spinning of the body on its own axis) will, for example, induce excessive afferent stimulation from the labyrinth of the inner ear and may cause nausea, vomiting and a depressor reflex. The *oculocardiac reflex* refers to bradycardia and hypotension induced by lateral pressure on the eyeball; the latter reflex, by virtue of its efferent vagal path, is sometimes effective in aborting attacks of cardiac arrhythmias such as atrial fibrillation (Chapter 5).

Figure 10.7. Blood pressure and coronary flow responses of patients with coronary artery disease (CAD) and normal subjects to the cold pressor test. *A* indicates similar arterial pressure response in the two groups, and *B*, a decrease in coronary flow in the patients. *Arrow* indicates start of 50-second cold pressor test. (Reprinted with permission from G. H. Mudge, W. Grossman, R. M. Mills, M. Lesch, and E. Braunwald, *N Engl J Med* 295:1333, 1976.)

Higher Center Influences

CNS Ischemic Response

Apart from the baroceptor response induced by a fall in blood pressure, severe hypotension, such as occurs in circulatory shock, will result in a profound, generalized vasoconstriction. Since the mechanism of this powerful reflex is probably hypoxia or ischemia of the brain stem, it is known as the "CNS ischemic response." It apparently represents a "last ditch" effort to maintain adequate perfusion of the CV medullary centers and is activated only when the arterial pressure is reduced to levels of about 50 to 70 mm Hg.

A similar mechanism is thought to be operative in the "Cushing reflex," which is a marked hypertension following acute elevation of cerebrospinal fluid (CSF) pressure; in this instance the flow of blood to the brain stem is decreased by the external pressure of CSF fluid on the blood vessels, thus activating the CNS ischemic response. The arterial blood pressure rises progressively in an effort to exceed the CSF pressure and maintain adequate blood flow to the brain.

Role of the Hypothalamus

The hypothalamus, as a midway point between the cerebral cortex and the medulla, provides a level of integration for a number of essential cardiovascular activities. Among these are the coordination of responses to *emotion, exercise* and *temperature change*. Experimental animals with lesions in the ventromedial hypothalamus will, upon relatively slight provocation, react with intense rage associated with high blood pressure, sweating and pupillary dilation. The hypothalamus plays a key role in determining the circulatory and other autonomic responses which accompany swings of mood and emotion.

The efficient and effective performance of *physical exercise* or work requires a close integration of the circulation and metabolism. That this is done by the hypothalamus is suggested by the fact that stimulation of the fields of Forel will, in the dog, produce a series of autonomic reactions closely resembling those which accompany physical exercise; these include highly coordinated responses of dilation of skeletal muscle vessels, constriction of nonmuscle beds and release of plasma catecholamines into the blood (Chapter 12, Physical Exercise).

The control center for *temperature regulation*, located in the preoptic region of the anterior hypothalamus, plays a key role in balancing heat production and loss. When the body (or the hypothalamus) is heated, sympathetic vasoconstrictor impulse traffic is decreased, vascular smooth muscles are relaxed, the cutaneous arteriovenous anastomoses

(AVAs) of exposed areas are opened and sweating occurs; all of these are essential to the preservation of heat balance. With cold the reverse response occurs in order to reduce heat loss (Chapter 11, Cutaneous Circulation).

Corticohypothalamic Patterns—Defense Reaction

From a circulatory standpoint, one of the more important behavior patterns involving the cerebral cortex and the hypothalamus is the "defense reaction." It has been shown that stimulation of a localized area in the ventral hypothalamus of the cat will produce circulatory reactions very similar to those invoked by the presence of actual danger or threat of danger to the animal. These reactions include sympathetic cholinergic vasodilation of skeletal muscle (to permit immediate maximum muscular effort), generalized sympathetic vasoconstriction and elevation of arterial pressure, increased plasma catecholamines and increased rate and contractility of the heart. These changes, similar to those mentioned as preparation for muscular exercise, instantly prepare the animal for full scale "fight or flight" reaction.

It has also been observed that stimulation of another hypothalamic site, the depressor area, located very near the defense center, calls forth a strong sympathetic inhibition involving hypotension and bradycardia; this sympathoinhibition resembles the "playing dead" reaction used by certain animals as a protective measure and is thought to be involved in psychogenic fainting. It has been suggested that in the face of overpowering stress, the corticohypothalamic depressor response may offer, in addition to fight or flight, a third option, *i.e.*, fainting and oblivion (Chapter 13, Fainting). The pathways involved in the defense reaction and the depressor reaction are shown in Figure 10.8.

Integrated CNS Control of the Circulation

The previous sections of this chapter have described specific control centers of the brain and important reflex patterns that govern the responses of the circulatory system to short-term environmental stresses. It has been stated, *e.g.*, that the medullary cardiovascular centers are indispensable and vital elements in circulatory control. These concepts are correct according to our present understanding.

There is, however, increasing evidence that in the constant interplay of these responses in the daily lives of higher animals and humans, the individual centers, particularly those of the medulla, are not the autonomous controlling forces they were once considered to be. As Hilton and others have pointed out, it now appears more than likely that a

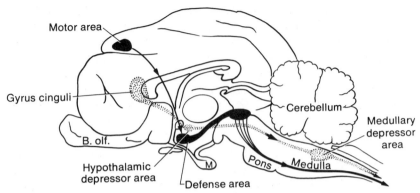

Figure 10.8. Illustration of the cortical and spinal connections of the defense center and "depressor area" of the hypothalamus. (Reprinted with permission from B. Folkow and E. Neil, *Circulation*. London: Oxford University Press, 1971.)

highly integrated cardio-respiratory-metabolic control is exercised by a hypothalamic-medullary complex.

While earlier views emphasized the primacy of the simple reflex patterns and medullary center controls, with higher center activity mainly in emergency situations, current evidence points to a more continuous regulation by the integrated "hypothalamic-medullary complex." This "complex" integrates the afferent reflex information at several different levels. In this integration process, certain hypothalamic systems appear of particular importance, *e.g.*, the defense center and its baroceptor inputs, and the temperature control center. In addition, there is increasing awareness of the importance of psychological factors in determining circulatory performance. Aside from the defense center responses to fear and rage, the cardiovascular system is undoubtedly influenced to a considerable degree by the cerebral cortex in response to more subtle forms of psychological stress. This is a large but still relatively undefined area for future research.

Finally, it should be recalled that entirely aside from nervous and humoral control mechanisms, individual organs and tissues have a considerable degree of circulatory autonomy. As previously described, the myocardium, *e.g.*, is capable of very significant intrinsic heterometric adjustments (Chapter 5) and individual organs are capable of highly important circulatory autoregulation. All of these are independent of nervous control (Chapter 9).

Long-Term Regulation of Arterial Blood Pressure

The previous portions of this chapter have been concerned with relatively short-term regulation of blood pressure. Guyton has recently advanced the concept that long-term control has a very different basis, namely the blood volume-urinary output balance, which in turn, is mainly influenced by the renin-angiotensin-aldosterone system. As indicated in Figure 10.9, an increase in arterial pressure, (1), causes increased fluid output through the kidneys, and a reduction in extracellular fluid volume, (3), blood volume, (4), and venous return, (6). The subsequent decrease in cardiac output will act to reduce the arterial pressure.

The continuous and overriding nature of this mechanism is due to two important factors: (a) only very small changes in body fluid volume are required to produce marked changes in arterial pressure; and (b) the kidney-body fluid control system has infinite gain. The latter implies that if atherosclerosis or some other process heightened renal vascular resistance, the arterial pressure would rise to whatever degree required to generate the necessary urinary output.

In Chapter 9, evidence was presented that both short- and long-term blood flow regulation are dictated by metabolic needs of the tissue and in the case of cardiac output, of the body as a whole. Thus the heart does not control its own output but merely pumps—within its capability—whatever blood is brought to it.

Guyton's interesting concept has the further implication that cardiac output and arterial pressure are separate entities, controlled by different mechanisms and are, in a sense, independent variables. Thus, an elevated blood pressure may be initiated by the need for ample perfusion

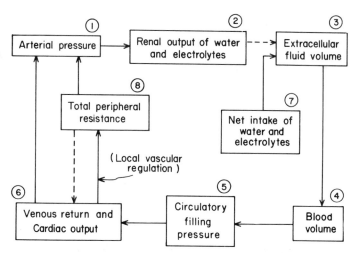

Figure 10.9. Renal-body fluid mechanism for long-term regulation of arterial blood pressure. (Reprinted with permission from A. C. Guyton, *Textbook of Medical Physiology*, 5th ed. Philadelphia: W. B. Saunders, 1976.)

through a renal bed in order to maintain urinary output; on the other hand, the hypertension may endure because of the increased peripheral resistance needed for the tissues to autoregulate their flow at an acceptably low level. Guyton's theory offers at present one of the more plausible explanations for long-term circulatory regulation of blood pressure.

References

Brown AM. Cardiac reflexes. In: *Handbook of Physiology*, Section 2: *The Cardiovascular System*, edited by RM Berne, N Sperelakis, and SR Geiger. Bethesda: American Physiological Society, 1979, Vol. I.

Cowley AW Jr, Liard JF, and Guyton AC. Role of the baroreceptor reflex in daily control of arterial blood pressure and other variables in dogs. *Circ Res* 32:564–576, 1973.

Donald DE and Shepherd JT. Autonomic regulation of the peripheral circulation. *Annu Rev Physiol* 42:429–439, 1980.

Estrin JA, Emery RW, Leonard JJ, Nicoloff DM, Swayze CR, Buckley JJ, and Fox IJ. The Bezold reflex: a special case of the left ventricular reflex. *Proc Natl Acad Sci USA* 76:4146–4150, 1979.

Fisher SJ and Malvin RL. Role of neural pathways in renin response to intravascular volume expansion. *Am J Physiol* 238:H611–617, 1980.

Fox IJ, Gerasch DA, and Leonard JJ. Left ventricular mechanoreceptors: a haemodynamic study. *J Physiol (Lond)* 273:405–425, 1977.

Guyton AC. Essential cardiovascular regulation—the control linkages between bodily needs and circulatory function. In: *Developments in Cardiovascular Medicine*, edited by CJ Dickinson and J Marks. Baltimore: University Park Press, 1978, pp. 265–302.

Hilton SM and Spyer KM. Central nervous regulation of vascular resistance. *Annu Rev Physiol* 42:399–411, 1980.

Kostreva DR, Hess GL, Zuperku EJ, Neumark J, Coon RL, and Kampine JP. Cardiac responses to stimulation of thoracic afferents in the primate and canine. *Am J Physiol* 231:1279–1284, 1976.

Randall WC. *Neural Regulation of the Heart*, New York: Oxford University Press, 1977.

Seagard JL, Pederson HJ, Kostreva DR, Van Horn DL, Cusick JF, and Kampine JP. Ultrastructural identification of afferent nerves of cardiac origin in thoracic sympathetic nerves in the dog. *Am J Anat* 153:217–232, 1979.

Shepherd JT. Reflex control of arterial blood pressure. *Cardiovasc Res* 16:357–383, 1982.

Thames MD, Miller BD, and Abboud FM. Baroreflex regulation of renal nerve activity during volume expansion. *Am J Physiol* 243:H810–814, 1982.

Uvnas B. Central cardiovascular control. In: *Handbook of Physiology*, Section 1: *Neurophysiology*, edited by J Field. Baltimore: Williams & Wilkins, 1960, Vol. II, pp. 1131–1162.

Zucker IH and Gilmore JP. Atrial receptor modulation of renal function in heart failure. In: *Disturbances in Neurogenic Control of the Circulation*, edited by FM Abboud, HA Fozzard, JP Gilmore and DJ Reis. Bethesda, Md: American Physiological Society, 1981, pp. 1–16.

chapter 11

Circulation to Special Regions

Cerebral Circulation

Anatomy

The main arteries to the cerebrum—the anterior, middle and posterior cerebral—come off the circle of Willis, which in turn is derived from the basilar and internal carotid arteries. Branches of the vertebrals and proximal basilar artery supply the cerebellum and base of the brain (Fig. 11.1).

The blood vessels traverse the subarachnoid space before penetrating

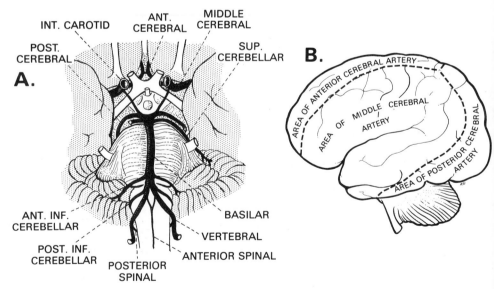

Figure 11.1.   Arterial supply to the brain. *A*, arterial circle of Willis at base of the brain is formed by the basilar and internal carotid arteries. *B*, approximate area of distribution of the three main arteries to the cerebral hemispheres. (Reprinted with permission from E. Gardner, *Fundamentals of Neurology*. Philadelphia: W.B. Saunders, 1963.)

the brain substance. Venous drainage is via the superficial venous intradural sinuses of the cranium which empty primarily into the internal jugular vein. The anatomical fixation of the dural sinuses to the skull, as well as the balance of intravenous and cerebrospinal fluid pressures (described below) prevent the collapse of the intracranial veins when subjected to negative transmural pressure upon standing.

Cerebrospinal Fluid

The cerebrospinal fluid (CSF) which in an adult has a total volume of about 100 to 160 ml, is formed in the choroid plexuses of the four ventricles at a rate of 400 to 600 ml/day; it circulates freely between the ventricles and cisterns of the brain, the subarachnoid space and the central canal of the spinal cord (Fig. 11.2). Originating as a plasma filtrate, it becomes CSF through facilitated diffusion, active transport and secretion, the last being an energy-requiring process of the choroidal epithelium (Fig. 11.2*B*); it differs from blood serum mainly in its very small protein content (20–40 mg/100 ml) compared to that of serum (5,500–8,000 mg/100 ml). Protein content of CSF is, however, diagnostically useful since it is increased in multiple sclerosis, spinal canal blockade and brain tumors.

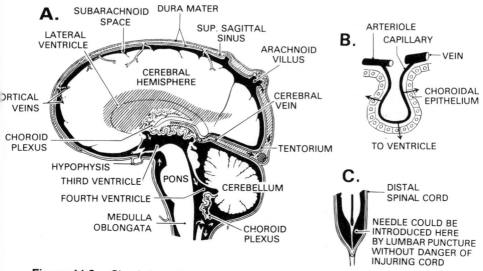

Figure 11.2. Circulation of cerebrospinal fluid (CSF). *A*, median section of the brain with projection of one lateral ventricle (*oblique lines*), the 3rd and 4th ventricles, central canal of the cord and subarachnoid space. CSF is formed from blood plasma and choroidal epithelium, *B*; passes into the ventricles and ultimately drains into the dural sinuses via the arachnoidal villi, *A*. (Reprinted with permission from E. Gardner, *Fundamentals of Neurology*. Philadelphia: W.B. Saunders, 1963.)

CSF is usually obtained via lumbar puncture (Fig. 11.2*C*). It has a normal pressure of 120 to 180 mm H_2O which represents a balance between its rate of formation and absorption back into the bloodstream. Reabsorption is mainly via arachnoidal villi which invaginate the dural sinuses (Fig. 11.2*A*). Interference with reabsorption will elevate both CSF as well as intracranial pressure (ICP) as shown, for example, by the pressure increase that occurs during lumbar puncture if both internal jugular veins are compressed. Similarly, a block of arachnoidal villi by infection, a severe head injury or a tumor may result in a progressive accumulation of CSF and an increase in ICP. ICP and CSF pressure are similar provided there is no interference with pressure transmission within the cranium and that proper corrections are made for the gravity effect (discussed later in this section).

In an infant, the cranial bones, which have unfused junctions (sutures), may be forced apart by such pressures so that the head may reach enormous size (hydrocephalus) with resultant brain compression, mental retardation and, if not arrested, death.

Acute elevation of CSF pressure will tend to reduce the cerebral blood flow; however, increased CSF pressure will activate the CNS ischemic reflex (Chapter 10) and arterial pressure will rise linearly to stay above CSF pressure (Cushing reflex). The heart rate then usually slows through baroceptor action; high pressure in the presence of bradycardia is suggestive of elevated CSF pressure. The rise in arterial pressure, along with the autoregulatory capacity of the cerebral vessels, will compensate, but only partially, for the increased resistance to flow induced by the heightened ICP. If cerebral autoregulation is maintained, ICP may reach pressures of 50 to 60 mm Hg before CBF is reduced sufficiently to produce ischemia; above this ICP level, blood flow may be drastically reduced and coma and death may follow quickly. Patients with severe head injury often have impaired autoregulation, and cerebral flow may fall to critical levels when the ICP reaches only 20 to 30 mm Hg.

Because the brain literally "floats" in CSF, its effective weight *in situ* is reduced from about 1,400 g to less than 50 g. This affords cushioning against trauma and reduces the risk of shearing or tearing of the brain tissue from its connections to extracranial tissues as they traverse the various foramina of the skull. Brain injuries may occur upon sudden rotational acceleration of the head, *e.g.*, from a blow to the side of the jaw, or severe linear acceleration which, because of brain inertia, may cause damage at the point opposite the impact (countrecoup).

Blood-Brain Barrier

The capillaries of the brain because of their selective permeability are frequently referred to as a "blood-brain barrier." Most proteins and high

molecular weight compounds, dyes, inulin, sucrose, mannitol and catecholamines pass with difficulty or not at all. However, some clinically
important precursors of neurotransmitters, *e.g.*, L-tryptophan and L-
dopa, can penetrate the blood-brain barrier and are useful in treating
neurological disorders. The relative impermeability to heavy metals and
certain antibiotics pose therapeutic problems in the treatment of brain
infections. On the other hand, anesthetics (volatile and nonvolatile),
ethanol, CO_2, O_2, urea and all lipids pass rapidly through brain capillaries. The barrier is partly morphological, *i.e.*, associated with its "tight"
endothelial junctions and basement membrane structure (Fig. 11.3).
The permeability barrier is in part also due to nonmorphological
factors, *i.e.*, different diffusion rates and transport mechanisms across
these capillaries. While the microstructure of the choroid plexus is unlike
that of the brain capillary, the former has a similar permeability barrier
so that some investigators refer to a blood-CSF barrier as well as a
blood-brain barrier; the similar composition of brain interstitial fluid
and CSF would tend to support such a concept.

The limited permeability of brain capillaries is diagnostically useful,
e.g., in "brain scans" in which a radioactive material such as technetium
(^{99}Tc) adsorbed onto a protein molecule, is injected intravenously; this
substance which would ordinarily not penetrate the brain may show up
as a darkened area on a gamma screen if the permeability mechanism
is damaged by a tumor or infarct.

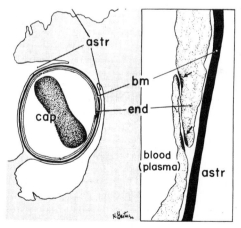

Figure 11.3. Microscopic view of a brain capillary containing an erythrocyte
and almost surrounded by the perivascular feet of an astrocyte (*astr*). The
capillary membrane consists of endothelial cells (*end*) (with a tight junction) and
a continuous basement membrane (*bm*). (Reprinted with permission from H.D.
Patton, J.W. Sundsten, W.E. Crill, and P.D. Swanson, *Introduction to Basic
Neurology*. Philadelphia: W.B. Saunders, 1976.)

Measurement of Cerebral Blood Flow

The widely used "inert gas" method involves inhalation of a subanesthetic dose of an indicator such as nitrous oxide (N_2O) with periodic measurement of arterial and venous (internal jugular) concentrations until equilibrium which is at about 10 minutes. At this point the arterial and venous N_2O concentrations are equal and that in brain tissue is about equivalent to the 10-minute venous blood sample concentration (Fig. 11.4).

Using the Fick equation (Chapter 7), the cerebral blood flow (CBF) is calculated as follows:

$$\text{CBF (ml/100 g brain tissue/min)} = \frac{100 \times N_2O \text{ uptake}}{(A\text{-}V) \; N_2O \text{ concentration}}$$

so that

$$\text{CBF (ml/100 g brain tissue/min)} = \frac{100 \times V_{10} \times S}{\int_0^{10}(A\text{-}V) \; dt}$$

in which

$$V_{10} = \text{venous } N_2O \text{ conc at 10 min}$$

and

S = partition coefficient of N_2O in blood and brain which equals one.

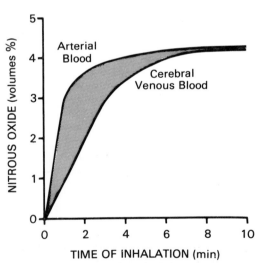

Figure 11.4.   Inert gas method for measuring cerebral blood flow (Kety-Schmidt method). N_2O concentrations in arterial and cerebral venous blood while breathing a 15% N_2O gas mixture for 10 minutes. (Reprinted with permission from S.S. Kety and C.F. Schmidt, *J Clin Invest* 27:476, 1948.)

Normal Values for CBF in Man. In the normal adult brain, which weighs 1,400 to 1,500 g, CBF is 50 to 60 ml/100 g brain tissue/min so that total brain flow is about 750 ml/min or 15% of the total cardiac output. The white matter (neuroglia) receives about one-half of the average figure but flow to the more vascular gray matter (neurons) is about two times the average.

There are a number of problems in the study of cerebral circulation. The difficulty stems from (a) the complex architecture of the brain, (b) the fact that regulatory mechanisms that govern cerebral and noncerebral tissues in the head are different and must be separated, and (c) the fact that the metabolic rate of brain tissue is heterogenous, *i.e.*, flow to gray and white matter varies widely. However, recent developments in methodology, such as the use of radionuclide-labeled microspheres, positron-emission tomography and radioautography, have greatly enhanced the study of cerebral blood flow.

Previous data have indicated that brain function, *e.g.*, mental arithmetic, produced only minimal changes in cerebral blood flow; however, newer methods such as radioautography have shown bursts of metabolic activity and flow in very small, localized brain areas coincident with brain activity. For example, simple voluntary contraction of hand muscle is accompanied by a sizable increase in CBF in the localized contralateral hand area of the motor cortex; a light stimulus to the retina will increase blood flow to the superior colliculus and occipital cortex, and during speech, local metabolic activation of the motor speech area of the cortex has been observed. Thus "function mapping" of the brain, using local flow and metabolism as indicators, has now become possible in animals and man and promises to add considerably to our understanding of neural function.

Characteristics and Control of Cerebral Circulation

Brain is the most vulnerable tissue of the body to ischemia; oxygen deprivation of only seconds may produce unconsciousness and in a few minutes irreversible damage. Fortunately, as many studies have shown, cerebral blood flow tends to remain remarkably constant under most physiological situations. This is due to a number of favorable factors that are protective of cerebral circulation.

Hydrostatic Factors and CBF

The CNS vascular bed is, *e.g.*, better protected against changes in hydrostatic pressure than any other in the body. Enclosed within the rigid confines of the skull and spinal canal, CSF is in a continuous fluid-filled chamber whose hydrostatic pressure at any point will, in a manner similar to that of blood vessels, vary directly with body position, *i.e.*, with the height of the vertical fluid column. Thus the intravenous and extravascular (essentially CSF) pressures are balanced at all points in the spine and cranium. In the upright position the CSF and venous pressures in the skull are both negative and in the lower spine are both positive. Thus venous collapse is prevented in the skull and venous distension in the lower spine, so the energy gradient is maintained across the CNS vascular bed regardless of position. This prevents the decrease in energy gradient that occurs, *e.g.*, in a hand lifted high over the head. In the latter situation there will be a hydrostatic fall in both arterial and venous pressures of 20 to 30 mm Hg, which in the veins will produce a negative pressure and collapse the walls, thereby effectively stopping blood flow. In spite of this protective feature, there is about a 20% reduction in CBF in the upright position.

Reflex Factors and Autoregulation

In addition, the cerebral circulation has other safeguards. These include autoregulation, the baroreflexes, the CNS ischemic reflex and specialized flow responses to P_{O_2} and P_{CO_2}. Autoregulation, an important protective mechanism (Chapter 9), is also effective in hypertensive patients (Fig. 11.5). Because of its heavy dependence on aerobic metabolism, there is a tight coupling between metabolism and blood flow, but the metabolite responsible for this coupling is unknown.

While older studies reported the presence of autonomic fibers in the walls of cerebral vessels, it has been the consensus that they play only a

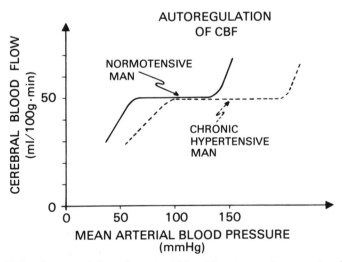

Figure 11.5. Autoregulation of cerebral blood flow in man in normotension and chronic hypertension. In hypertension the autoregulation persists but the curve is shifted to the right. In this study, intracranial pressure, P_{CO_2} and P_{O_2} were maintained constant. (Reprinted with permission from N.A. Lassen, *Peripheral Circulation*, edited by P.C. Johnson. New York: John Wiley & Sons, 1978.)

minor role in normal cerebrovascular control. However, more recent studies have indicated wide species differences in this regard as well as the complicating effects of anesthesia. In monkeys and rabbits, *e.g.*, constrictor responses to nerve stimulation have been reported. There currently remains, therefore, a serious difference of opinion regarding the neural control of cerebral circulation in normal subjects. Recent reports have indicated that in hypertension, vasoconstriction does occur and that it may play a role in attenuating the passive increase in CBF which would otherwise occur. Thus, it apparently acts to minimize the disruption of the blood-brain barrier and thereby may exert a protective effect in hypertension.

P_{O_2}, P_{CO_2} and Cerebral Blood Flow

The cerebral circulatory response to hypoxia is different than that of other beds. Resistance vessels in kidney and skeletal muscle, *e.g.*, reflexly constrict during systemic hypoxia, a sympathetic reflex response induced by activation of the arterial chemoreceptors. In contrast, the cerebral and coronary circulations dilate in response to hypoxia, a direct local tissue response due to dilation of distal intraparenchymal vessels. This protects the brain and myocardium, the tissues most dependent on aerobic metabolism. The CBF responds, however, only to rather severe hypoxia, *i.e.*, to P_{O_2} levels below 50 mm Hg.

Arterial P_{CO_2} is an important regulator of cerebral flow and P_{CO_2} alterations exert a profound influence on CBF; hypercapnia causes intense cerebral vasodilation, and hypocapnea is the cause of a marked vasoconstriction (Fig. 11.6*A*). The CO_2 effect is probably mediated by

Figure 11.6.   Effect of P_{CO_2} (*left*) and P_{O_2} (*right*) on cerebral blood flow. *Left*, note that the steepest part of the P_{CO_2} curve is near 40 mm Hg indicating high sensitivity of CBF to P_{CO_2} at physiological levels. *Right*, at the normal P_{O_2} levels of 80 to 120 mm Hg, the effect on CBF is practically nil. (Reprinted with permission from N.A. Lassen, *Peripheral Circulation*, edited by P.C. Johnson. New York: John Wiley & Sons, 1978.)

pH variations in cerebrospinal fluid and apparently serves primarily to maintain the pH of brain tissue; this objective is, in turn, probably associated with the fact that a decreased pH profoundly depresses neuronal activity. Arterial Po_2 changes within the physiological ranges have relatively little effect on CBF (Fig. 11.6B).

Pathophysiology of Cerebral Blood Flow

CBF is decreased in sleep, surgical anesthesia (as much as 50%) and in cerebral arteriosclerosis. The prevalence of the latter has important clinical implications since cerebral vascular disease is first in frequency among all neurological diseases and furthermore comprises 50% of all neurological hospital admissions to adult wards; the most serious consequence of cerebral arteriosclerosis is "cerebral vascular accident" (CVA or stroke). Whether the decrease in CBF is involved in the etiology of dementia or simply results from the decreased metabolic demand is debatable. Vascular stroke is the most common and devastating disease affecting the CNS and in developing countries is the third leading cause of death, ranking behind heart disease and cancer.

Vascular stroke may be due to a thrombus, embolus or rupture of a cerebral artery, which can result in infarction of brain tissue or to a mass effect from a hematoma (tissue hemorrhage). The most common vascular distribution affected is that of the middle cerebral artery; the clinical results, depending on the branch affected and extent of the infarction, are varying degrees of paralysis and fine sensory loss over the contralateral half of the body (hemiplegia and hemianesthesia) as well as speech (if the dominant hemisphere is involved) and visual problems. While flow to the infarcted area is diminished, that adjacent to the infarction may have increased flow, presumably due to the accumulation of metabolites at the periphery of the lesion.

In a recent investigation, Doppler ultrasound flowmeters were used to study cardiac output (CO) and common carotid blood flow in normal adults and cerebrovascular disease patients with more than a 50% reduction in diameter of their internal carotid arteries. In this study, the patients showed a 15% *increase* in common carotid flow (CCF) in the upright position and increases in their common carotid flow/cardiac output (CCF/CO) ratios in the upright position and in upright exercise. This was in contrast to normal adults who showed the expected 20% decrease in CCF in the upright position and during upright exercise. It was concluded that patients with cerebrovascular disease have a diminished autoregulatory capacity resulting in abnormal augmentation of cerebral blood flow with increases in CO. While the clinical significance of this flow aberration is not yet clear, it is anticipated that such studies will lead to a better understanding of the dynamics of CBF in stroke patients.

Coronary Circulation

Coronary circulation is critical not only because of the obvious central role of the heart but also because coronary artery disease (*i.e.*, ischemic heart disease) is the leading single cause of death in most of the "developed" countries of the world. There are special difficulties in the study of coronary circulation, *e.g.*, the marked anatomical vagaries of coronary arterial and venous vessels, the problem of high-fidelity recording on a constantly moving organ, and the significant species differences in the response of this bed. Moreover, the study of responses, *e.g.*, to a drug on the coronary circulation, is complicated by the indirect effect of the drug on the heart itself, whose altered activity will strongly affect the coronary circulation. In this chapter, the anatomy, characteristics and control of the normal coronary circulation will be considered. Two of the most important manifestations of coronary pathophysiology, *i.e.*, ischemic heart disease and congestive heart failure, are discussed in Chapter 14.

Anatomy

The adult human heart, which has a mass of 250 to 300 g, has three main arteries, the right coronary, supplying the right ventricle and a portion of the posterior left ventricle, and the left anterior descending and circumflex which are the terminal branches of the left coronary and supply primarily the left ventricle (Fig. 11.7). A limited number of small arteries (arterioluminal) run from the main coronary arteries into the ventricles.

The "dominant" supply to the heart is usually determined by that artery which forms the posterior descending; the latter derives from the left circumflex in 85% of the cases in the dog (left dominance) but in man it is a continuance of the right coronary in about 90% of cases (right dominance). The conventional term "dominant" refers to the vessel which furnishes the major arterial supply to the inferior wall of the left ventricle and to the AV node; thus the term does not relate to the proportional mass of total myocardium supplied. From a functional standpoint, the anterior descending branch of the left coronary supplies the largest portion of the most important ventricle, *viz.*, the left, and in this sense is the predominant vessel.

The anterior cardiac vein from the right ventricle carries about 15 to 20% of the venous blood and drains into the right atrium. Most of the blood from the left ventricle empties into the great cardiac and other veins and finally into an expanded venous chamber, the coronary sinus; the coronary sinus, which carries 65 to 75% of coronary venous blood, drains into the right atrium. A few small Thebesian veins, carrying about 3 to 5% of the total venous blood, drain directly into the cardiac chambers, mainly the right ventricle (Fig. 11.8).

Figure 11.7.   Coronary vessels of the human heart. Anterior view (*left*) shows the right coronary artery and anterior descending artery; posterior view (*right*) shows the left circumflex artery and the posterior descending artery. The latter may be formed by the right coronary or left circumflex artery. The anterior cardiac veins from the right ventricle and the coronary sinus, draining primarily the left ventricle, empty into the right atrium.

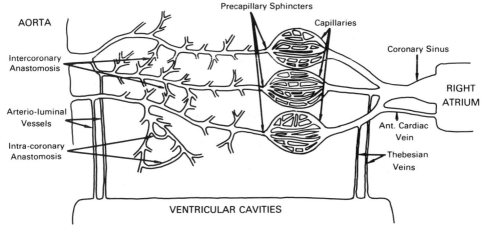

Figure 11.8. Diagrammatic sketch of the coronary vasculature showing arterioluminal vessels, thebesian veins, collateral arteries and precapillary sphincters.

Capillary and Collateral Circulation

As arteries pass across the surface of the heart, small branches come off at right angles to penetrate the myocardium and end in a rich network of arteries and capillaries. There are precapillary sphincters which play an important role in opening up additional exchange beds during exercise (Fig. 11.8).

Since regional blood flow is highly important in the study of coronary disease, the development and validation of accurate methods assumes special significance. Recent studies have shown good agreement between the tritiated water and microsphere techniques, two of the most reliable of the regional flow methods.

Because coronary occlusion is a common clinical entity, the potential for development of collateral vessels becomes very important. Collaterals are anastomotic channels, usually small, preexisting arterial connections without intervening capillaries. These connections may be between main coronary arteries (intercoronary) or between branches of the same coronary artery (intracoronary) (Fig. 11.8).

The ability to develop collateral vessels varies with different species. In the dog, collateral vessels are located mainly near the epicardium and are relatively plentiful. In man, they are mainly subendocardial and less well developed; in man and in some animal species such as the pig (which has few collaterals), sudden occlusion of a large vessel usually results in a significant infarction (necrosis) with possible cardiac arrest and death. However, with gradual occlusion of even 90% of the lumen of a large vessel (*e.g.*, in the dog), the collaterals open, there is proliferation of the vascular endothelium and smooth muscle cells and within 4 to 8 weeks coronary flow may return almost to the preocclusion level.

A number of studies have suggested that after partial coronary artery occlusion, collateral vessels and myocardial capillary density will increase more rapidly in chronically exercised animals than in nonexercised animals. It is interesting that this enhanced capillarization seems to be related to the bradycardia of exercise since it will apparently occur also in nonexercised animals subjected to chronic bradycardic pacing. Whether this response is likely to occur in human coronary patients (many of whom are elderly) is not known. Collateral vessels apparently develop either because of (a) increased physical stress on the wall of the blood vessels due to heightened pressure gradients, or (b) the stimulating effect of hypoxia or other metabolites resulting from the ischemia.

Normal Values and General Characteristics

In man, coronary flow is usually measured either by the inert gas method (previously described) involving catheterization of the coronary sinus, or by a "washout" technique following injection of a radioactive agent such as ^{133}Xe or ^{85}Kr into the catheterized coronary artery. Direct measurement with an electromagnetic or ultrasonic flowmeter in an experimental animal permits the recording of phasic flow as shown in Figure 11.9.

The smaller flow in the left coronary during systole (one-fifth of the total) is due to the external compression of the artery; the lesser pressures of the right ventricle produce less throttling and permit a proportionately

Figure 11.9. Right and left coronary arterial flow during systole and diastole. Note the greater effect of external compression on systolic flow to the left coronary as compared to the right. (Reprinted with permission from B. Folkow and E. Neil, *Circulation*. London: Oxford University Press, 1971.)

greater systolic flow into the right coronary artery. The normal adult heart has a coronary blood flow of 70 to 80 ml/100 g/min and a total flow of about 250 ml/min, *i.e.*, 4 to 5% of the cardiac output.

How much reduction in coronary flow is required to impair myocardial contraction? While a full answer to this key question is not available, a recent study of experimental coronary stenosis in conscious dogs indicated that a 10 to 20% reduction in myocardial blood flow will cause significant impairment of regional myocardial contractility. Larger reductions in flow induce progressively greater decrements, but a 95% flow reduction was required to stop contractility entirely in the affected region. The investigators reported that this regional ischemia did not significantly affect general ventricular performance.

During these procedures, arterial blood pressure, heart rate and LV systolic pressure were maintained, thus indicating that the nonischemic portions of the myocardium were able to compensate for the loss of regional contractility. In human patients, the clinical result of a coronary occlusion will depend on several factors including the rapidity of the occlusion, the area of the myocardium involved, the age and physical condition of the patient, etc. The pathophysiological effects of human coronary occlusion are further discussed in Chapter 14 (Ischemic Heart Disease).

Control of Coronary Circulation

The three main factors influencing flow are (a) *mechanical,* mainly external compression and perfusion pressure, (b) *metabolic* and (c) *neural.*

Mechanical Factors and Coronary Flow

The compression effect is responsible for 25% of coronary flow resistance in the left ventricle at normal heart rates. For reasons which are not understood, resistance is significantly higher in the right ventricle. During tachycardia, when systole occupies an increasing percentage of the cycle, it can account for as much as 55% of vascular resistance. But external compression also affects intramyocardial flow distribution; as the left ventricle contracts, the pressure inside the muscle increases to a level comparable and even higher than the intraventricular pressure (Fig. 11.10). Furthermore, the myocardial pressure is graded, being very low on the epicardial side and at its peak near the endocardium so that subendocardial vessels are compressed the most. As a result, subendocardial flow is primarily diastolic. In spite of this, injection of microspheres and other studies indicate that in the normal myocardium, subendocardial and subepicardial flow are about equal. However, when diastolic pressure is low such as in shock, aortic stenosis or coronary occlusion, subendocardial flow decreases disproportionately so that this

Figure 11.10. Simultaneous intraventricular and intramyocardial pressures from left ventricle of the dog. (Reprinted with permission from H. Kreuzer and W. Schoeppe, *Pfluegers Arch* 278:181, 1963.)

area is more vulnerable to ischemia. This seems to be borne out by the fact that after coronary occlusion, infarcts are more common in the subendocardial area.

Since at normal rates, about 80% of coronary flow occurs in diastole, it follows that aortic diastolic pressure becomes the primary determinant of coronary perfusion pressure. Theoretically, coronary flow would, therefore, fluctuate with the diastolic pressure; however, as discussed in Chapter 9, the coronary vessels show a high degree of "autoregulation," *i.e.*, between perfusion pressures of 60 to 180 mm Hg, flow remains relatively constant. Thus the increase in coronary flow which occurs in conditions in which diastolic pressure is elevated is due mainly to the increase in flow accompanying the increased afterload work and increased cardiac metabolism (as described below) rather than from the elevated perfusion pressure.

Cardiac Metabolism and Coronary Flow

One of the most striking features of myocardial physiology is the close parallelism between metabolic rate and coronary flow; as previously discussed (Chapter 9) a general correlation exists in all tissues. Because of this close coupling, any increase of cardiac work as a result of exercise (Fig. 11.11), excitement or administration of inotropic agents will induce a corresponding increase in coronary flow. The precise mechanism of this metabolic rate-blood flow coupling is not certain. Both increased

Figure 11.11. Effect of treadmill exercise on coronary flow in the dog. There is a large increase in coronary flow associated with the increased heart rate, blood pressure and cardiac output. (Reprinted with permission from E.M. Khouri, D.E. Gregg, and C.R. Rayford, *Circ Res* 17:427, 1965.)

P_{CO_2} and reduced pH will increase local flow but unquestionably, hypoxia, *i.e.*, decreased P_{O_2}, is the most potent stimulus of all to coronary flow. The available evidence suggests that the chief metabolic mediator of the hypoxic vasodilation in the coronary bed is adenosine. Other factors, such as K^+, CO_2, pH and prostaglandins, contribute to an unknown degree.

Neural Control of Coronary Flow

In order to study neural effects on myocardial blood flow, it is necessary to differentiate the direct effect on coronary vessels from an indirect effect that is secondary to stimulation of the myocardium. This is particularly important in the study of agents to counteract coronary vasospasm. Certain drugs as well as sympathetic stimulation, will, *e.g.*, increase the myocardial work and with it increase local accumulation of metabolites, which will in turn produce a secondary vasodilation of the coronary vascular bed. This will complicate any direct action the drug or neural stimulation may have on the coronary vessels themselves. This problem is usually circumvented by studying blood flow in the K^+ arrested, fibrillating heart or by using selective sympathetic and parasympathetic blocking agents (Chapter 9).

Studies using such procedures indicate that the main neural effects on coronary circulation are sympathetic. In the dog, cardiac sympathetic (stellate) stimulation usually results in increased myocardial blood flow. However, if the inotropic and chronotropic effects are blunted by β-blockade, a widespread adrenergic vasoconstriction, particularly to left stellate stimulations, is unmasked. It appears, therefore, that while the metabolic vasodilator effect is a dominant influence in controlling coronary flow, it is modulated by the α-adrenergic vasoconstrictors. β_2- and cholinergic receptors probably have only a secondary role in the normal regulation of coronary flow in the intact organism.

Renal Circulation

The kidneys have two major functions: (a) they excrete the primary end-products of bodily metabolism; and (b) they control the concentrations of most constituents of body fluids. Through these activities, they play a vital role in regulating the salt and water balance of the body. This section on renal circulation is mainly concerned with (a) the renal circulatory architecture and how it is adapted to kidney function, (b) some general characteristics of renal blood flow, and (c) the mechanisms affecting neurohormonal control of the kidney. The relationship of circulatory control mechanisms to plasma volume and to the genesis of hypertension are discussed in Chapters 10 and 15, respectively.

Functional Anatomy

The basic functional unit of the kidney, the nephron, is composed of (a) the glomerulus, which consists of a tuft of capillaries through which the plasma is filtered, and (b) long tubules adapted for reabsorption in which the filtered plasma is converted to urine. In man, about 85% of the nephrons are in the outer part, or cortex, of the kidney (cortical nephrons); some of these, *i.e.*, juxtamedullary nephrons, lie close to the inner portion, or medulla, of the kidney (Fig. 11.12). Huge quantities of plasma, about 180 L/day, are filtered through the porous walls of the glomerular capillaries; the main elements retained are the plasma proteins. In all, 98% to 99% of this plasma fluid is reabsorbed back into the blood through the renal tubules; the remaining 1.5 to 2.0 L/day passes through as urine.

From the renal artery, interlobar arteries ascend between the pyramids and divide into arcuate arteries that, in turn, subdivide into interlobular vessels and thence into thick-walled afferent arterioles. The latter supply the glomerular capillaries (Fig. 11.12, *left*). The shorter, thin-walled, efferent arterioles subdivide to form the peritubular capillary plexuses that surround the cortical convoluted tubules. The efferent arterioles from the juxtamedullary nephrons drain downward into vasa recta in

Figure 11.12. Renal circulation. *Left*, blood supply to cortical and juxtamedullary nephrons. *Right*, juxtaglomerular complex including JG cells and macula densa. (Reprinted with permission from R.F. Pitts, *Physiology of Kidney and Body Fluids*, 3rd ed. Chicago: Year Book Medical Publishers, 1974; A.M. Ham and T. Leeson, *Histology*, 4th ed. Philadelphia: J.B. Lippincott, 1961.)

the proximity of the loops of Henle before turning back upward to empty into the cortical veins.

Near the glomerulus, the afferent arteriolar wall is thickened asymmetrically and contains small specialized juxtaglomerular (JG) cells that are the site of renin formation; the portion of the distal tubule lying adjacent to the JG cells forms a small cellular plaque called the macula densa, which together with the JG cells is termed the juxtaglomerular apparatus, or JGA (Fig. 11.12, *right*), which constitutes an important regulatory system.

Characteristics and Control of Renal Circulation

As described in Chapter 9, the kidneys are highly vascular organs. Although weighing only 300 g, they receive a blood flow of 1,000 to 1,200 ml/min, about 20% of the total cardiac output. Of this very large flow, only a modest portion is for metabolic needs, so the renal $(A-V)o_2$ difference is relatively small. The great part of the flow becomes glomerular filtrate and serves as the main regulator of the body's water and electrolyte balance. The renal circulation consists of two capillary beds arranged in series, the glomerular and the peritubular beds.

In passing through the afferent arterioles, the mean arterial pressure falls from 100 mm Hg to about 60 mm Hg in the glomerular capillaries. Passage through the efferent arterioles results in a further decrease of pressure to about 15 mm Hg in the peritubular capillaries. This pressure then further declines to about 8 mm Hg in the renal venules. The high pressure glomerular bed is adapted for filtration; the peritubular bed, with a relatively low hydrostatic pressure and high osmotic pressure, is well adapted for reabsorption.

Intrinsic (Local) Control of Renal Circulation

The glomerular filtration rate (GFR) of the kidney remains very constant. This ability to maintain a relatively constant GFR protects the body from large fluctuations in water and solute excretion that would otherwise occur with the fluctuations in arterial pressure. The evidence indicates that this GFR control takes place mainly in the efferent arterioles.

The mechanism responsible for this close relation between renal circulation and renal excretory function is not known. One of the proposed theories is tubuloglomerular feedback, which suggests that increased volume delivery to the distal tubule causes a direct decrease in GFR and a restoration of normal filtration. It has also been proposed that when arterial pressure, GFR, and distal delivery of electrolytes are reduced, activation of the renin-angiotensin system causes constriction of efferent arterioles restoring glomerular perfusion pressure and GFR.

Renal blood flow shows a high degree of autoregulation, and changes in arterial pressure over a range of 80 to 200 mm Hg cause remarkably little change in renal blood flow. The mechanism responsible for the autoregulation is not certain. The two most likely explanations appear to be a myogenic mechanism (Chapter 9) or the participation of the JGA, *i.e.*, a mechanism similar to the regulation of GFR as described above.

Extrinsic Control of Renal Circulation

While the intrinsic control mechanisms provide considerable stability to the renal circulation, they do not prevent large variations in renal blood flow and GFR from occurring during activation of the sympathetic nervous system. Strong renal arterial vasoconstriction can result from emotional stress, the defense reaction (Chapter 10), exercise (Chapter 12), or as reflex responses to decreased central blood volume, hypotension (Chapter 10), hemorrhage (Chapter 13) or shock (Chapter 15). The renal vasoconstriction lowers glomerular capillary hydrostatic pressure and filtration rate and thus tends to retain water and increase plasma volume. The renal vasoconstriction affects primarily the outer cortex, where most of the glomeruli are located. Vasodilators, *e.g.*, histamine, dopamine, and prostglandins of the A and E series generally induce greater fractional flow to the inner cortex and medulla. It is thought that PGE_2, a particularly potent renal vasodilator which is synthesized in the renal medulla, protects the renal parenchyma against the excessive salt and water-conserving action of the renin-angiotensin system. It has been suggested that PGE_2 deficiency may play a role in the genesis of essential hypertension, but the evidence thus far is only fragmentary.

Neurohormonal Control of Plasma Volume

There are two neurohormonal mechanisms that can significantly influence renal blood flow and plasma volume: (a) the renin-angiotensin-aldosterone (RAA) system concerned with the renal control of Na^+; and (b) the antidiuretic hormone or ADH (vasopressin) system concerned with the renal control of free water.

In this section, these neurohormonal mechanisms are briefly described from the standpoint of the involvement of the circulatory system. Other important factors in fluid-volume control, such as thirst, other diuretic and saluretic hormonal mechanisms and the interactions between the ADH and renin-aldosterone systems, have been omitted.

Renin-Angiotensin-Aldosterone System

The enzyme renin, produced by the modified smooth muscle cells, *i.e.*, the JGA cells, acts on the circulating α_2-globulin (renin substrate) and splits off a decapeptide, angiotensin I. Additional amino acids are subsequently split off (mainly in the lung) by converting enzyme to yield the octapeptide angiotensin II. Although angiotensin II is a potent vasoconstrictor, its most important action is to stimulate aldosterone production and secretion by the cells of the zona glomerulosa of the adrenal cortex. An increased renin release by the kidney will therefore lead to greater release of aldosterone and to an increased reabsorption of Na^+ into the renal collecting tubule (and greater excretion of K^+). The reabsorbed Na^+ will carry water with it and thus increase plasma

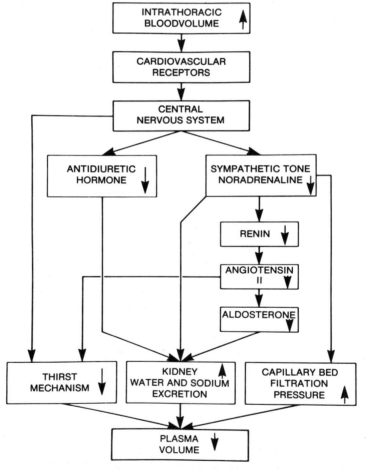

Figure 11.13. Major pathways for the reflex control of plasma volume following expansion of intrathoracic blood volume. (Reprinted with permission from O.H. Gauer and J.P. Henry, Neurohormonal Control of Plasma Volume. In: *Cardiovascular Physiology II, International Review of Physiology*. Baltimore: University Park Press, 1976, Vol. 9, p. 165.)

volume (Fig. 11.13). As with other self-correcting systems, when the volume deficit has been corrected, the RAA system is shut off.

The primary stimuli for renin secretion appear to be (a) increased sympathetic nerve activity, which may be produced reflexly by decreased central blood volume or arterial pressure or by other causes as described above, (b) decreased plasma Na^+ (probably sensed by the macula densa), or (c) decreased distension of renal arterioles. It should be noted that aldosterone is stimulated not only by angiotensin II but also by ACTH as well as other factors.

In the early hypovolemic stage of congestive heart failure, there is a suppression of the RAA mechanism, probably due to the continued elevation of central blood volume. However, in the later stages there appears to be an adaptation of the vagal endings with the resultant increase in the neurohormonal drive usually seen in chronic heart failure. This question is discussed further in Chapter 14 (Congestive Heart Failure).

ADH (Vasopressin) Mechanism

Antidiuretic hormone, or ADH (also called vasopressin), is an octapeptide synthesized in the hypothalamus and transported to and released from the posterior pituitary gland. As a messenger between the CNS and kidney, it plays a key role in maintaining the volume and osmolality of body fluids.

ADH is released from the posterior pituitary gland in response to a number of stimuli including: (a) activation of the sympathetic nervous system by emotion or decreased plasma volume as sensed by cardiopulmonary receptors, particularly of the left atrium; (b) increased osmolality of interstitial fluid of brain (as sensed by osmoreceptors); and (c) increased plasma concentrations of angiotensin II. ADH acts on the collecting tubules of the kidney to increase reabsorption of free water, inhibit diuresis and increase plasma volume (Fig. 11.13). As described in Chapter 10, increased distension of CP receptors will inhibit the secretion of ADH, and decreased distension will increase it. Diabetes insipidus, a rare disorder characterized by polyuria (excessive diuresis) and polydipsia (excessive thirst), is an ADH deficiency disease but usually has no primary blood pressure abnormality.

In its second role, in which it is more commonly known as vasopressin, this hormone acts as an arterial vasoconstrictor, and its importance in circulatory physiology is becoming increasingly recognized. It is released in increasing quantities by the posterior pituitary gland during hemorrhage in which its constrictor action exerts a pressor effect adjunctive to that resulting from the arterial and cardiopulmonary baroceptor reflexes. It is now available as a highly purified synthetic arginine vasopressin (AVP) standard. A normal concentration in human plasma is about 4 to 6 picograms (pg) per ml of plasma. Its arteriolar vasocon-strictor action, which is significant at low concentrations, is increased 50- to 100-fold after baroceptor denervation and 2,000- to 8,000-fold after ablation of the CNS. Cowley and his colleagues have presented increasing evidence that AVP may be importantly concerned with long-range regulation of arterial pressure.

Splanchnic Circulation

Functional Anatomy

Splanchnic circulation is actually a collection of several grossly differ-ent circulations serving organs with very dissimilar functions. In the human adult, the total splanchnic blood flow (SBF) is about 1,500 ml/min, *i.e.*, approximately 25% of the cardiac output. The splanchnic vasculature has some unique characteristics, *e.g.*, the portal circulation is coupled with that of the gastrointestinal tract in series and with the hepatic artery in parallel. The arteries to the various splanchnic organs have many interconnecting branches. About 70% of the liver blood flow is from the portal vein and about 30% travels via the hepatic artery. All SBF ultimately drains via the hepatic veins. Thus, in spite of providing blood flow to a great diversity of organs, the splanchnic circulation has an anatomical commonality of final flow and, in this sense, can be considered as a single hypothetical flow tract (Fig. 11.14).

Characteristics and Control

Most arterial beds in the splanchnic circulation have approximately normal arteriovenous pressure relations. The portal bed, however, is a low-pressure, low-resistance system with a portal pressure of about 8 to 10 mm Hg and a hepatic venous pressure of about 0 to 2 mm Hg. Pressure flow studies of the portal circuit indicate that it is a relatively "passive" bed, *i.e.*, it generally imposes little active resistance to flow. There is a partial reciprocity between hepatic artery and portal vein that tends to maintain a constant total liver blood flow. The hepatic sinuses are lined with a very porous, "discontinuous" type of endothelium that offers little resistance to either proteins or fluid. As a consequence, the volume flow of hepatic lymph is great, and its protein content is almost as high as that of plasma. The normal O_2 extraction of splanchnic blood is low, *i.e.*, only about 15 to 20%, so there is a considerable oxygen reserve available in low flow states.

All splanchnic organs are richly innervated with sympathetic α-receptors which receive innervation primarily from the splanchnic nerves. Sympathetic stimulation, either as a response to exercise, in-creased temperature or through baroceptor stimulation (as a result of

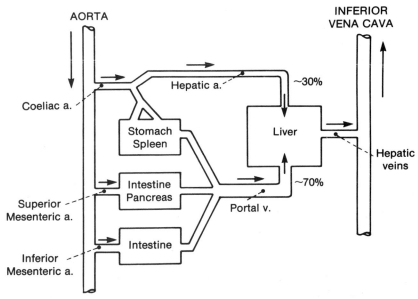

AORTA

INFERIOR
VENA CAVA

Hepatic a.

~30%

Coeliac a.

Stomach
Spleen

Liver

Hepatic
veins

Intestine
Pancreas

~70%

Superior
Mesenteric a.

Portal v.

Intestine

Inferior
Mesenteric a.

Figure 11.14. Simplified schema of splanchnic vascular bed showing the parallel arrangement of the circulation of the various gastrointestinal organs and their series arrangement with the portal circulation to the liver. Also the dual blood supply to the liver and the common venous drainage of all these organs. (Reprinted with permission from L.B. Rowell, The splanchnic circulation. In: *The Peripheral Circulations*, edited by R. Zelis. New York: Grune & Stratton, 1975.)

hemorrhage, upright posture or lower body negative pressure), will invoke strong splanchnic vasoconstriction. This serves to redistribute the splanchnic flow and is a key factor in maintaining arterial pressure during low cardiac output states. Splanchnic venous constriction in response to sympathetic stimulation is also a very effective aid in hypotensive states since about 20 to 25% of the total blood volume is contained in the splanchnic region.

There is no evidence of neural vasodilators in the splanchnic bed and very little indication of autoregulation in the intact, innervated organism. During gastric and intestinal digestion, there is hyperemia, which indicates a close coupling of blood flow and functional state. The mechanism of this effect is not known but has been ascribed to neural influences, to the action of gastrointestinal hormones such as secretin or gastrin, or to other agents such as serotonin or bradykinin.

Pathophysiology

During *hemorrhage*, the splanchnic circulation plays an important role. A strong splanchnic vasoconstriction is initiated by the low-pressure cardiopulmonary baroceptors and, as arterial pressure falls, is strengthened by the arterial baroceptors. In severe shock this response is further reinforced by the reflex effect of the chemoreceptors. Venous constriction is an important part of this response, and it has been estimated that as much as 50% of additional blood volume mobilized from "blood reservoirs" in shock may come from the splanchnic region. Some venoconstriction is "active," but a significant portion is "passive," *i.e.*, it is due to the recoil of veins onto the smaller venous volume, which is, in turn, a result of constriction of the precapillary resistance vessels. Vasoconstriction can persist unabated for prolonged periods.

In *physical exercise* there is a constriction of both arteries and veins in the splanchnic area. The venous constriction is primarily responsible for the 35% decrease in splanchnic blood volume that occurs during mild supine exercise. SBF decreases in proportion to the intensity of the exercise. Rowell has made the interesting observation that in normal subjects, trained athletes and mitral stenosis patients the rate of decrease of SBF with increasing intensity of exercise ($\dot{V}_{O_2}/\dot{V}_{O_2}$max) was similar, *i.e.*, had the same slope and similar intercepts. Although the patients, normal subjects and athletes had, in that order, progressively larger $\dot{V}_{O_2}$max values, they all reduced their SBF by about 80% at their $\dot{V}_{O_2}$max. The $\dot{V}_{O_2}$max, in effect, diverts this flow, *i.e.*, about 250 to 300 ml O_2/min, into the general circulation. However, this O_2 transport capacity represents a much higher fraction of $\dot{V}_{O_2}$max in the patients with a limited cardiac output than in normal subjects or athletes. As a consequence, this capacity provides to these patients a substantial boost to their O_2 transport.

The importance of the sympathetic vasoconstrictor mechanism, particularly in cardiac patients, is demonstrated by Rowell's estimate that constriction of the combined splanchnic, renal, cutaneous and non-working muscle bed provides 42% of the total capacity for O_2 delivery in mitral stenosis patients at their $\dot{V}_{O_2}$max. The vasoconstrictor response obviously has its greatest significance in patients with low cardiac output.

Heat stress with increase in body temperature also causes a splanchnic vasoconstriction and diminished SBF. With combined heat and exercise stress the tendency toward splanchnic vasoconstriction in the two stresses is additive so that there is a tendency toward an even greater shunting of splanchnic blood into the general circulation. However, additional skin blood flow is now needed to dissipate the added heat. Cardiac patients with a limited myocardial reserve are often unable to increase cardiac output to supply this additional need and so must try to divert flow from other sources. When they become unable to do this they reach the point of decompensation.

This vasoconstrictor capacity of the splanchnic, renal and nonworking muscle bed provides a most important reserve. However, additive stresses, *e.g.*, exercise and heat, may rapidly deplete these reserves in patients whose cardiac output is compromised.

One of the most serious of liver diseases is cirrhosis, an irreversible alteration of liver architecture consisting of diffuse fibrosis with widespread necrosis of liver parenchyma and areas of nodular regeneration. It is usually the aftermath of chronic chemical (usually alcoholic), bacterial or other toxic damage to the liver. Portal venous hypertension (up to 20 or 25 mm Hg) may occur with ascites (accumulation of intraperitoneal fluid). In an effort to bypass the hepatic circulatory obstruction, many portal-systemic collaterals develop, among them, large vessels in the esophageal mucosa called esophageal varices. Hemorrhage from an esophageal varix with hemoptysis (spitting up of blood) and massive bleeding into the stomach is a major complication of portal hypertension, with a mortality rate as high as 50 to 60% for each bleeding episode.

Cutaneous Circulation

The main function of skin circulation is to maintain temperature balance by providing (a) insulation against cold and (b) efficient heat transfer between the body core and the periphery. This heat-regulating mechanism, aided by sweat production and evaporative cooling, is much better adapted to protect against overheating than against excessive cold.

Anatomy of Skin Vasculature

Skin has a variable thickness, generally 1 to 3 mm, a surface area in the 70-kg adult of 1.7 to 1.8 m^2 and an aggregate mass of 2 to 2.5 kg, about 4% of the total body weight. From a functional standpoint, the vasculature is of two general types. The first is an extensive, superficial arteriolar-capillary-venular network of the usual architecture with an extensive, slow-flowing subcutaneous venous plexus; this general structure prevails over most of the body with particularly rich networks in the forearm, legs and thighs. The second vascular arrangement, which is found in palms of the hands, soles of the feet and in the face (especially the ears, nose and lips), is similar to the above but has, in addition a large number of unique arteriovenous anastomoses (AVAs); skin in these areas is studded with numerous such capillary bypasses which consist of coiled arterial vessels about 50 μm in diameter with thick muscular walls, well supplied with sympathetic nerve fibers. These vessels do not have capillary exchange surfaces and by virtue of their unusual vascularity are capable of large heat exchanges (Fig. 11.15).

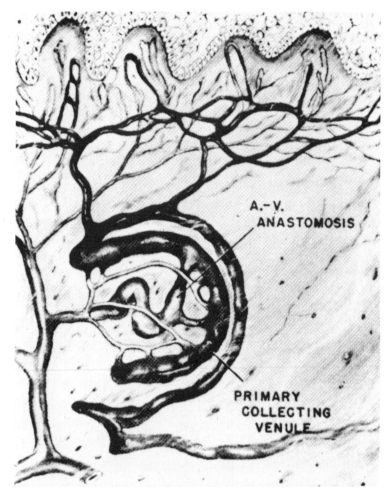

Figure 11.15. Schematic drawing of blood vessels of the finger showing superficial plexus and an AV anastomosis which connects directly to a venule of the subcutaneous plexus. When dilated, the AVAs are capable of huge increases in flow. (Reprinted with permission from A.C. Hseih. In: *The Peripheral Circulations*, edited by R. Zelis. New York: Grune & Stratton, 1975.)

Normal Values and Response Range

Skin blood flow is commonly determined in man with the venous occlusion plethysmograph (Chapter 6). Such studies have shown that this tissue is capable of extreme flow ranges; under maximum heat stimulation, hand skin flow can increase about 30-fold from the normal values of 3 to 5 ml/100 g tissue/min and with cold application of 15°C,

10-fold decreases to 0.3 to 0.5 ml/100 g/min. With further cooling (*e.g.*, to 10°C) there follows, however, a cold-induced vasodilation, a protective, local, nonneurogenic reaction, sometimes called the "hunting response." Its mechanism is unknown.

Control of Skin Blood Vessels

While there are direct blood flow effects of heat and cold on skin, as described above, by far the main mechanism is an "indirect" sympathetic reflex response. This is due to a stimulation of heat-sensitive thermoreceptors in the skin and in the hypothalamus (via warmed blood) which markedly vasodilate resistance vessels (*i.e.*, arterioles and AVAs) as well as capacitance vessels. The result is a large increase in both arterial flow and in the slow-velocity, subcutaneous venous flow, the latter being especially well adapted to transfer heat to the environment. Vasodilation in the hands, feet and face is "passive," *i.e.*, due to reduction in sympathetic tone, but in other areas is mainly "active" (Fig. 11.16).

This active vasodilation is carried out by arterioles, but not by AVAs; some investigators have proposed that this dilation mechanism is similar to that prevailing in certain glandular tissues and sweat glands and that it involves the local release of an enzyme which acts on a globulin substrate to liberate bradykinin, a potent vasodilator.

The reflex response to cold, while less marked, is significant and includes not only reduction of arterial flow but also venoconstriction, with a resultant decrease in subcutaneous venous volume and an increase in velocity of venous blood flow, a distinct advantage in minimizing heat loss. During severe and prolonged cold, the direct effects, added to the indirect reflex effects, may so reduce skin flow that it is almost immeasurable, with the distinct risk of frostbite and severe tissue damage. Frostbite was previously discussed in Chapter 2 under blood viscosity.

Pathophysiological Responses

Inflammation of the skin or pressure on the skin surface induces a vascular reaction depending on the intensity of the stimulus. After light stroking there is pallor and after a heavier stroking a red line due to venular dilation. Upon repeated or heavier pressure, the reddening or "flare" will occur and spread because of arteriolar involvement; with still greater trauma, wheals will result. This sequence has been called the "triple response" and is ascribed to the local production and spread of histamine; it involves a local vascular mechanism and is thought to be an axon reflex.

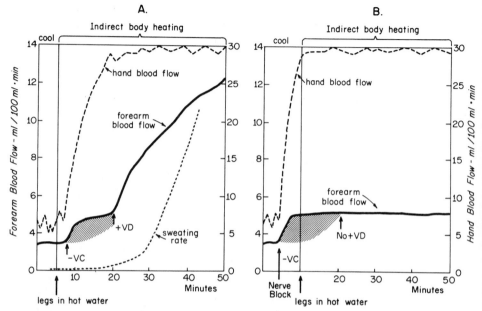

Figure 11.16. Reflex effects of indirect heating on skin blood flow in normal hand and forearm, *i.e.*, changes in finger and forearm blood flow when legs were put in hot H_2O. *A*, vasodilation in the hand is mediated only by release of tonic sympathetic vasoconstrictor tone (−VC); this "passive" vasodilation accounts, however, for only a small part of the blood flow in the forearm (−VC to +VD). The remainder, as well as the sweating, is due to active sympathetic vasodilation and can be prevented by sympathetic blockade, *B*; note in *B* the abrupt increase in hand (skin) blood flow after nerve block illustrating the neurogenic control of skin blood flow. However, (in *B*) the nerve block prevented the increase in forearm blood flow. (Reprinted with permission from J.T. Shepherd, *Physiology of Circulation in Human Limbs in Health and Disease*. Philadelphia: W.B. Saunders, 1963.)

Blood vessels of skin are unusually sensitive to central nervous and hormonal influences. Fear may be marked by vasoconstriction and pallor; cold sweats may occur due to nervous tension, and blushing will follow certain emotional stimuli, although the latter response is reportedly becoming extinct in Western civilization.

The unusual sensitivity of skin vessels to nervous and hormonal influences makes this tissue vulnerable to certain vasospastic disorders of the extremities. *Raynaud's disease*, a chronic condition of this type, affects the hands and occurs particularly in women in colder climates. It is characterized by frequent vasospasms and blanching of the fingers of both hands followed by vasodilation, ischemic pain and in some cases eventual tissue necrosis. The condition is thought to be an exaggerated vasoconstrictor response to continued sympathoadrenal stimulation associated with nervous tension. Bilateral upper thoracic sympathec- tomy is sometimes helpful but usually does not afford lasting relief.

Circulation in Skeletal Muscle

The primary function of these vessels is to serve the metabolic needs of skeletal muscle, needs which can increase as much as 100-fold over the resting level. Because of the great muscle mass, a secondary role is to provide a reserve of vascular resistance for certain emergencies such as circulatory shock. Muscle circulation has two quite different mecha- nisms to discharge these two different functions, *i.e.*, a local metabolic and central neural control system.

General Flow Characteristics and Normal Values

As mentioned in Chapter 9, at rest 20 to 25% of the cardiac output supplies the skeletal muscles with about 4 to 6 ml of flow per 100 g/min; however, at maximal exercise almost 90% of the cardiac output may be diverted to the working muscles (Chapter 12, Exercise). Rapid, phasic (white) fiber units, which comprise 80 to 85% of the muscle mass, may upon contraction increase their flow 10-fold from a resting level of 2 to 4 ml/100 g/min while the slow, tonic (red) fibers, may experience a 4-fold increase from somewhat higher resting values of 20 to 30 ml/100 g/min. In experimental animals such flow determinations are usually made by direct flowmetering of the arteries and in man by means of venous occlusion plethysmography (Chapter 6).

Muscle arterioles have a high resting tone, most of which is inherent in the vascular muscle itself (myogenic tone) and the remainder due to a tonic sympathetic vasoconstrictor outflow with a frequency of about 1 impulse/sec. An increase in the stimulation frequency to 4 to 5 impulse/sec produces about a 70% reduction in flow but has a lesser effect on exercising muscle (Fig. 11.17). An important advance in flow dynamics has been the development of methods to study regional circulation and the degrees of nonuniformity of flow, *i.e.*, perfusion heterogeneity using tritiated water.

Local (Metabolic) Control of Muscle Circulation during Exercise

At rest the neural factors are primary but during muscle contraction the local metabolism becomes practically the exclusive regulator of the muscle flow; skeletal muscle has well-developed autoregulatory and reactive hyperemic properties, a further manifestation of the link be- tween metabolism and flow in this bed. During physical exercise the skeletal muscles achieve their tremendous increase in oxygen exchange

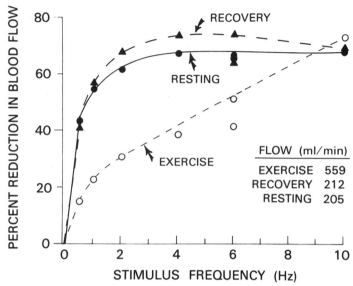

Figure 11.17. Effect of frequency of electrical stimulation of the lumbar sympathetic chain on limb flow in the dog. At rest there was marked flow reduction with increase in frequency. During exercise the stimulation was less effective because the bed was under metabolic control. (Reprinted with permission from D.E. Donald, D.J. Rowlands, and D.A. Ferguson, *Circ Res* 26:185, 1970.)

through (a) extreme metabolic dilation of the microcirculation, (b) increase in the number of perfused capillaries (recruitment), and (c) increased oxygen extraction in the capillary bed.

During rhythmic exercise, flow is intermittent because of the mechanical compression effect on the vasculature. Flow interference begins at about 30% of maximum tension with complete stoppage at about the 70% level; this deprives the fiber of oxygen at its time of greatest need although the myoglobin of red muscles provides some assistance through its oxygen "accumulator" and release action. On the venous side, this intermittent compression of veins in conjunction with venous valves, produces a strong phasic milking action (Chapter 6, Venous Return); the resultant lowering of net venous pressure is thought to play an important role in increasing perfusion through lower extremity muscles during exercise such as running.

As with other vascular beds, considerable effort has been directed to the study of the possible mechanism of the hyperemia during increased metabolism. A number of vasodilator substances has been proposed, most prominently Po_2, H^+, K^+ and adenosine; as yet there is no agreement on any one agent.

Some investigators believe that local hyperosmolality may be a factor, at least in initiating the hyperemic response. With exercise there is known to be a metabolic breakdown within the muscle cell of many large molecules into smaller ones, which increases osmolality and causes transfer of water into the cell; this is probably responsible for the 10 to 15% decrease in plasma volume which is usual after exercise.

Central (Neural) Control of Muscle Circulation

Sympathetic vasoconstriction is the primary circulatory control mechanism of skeletal muscle in nonexercise situations. Vasodilation can be brought about either passively by decreased stimulation of vasoconstrictors (which is the most common mechanism) or actively via sympathetic cholinergic or β-adrenergic vasodilators. Cholinergic vasodilation mainly results from cerebral activity such as mental effort or emotion; it is thought that these descending impulses from the higher centers may bypass the medullary cardiovascular centers.

Skeletal muscle vessels are also important participants in reflex response. Increased stimulation of arterial baroceptors and certain cardiopulmonary receptors will result in decreased sympathetic tone and passive vasodilation of skeletal muscle resistance vessels; it is also thought that some active vasodilation also occurs, at least initially. Conversely, decreased stimulation of arterial and cardiopulmonary receptors will result in reflex sympathetic vasoconstriction in skeletal muscle (Fig. 11.18).

Stimulation of aortic and carotid body chemoreceptors, *e.g.*, during hypoxia or shock, will also induce reflex vasoconstriction in skeletal muscle. If, however, a vasodilation stimulus is imposed on a bed previously vasoconstricted, *e.g.*, by hemorrhage or hypoxia, such sudden inhibition—accompanied as it sometimes is by vagal bradycardia—can lower peripheral resistance sharply and result in fainting (Chapter 13).

It should also be mentioned that muscle veins, in sharp contrast to splanchnic and cutaneous veins, are practically devoid of adrenergic nerve endings in their walls and as a consequence these veins react little if at all to sympathetic vasomotor constriction and so do not serve a significant reservoir function.

Neurohormonal Effects

Under certain circumstances, catecholamines may influence muscle vasculature. As described in Chapter 9 (Neural Control of Flow) the arterioles of skeletal muscle contain sympathetic α-, β- and cholinergic receptors so that the result of sympathetic stimulation is usually a

Figure 11.18. Response of forearm skeletal muscle blood flow to decreased (*A*) and increased (*B*) cardiopulmonary receptor stimulation due to intrathoracic blood volume changes. These changes were produced by head-up tilt and leg raising, respectively. Sympathetic blockade in the control arm prevented the flow changes. Arterial baroceptors were not involved since arterial pressure did not change. (Reprinted with permission from J.T. Shepherd, *Physiology of the Circulation in Human Limbs in Health and Disease.* Philadelphia: W.B. Saunders, 1963.)

balance between two or more effects. Norepinephrine (NE) injection has a small β-dilator, but a much stronger α-constrictor action; a moderate intravenous dose of NE in the intact organism will, therefore, raise the blood pressure and thereby activate the arterial baroceptors, producing a subsequent reflex vasodilation and corrective fall in pressure. Epinephrine usually induces a marked but transitory β-dilator action which is enhanced if its secondary effect, an α-constrictor action, is blocked (Chapter 9).

Pulmonary Circulation

Anatomy

The pulmonary and systemic circuits are in series and in the normal resting adult, each ventricle has an output of about 70 ml/kg/min or 5 L/min. The pulmonary circulation, with only one-tenth the capacity of the systemic, must, in the same time period, accommodate the same ejected volume. The pulmonary vessels, which are much shorter, accommodate this volume without excessive pressure fluctuations because of thinner walls and greater compliance. The pulmonary capillaries form a very thin, rich, vascular network around the alveoli which facilitates blood-gas exchange.

The blood supply to the lung itself, the bronchial circulation, constitutes only 1 to 2% of the left ventricular output. Venous drainage is mainly via the azygous system. Bronchial veins form a latticework in the adventitia and submucosa of the bronchial tree. In the presence of post-pulmonary capillary hypertension, *e.g.*, in mitral stenosis, the bronchial veins become congested and frequently form varicosities. With sudden, strong respiratory movements, damage to these venous walls may result in hemoptysis (spitting up of blood).

Pressure and Flow in the Pulmonary Vessels

The mean pressures in the right ventricle and pulmonary artery are about one-sixth as great as those of the left ventricle and aorta (Fig. 11.19). Since the total flows are equal, the pulmonary vascular resistance is only one-sixth that of the systemic. However, the pressure waves, flow patterns and cardiac valvular movements of these two circuits are quite similar. The normal mean pressure in the pulmonary artery is about 15 mm Hg, in the capillaries about 10 mm Hg and in the pulmonary veins and left atrium about 5 mm Hg. Thus the pulmonary arterial-capillary gradient is about equal to the pulmonary capillary-venous gradient (about 5 mm Hg) indicating that these two segments contribute about equally to pulmonary vascular resistance, a very different situation than in the systemic circuit. The mean pulse pressures in the left atrium are somewhat higher than those of the right (Fig. 11.19) because of the more forceful contractions of the left atrium and ventricle.

The total thoracic blood volume (TBV), which in the normal 70-kg adult is about 1,200 ml, includes the pulmonary blood volume, *i.e.*, within the lung, which is about 500 ml. In the discussion on vascular volumes and pressures (Chapter 1), it was mentioned that the TBV (also called central blood volume) represents about a quarter of the total blood volume and provides an important reserve filling pressure for the ventricles. The volume contained in the vena cavae and right heart, (about 350 ml) constitutes right heart reserve, and that in the pulmonary artery, lungs and pulmonary veins (about 900 ml) serves as left heart reserve.

As a low-pressure system, about one-half of the TBV (*i.e.*, about 500 ml) is readily dislocated into the lower extremities upon assumption of the upright position; a substantial fraction of the TBV is also displaced

Figure 11.19. Representative pressures (mm Hg) in normal adult pulmonary and systemic circulation. (Reprinted with permission from J.H. Comroe, *Physiology of Respiration*, 2nd ed. Chicago: Year Book Medical Publishers, 1974.)

into the general venous circulation during hemorrhage, dehydration or other vascular stress in which there is a fall in systemic venous pressure. Conversely, thoracic blood volume and pressure rise in the supine position, in exercise, during generalized systemic vasoconstriction, water immersion in the upright position, or left heart failure, *i.e.*, any condition in which extrathoracic venous volume and pressure rise. It should also be noted that TBV fluctuates during each breathing cycle because of rhythmic alterations of intra- and extrathoracic pressure. During inspiration there is a net increase of about 250 ml of blood in the chest and during expiration a similar decrease (Venous Return, Chapter 6).

Distribution of Blood Flow in the Lung

In order to carry out its primary mission of blood-gas exchange, it is necessary that the oxygen-poor blood delivered via the pulmonary arteries be maximally exposed to oxygen-rich air of the alveoli, *i.e.*, that perfusion and ventilation be kept in balance. An imbalance between these two is, however, a common occurrence and is responsible for most gas exchange problems in pulmonary disease. One factor contributing to the ventilation-perfusion imbalance is the effect of posture on flow distribution; in the upright position, there is minimal flow to the lung apex and a progressively increasing rate of flow toward the base. What is the reason for this inequality?

As described in Chapter 6 (Respiratory Pump), respiratory excursions induce fluctuating negative intrathoracic pressures; these pressures are exerted, however, mainly on the pulmonary arterial and pulmonary venous vessels. Pulmonary capillaries on the other hand are more strongly influenced by alveolar pressures. Because the alveolocapillary membrane is thin and pliant, the effective extravascular capillary pressure normally approximates the alveolar pressure (P_A) rather than the more negative intrathoracic pressure. But in the upright position there may be a hydrostatic pressure difference of 30 cm H_2O (23 mm Hg) between the apex and base of the lung. Since the normal pulmonary artery pressure is only about 20 cm H_2O, this hydrostatic pressure difference has important pulmonary hemodynamic consequences.

Since at the lung apex, *i.e.*, above the heart, the pulmonary intracapillary pressure may be lower than alveolar pressure, some of the capillaries may collapse and flow at the apex will be less than that at the base (Fig. 11.20, zone 1). However, at the base (Fig. 11.20, zone 3), the added hydrostatic pressure increases the capillary transmural pressure well beyond the alveolar pressure so the vessels will not only remain patent but are distended and flow will be increased. In this situation it is seen that flow depends not only on the usual longitudinal driving pressure gradient but also on the transmural pressure gradient which must be positive in order to prevent collapse.

In the upright subject the ventilation-perfusion ratio is greater than one at the apex and decreases to values below one at the base. In the normal individual this is not a serious handicap to gas exchange; however, if there is a pathological deficiency of either ventilation or perfusion, this potential handicap can be exaggerated and present a serious threat to possible gas exchange.

Control of Pulmonary Vessels

The pulmonary circulation acts mainly as a passive, compliant, vascular bed, adapting to the demands of the circulation at large. Most studies indicate that although the vessels are well supplied with vagal and sympathetic fibers, these apparently have little functional role. Pulmonary vessels will, however, constrict strongly under the influence of hypoxia. This is a regional phenomenon which occurs in the area of

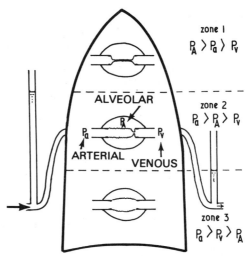

Figure 11.20. Illustration of hydrostatic effect of body position on pulmonary capillary flow. In zone 1 above heart level, the extramural pulmonary alveolar pressure (P_A) may be greater than the pulmonary capillary pressure and some capillaries may collapse. In zone 2, flow may be intermittent; in zone 3 below the heart, with increased hydrostatic pressure, the capillaries distend and flow is increased. (Reprinted with permission from J.B. West, C.T. Dollery, and A. Naimark, *J Appl Physiol* 19:713, 1964.)

the hypoxia and may be due to local release of a vasoconstrictor substance. It should be noted that this pulmonary vasoconstrictor response is directly opposite to the usual vasodilator effect of hypoxia in all other circulatory beds. The hypoxic vasoconstriction is reinforced by similar vasoconstrictor action of decreased pH which often coexists. Hypoxic vasoconstriction serves a useful purpose in diverting the flow from poorly ventilated regions to other lung areas with more abundant oxygen, thus improving the overall gas exchange. Hypoxic vasoconstriction, which may occur at altitude or in patients with chronic obstructive pulmonary disease, can—if prolonged—lead to pulmonary hypertension.

Drugs which constrict pulmonary vessels include norepinephrine, serotonin, histamine and a number of the prostaglandins. Isoproterenol and acetylcholine are vasodilators.

Pulmonary Capillary Dynamics and Edema

The combination of a plasma osmotic pressure of about 28 mm Hg and a low pulmonary capillary hydrostatic pressure of 10 mm Hg results in a rather unusual net inward force of about 18 mm Hg. This factor coupled with a rather "tight" capillary endothelium helps to maintain narrow interstitial spaces between the capillary and alveolar surfaces which in turn expedite gaseous diffusion. This negative pressure gradient represents a safety factor reducing the chances of interstitial fluid accumulation; pulmonary edema will, for example, usually not occur in experimental animals until left atrial pressure exceeds 20 mm Hg.

However, in case of severe left ventricular failure or mitral stenosis, left atrial pressure and volume will steadily increase with an eventual damming effect and an increase in pulmonary venous and capillary pressures; interstitial edema will then develop and if the process continues, fluid will also accumulate in the alveoli resulting in progressive interference with oxygenation, shortness of breath and difficulty in breathing, *i.e.*, dyspnea (see Congestive Failure, Chapter 14).

Pulmonary edema may also develop in certain cases of elevated cerebrospinal fluid pressure (P_{CSF}), *e.g.*, following head injury. When P_{CSF} reaches levels sufficient to induce large increases in systemic arterial pressure, pulmonary capillary pressure rises along with left atrial pressure and cardiac output. Recent studies by Maron and Dawson have shown that the pulmonary hypertension in this condition is probably the result of a strong pulmonary venous constriction due to adrenal catecholamines liberated during the elevation of P_{CSF}.

References

General

Abboud FM, Fozzard HA, Gilmore JF, and Reis DJ. *Disturbances in Neurogenic Control of the Circulation*, Bethesda, Md: American Physiological Society, 1981.
Donald DE and Shepherd JT. Autonomic regulation of the peripheral circulation. *Annu Rev Physiol* 42:429–439, 1980.
Johnson PC. *Peripheral Circulation*. New York: John Wiley & Sons, 1978.
Korner PI. Control of blood flow to special vascular areas: brain, kidney, muscle, skin, liver and intestine. In: *Cardiovascular Physiology, MTP International Review of Science*, edited by AC Guyton and CE Jones. Baltimore: University Park Press, 1974.
Mellander S and Johansson B. Control of resistance, exchange and capacitance functions in peripheral circulation. *Pharmacol Rev* 20:117–196, 1968.
Olsson RA. Local factors regulating cardiac and skeletal muscle blood flow. *Annu Rev Physiol* 43:385–395, 1981.
Paradise NF and Fox IJ. Regional blood flow measurement. In: *Dye Curves: The Theory and Practice of Indicator Dilution*, edited by DA Bloomfield. Baltimore: University Park Press, 1974.
Rowell LB. Human cardiovascular adjustment to exercise and thermal stress. *Physiol Rev* 54(1):75–159, 1974.
Shepherd JT. *Physiology of the Circulation in Human Limbs in Health and Disease*. Philadelphia: W.B. Saunders, 1963.
Zelis R. *The Peripheral Circulations*. New York: Grune & Stratton, 1975.

Cerebral Circulation

Cagle G, Greene ER, Miranda JP, Miranda FG, and Reilly PA. Non-invasive ultrasound measurements of cardiac output and common carotid blood flow in cerebrovascular disease patients as a function of posture and exercise. *Physiologist* 25:323, 1982.
Kety SS and Schmidt CF. The nitrous oxide method for the determination of cerebral blood flow in man: theory, procedure and normal values. *J Clin Invest* 27:476, 1948.

Kontos HA. Regulation of the cerebral circulation. *Annu Rev Physiol* 43:397–407, 1981.
Lassen NA. Brain. In: *Peripheral Circulation*, edited by PC Johnson. New York: John Wiley & Sons, 1978.
Patton HD, Sundsten JW, Crill WE, and Swanson PD. *Introduction to Basic Neurology.* Philadelphia: W.B. Saunders, 1976.
Strandness DE and Sumner DS. *Hemodynamics for Surgeons.* New York: Grune & Stratton, 1975.
Symposium on Cerebral Circulation: Chairmen—FM Abboud and DD Heistad. *Fed Proc* 40:2296–2334, 1981.

Coronary Circulation

Berne RM and Rubio R. Coronary circulation. In: *Handbook of Physiology*, Section 2: *The Cardiovascular System*, edited by RM Berne, N Sperelakis and SR Geiger. Bethesda, Md: American Physiological Society, 1979, Vol. I, pp. 873–952.
Braunwald E, Ross J, and Sonnenblick EH. Regulation of coronary blood flow. In: *Mechanisms of Contraction of the Normal and Failing Heart.* Boston: Little, Brown, 1976.
Cohen MV, Yipintosi T, and Scheuer J. Coronary collateral stimulation by exercise in dogs with stenotic coronary arteries. *J Appl Physiol* 52:664–671, 1982.
Feigl EO. Coronary physiology. *Physiol Rev* 63:1–205, 1983.
James TN. *Anatomy of the Coronary Arteries.* New York: Hoeber Medical Division, Harper & Row, 1961.
Rinkema LE, Thomas J, and Randall WC. Regional coronary vasoconstriction in response to stimulation of stellate ganglia. *Am J Physiol* 243:H410–415, 1982.
Rubio R and Berne RM. Myocardium. In: *Peripheral Circulation*, edited by PC Johnson. New York: John Wiley & Sons, 1978, pp. 231–253.
Santamore WP and Bove AA. *Coronary Artery Disease.* Baltimore: Urban and Schwarzenberg, 1982.
Sarnoff SJ, Braunwald E, Welch GH, Case RB, Stainsby WN, and Macruz R. Hemodynamic determinants of oxygen consumption of the heart with special reference to the tension-time index. *Am J Physiol* 192:148–156, 1958.
Tripp MR, Meyer MW, Einzig S, Leonard JJ, Swayze CR, and Fox IJ. Simultaneous regional myocardial blood flow by tritiated water and microspheres. *Am J Physiol* 232:H173–190, 1979.
Wright AJA and Hudlicka O. Capillary growth and changes in heart performance induced by chronic bradycardial pacing in the rabbit. *Circ Res* 49:469–477, 1981.
Vatner SF. Correlation between acute reductions in myocardial blood flow and function in conscious dogs. *Circ Res* 47:201–207, 1980.

Renal Circulation

Cowley AW Jr. Vasopressin and cardiovascular regulation. In: *Cardiovascular Physiology IV, International Review of Physiology*, Baltimore: University Park Press, 1982, Vol. 26, pp. 189–242.
Echtenkamp SF, Zucker IH, and Gilmore JP. Characterization of high and low pressure baroceptor influences on renal nerve activity in the primate macaca fascicularis. *Circ Res* 46:726–730, 1980.
Gauer OH and Henry JP. Neurohormonal control of plasma volume. In: *Cardiovascular Physiology II, International Review of Physiology*, edited by AC Guyton and AW Cowley. Baltimore: University Park Press, 1976, Vol. 9, pp. 145–190.
Hall JE. Regulation of renal hemodynamics. In: *Cardiovascular Physiology IV, International Review of Physiology*, edited by AC Guyton and JE Hall. Baltimore: University Park Press, 1982, Vol. 26, pp. 243–321.
Hollenberg NK. The renal circulation. In: *The Peripheral Circulations*, edited by R Zelis. New York: Grune & Stratton, 1975, pp. 131–150.
Thames MD. Contribution of cardiopulmonary baroceptors to the control of the kidney. *Fed Proc* 37:1209–1213, 1978.

Splanchnic Circulation

Granger DN and Kvietys PR. The splanchnic circulation: intrinsic regulation. *Annu Rev Physiol* 43:409–418, 1981.

Jacobson ED and Tepperman BL. (eds.). Splanchnic circulation (Symposium). *Fed Proc* 41:2079–2116, 1982.

Rowell LB. The splanchnic circulation. In: *The Peripheral Circulations*, edited by R Zelis. New York: Grune & Stratton, 1975, pp. 163–192.

Cutaneous and Skeletal Muscle Circulation

Greenfield ADM: The circulation through the skin. In: *Handbook of Physiology*, Section 2: *Circulation*, edited by WF Hamilton and P Dow. Washington, D.C.: American Physiological Society, 1963, Vol. II, pp. 1325–1351.

Heistad DD and Abboud FM. Factors that influence blood flow in skeletal muscle and skin. *Anesthesiology* 41:139–156, 1974.

Hseih ACL. The cutaneous circulation. In: *The Peripheral Circulations*, edited by R Zelis. New York: Grune & Stratton, 1975, pp. 79–94.

Paradise NF, Swayze CR, Shin DH, and Fox IJ. Perfusion heterogeneity in skeletal muscle using tritiated water. *Am J Physiol* 220:1107–1115, 1971.

Rowell LB. The cutaneous circulation and circulation to skeletal muscle. In: *Physiology and Biophysics*, edited by TC Ruch, HD Patton and AM Scher. Philadelphia: W.B. Saunders, 1974, 20th ed., pp. 185–214.

Rowell LB. Human cardiovascular responses to exercise and thermal stress. *Physiol Rev* 54:75–159, 1974.

Shepherd JT. *Physiology of the Circulation in Human Limbs in Health and Disease.* Philadelphia: W.B. Saunders, 1963.

Sparks HV. Skin and muscle. In: *Peripheral Circulation*, edited by PC Johnson. New York: John Wiley & Sons, 1978, pp. 193–230.

Pulmonary Circulation

Cumming G. The pulmonary circulation. In: *Cardiovascular Physiology, MTP International Review of Science*, edited by AC Guyton and CE Jones. Baltimore: University Park Press, 1974.

Green, JF. The pulmonary circulation. In: *The Peripheral Circulations*, edited by R Zelis. New York: Grune & Stratton, 1975, pp. 193–210.

Maron MB and Dawson CA. Pulmonary venoconstriction caused by elevated cerebrospinal fluid pressure in the dog. *J Appl Physiol* 49:73–78, 1980.

Schreiner BF Jr and Yu PN. Pulmonary circulation, congestion and edema: anatomic and physiologic conditions. In: *Clinical Cardiovascular Physiology*, edited by HJ Levine. New York: Grune & Stratton, 1976, pp. 635–706.

Slonim NB and Hamilton LH. *Respiratory Physiology.* St. Louis: C.V. Mosby, 1981, 4th ed.

West JB. *Respiratory Physiology.* Baltimore: Williams & Wilkins, 1979, 2nd ed.

chapter 12

Physiology of Exercise and the Effect of Aging

Physical exercise is one of the most physiologically demanding activities engaged in by man. Even upon anticipation, there occurs a strong sympathoadrenal activation, particularly if there is an emotional element involved. When muscular activity begins, there rapidly follows a complex and highly integrated series of neuromuscular, respiratory, circulatory and metabolic events which permit the transformation of chemical energy into muscular work. During recovery there is an orderly payback of the oxygen debt which has been accumulated.

While many systems are involved, emphasis in this chapter is on cardiovascular response to exercise (both isotonic and isometric), on physical training and on exercise stress testing. Because of the increased interest in the effects of aging on cardiovascular performance, we have also incorporated a brief account of some recent studies in this field.

Dynamic (Isotonic) Exercise

Dynamic exercise refers to repeated voluntary muscle movements in which there is alternate contraction and relaxation of the muscle, as distinct from isometric (static) exercise, in which the muscle is kept in a state of continued contraction.

General Circulatory Response to Exercise

With the rapid increase in energy requirements, equally rapid circulatory adjustments are essential in order to meet the increased need for O_2 and nutrients by the exercising muscle. Also important is the need to remove the end products of metabolism such as CO_2 and lactic acid and to dissipate the excess heat produced by the reactions. The emphasis in this section is on how the circulatory system meets these increased demands.

The increase in oxygen consumption ($\dot{V}O_2$) during exercise is directly proportional to the work performed up to maximal work capacity ($\dot{V}O_{2max}$). The increased oxygen demand is met through an increase both in cardiac output (CO) and in O_2 extraction from the blood. $\dot{V}O_2$ is the best measure of exercise intensity and $\dot{V}O_{2max}$ is the best single measure of cardiovascular reserve and physical fitness. With a typical 4- to 5-fold increase in CO and a 2- to 3-fold increase in (A-V)O_2 difference, $\dot{V}O_2$ can be increased 8 to 15 times during exercise. Exceptional athletes may achieve values of $\dot{V}O_{2max}$ between 5 and 6 L/min, a 20-fold increase over resting levels.

How is this extraordinary shift in body metabolism brought about? Mainly through the greatly increased and superbly coordinated activity of almost all systems of the body, *i.e.*, neuromuscular, respiratory, cardiovascular, metabolic and hormonal.

In normal individuals, there is an approximately linear relationship between total oxygen consumption ($\dot{V}O_2$) and heart rate (HR), cardiac output (CO) and minute ventilation ($\dot{V}_E$) (Fig. 12.1). At or near maximal working capacity ($\dot{V}O_{2max}$), CO and HR tend to plateau, whereas $\dot{V}_E$, beginning at about 50% $\dot{V}O_{2max}$ rises more rapidly than $\dot{V}O_2$. Some investigators have suggested that the tight coupling between CO and $\dot{V}O_{2max}$ may be due to central chemoreceptors.

The increased cardiac output is accomplished through increases in both heart rate and stroke volume (SV). Cardioacceleration at low levels of exercise is due to vagal release but at high levels is due to combined vagal release and sympathetic activation. The maximal heart rate (HR_{max}), which is usually achieved at $\dot{V}O_{2max}$, is an important limiting

Figure 12.1. Effect of progressive exercise on heart rate, cardiac output (CO), ventilation and venous HbO_2 saturation. (Reprinted with permission from E.H. Starling and L. Evans, *Principles of Human Physiology*, 14th ed. Philadelphia: Lea & Febiger, 1968.)

factor in cardiovascular performance. HR_{max} decreases progressively with age. Although there is considerable individual variability, it can be approximated by the formula $HR_{max} = 220 - $ age(in years).

The increase in SV is due to increased filling of the ventricles (Frank-Starling mechanism) and heightened myocardial contractility induced by sympathetic stimulation. Some of the past controversy regarding SV response to exercise is now known to have been due to postural effects. In supine exercise, because of increased filling pressure, SV is greater (than in the upright) and with increasing exercise is maintained nearly constant, so that the CO increase in the supine is achieved mainly through increase in HR.

In the sitting or standing position, SV is about one-third less than in the supine position. Thus, in upright exercise SV is initially smaller but increases progressively at increasing work levels until about 40% of $\dot{V}O_{2max}$, at which point it reaches its maximal value (for the upright position) and plateaus. However, the SV at $\dot{V}O_{2max}$ is still less in upright than in supine exercise. Final CO levels are very similar at equivalent work loads in the two positions.

Thus, at submaximal workloads the increase in CO is due to increases in both HR and SV. But at high work levels—because of earlier leveling off of SV—the increase in $\dot{V}O_2$ is achieved mainly by the increase in HR.

During exercise, there is a pronounced rise in systolic pressure (SP), which reaches levels of 170 to 200 mm Hg at $\dot{V}O_{2max}$. In spite of a 4- to 5-fold increase in CO, diastolic pressure is changed little, mainly because of the decreased vascular resistance in exercising muscle. The result is an increase in pulse pressure that parallels the rise in systolic pressure and a moderate increase in mean arterial blood pressure.

The primary mechanism of this circulatory response has been termed the "exercise pressor response" by Mitchell et al. Physical exercise (either dynamic or static) stimulates small myelinated (group III) and unmyelinated (group IV) fibers in skeletal muscle, which invoke a sympathetic response of peripheral vasoconstriction, tachycardia, increased myocardial contractility and hypertension. The degree of response is approximately proportional (in both dynamic and static exercise) to the muscle mass involved and the intensity of the exercise. Similar responses can be induced in experimental animals by electrical stimulation of skeletal

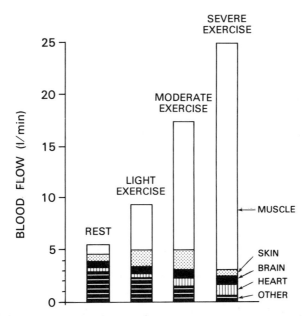

Figure 12.2. Distribution of blood flow with increasing levels of exercise in man. In severe exercise there is about a 20-fold increase in skeletal muscle flow and a 4-fold increase in coronary flow with little change in brain blood flow and a marked decrease to almost all remaining tissues. (Reprinted with permission from E.H. Starling and L. Evans, *Principles of Human Physiology.* Philadelphia: Lea & Febiger, 1968.)

muscles (particularly fast twitch fibers) or of the group III or group IV afferent fibers from these muscles. The central pathways of the exercise pressor reflex are not yet known.

Distribution of Blood Flow in Exercise

A rise in blood flow to the exercising muscles is brought about through both an increase and a redistribution of CO. At rest, only about 15 to 20% of CO is distributed to skeletal muscle in contrast to 85 or 90% during maximal exercise. This represents a 15- to 20-fold increase in flow to the skeletal muscles and a 3- to 4-fold increase to the myocardium (Fig. 12.2); muscle is the only tissue in the body that can markedly increase its own blood flow.

In skeletal muscle, the increased flow is initiated by the anticipatory sympathetic cholinergic vasodilation and is reinforced by the metabolic hyperemia. As the exercise continues, the general tendency to sympathetic vasoconstriction is, in skeletal muscle, overwhelmed by metabolic vasodilation, thereby resulting in a massive increase in blood flow to this tissue. The vasodilation in the capillary bed of working muscle is

Figure 12.3. Changes in forearm blood flow during severe leg exercise in human subjects. After a temporary increase in forearm (muscle) flow during leg exercise, there was a constriction and flow reduction to about 50% of control. (Reprinted with permission from B.S. Bevegard and J.T. Shepherd, *J Appl Physiol* 21:123, 1966.)

probably due to the direct action of metabolites, particularly increases in P_{CO_2}, K^+ and H^+.

The redistribution of flow, which is highly important in the shunting of oxygenated blood to active muscle, results not only from a decreased vascular resistance in skeletal muscle but also from strong sympathetic vasoconstriction in other tissues such as kidney, splanchnic area and nonexercising muscle. Blood flow to the vasculature of the brain and myocardium (which have few α-receptors) is unchanged or increased (Fig. 12.2).

Thus, as might be expected, during leg exercise, blood flow to the nonexercising forearm muscles is decreased (Fig. 12.3). However, this normal forearm response to leg exercise may be reversed in certain disorders. Mark et al. reported that during leg exercise, vasodilation (instead of vasoconstriction) occurs in the forearm (and perhaps in other muscle tissue as well!) in aortic stenosis patients. They suggested that this altered response may be due to reflexes from left ventricular baroceptors stimulated by the dilated ventricle and theorized that this reaction may be responsible for the exertional dyspnea and syncope that may occur in aortic stenosis and pulmonary hypertension patients. This vasodilator reaction of the forearm to exercise will usually revert to the normal vasoconstrictor response after surgical implantation of an efficient valve.

Although there is wide vasodilation of skeletal muscle arterioles, the veins of both exercising and nonexercising tissues are constricted, particularly those of the splanchnic venous bed. This is a sympathetic effect that assists in shunting blood into the central circulation, thereby aiding cardiac output.

During running there is a remarkable decrease in venous pressure at the ankle because of muscle pump action (Chapter 6, Skeletal Muscle Pump). However, pressure in the common femoral veins and inferior vena cavae increases to levels of 20 to 25 mm Hg, probably due to the high abdominal pressure that is mechanically necessary to fix and hold the pelvis, a condition which is essential to the running motion. This heightened intraabdominal venous pressure is a significant energy barrier for the heart.

Thermoregulatory adjustments are essential in any exercise which lasts more than a few minutes since 80% of the total energy produced is thermal and must be carried to the skin surface to be dissipated. In moderate exercise, skin blood flow usually increases 3- to 4-fold. In severe exercise a constrictor tendency manifests itself and flow returns toward baseline levels apparently in an effort toward maximum conservation of flow for skeletal muscle exchange (Fig. 12.2). The hypothalamus is the essential integrator for both the vasomotor and the thermoregulatory changes (Chapter 10, Role of Hypothalamus).

Arm vs. Leg Exercise

At submaximal work intensities, the $\dot{V}O_2$ for arm and leg work is not significantly different. However, the achievable $\dot{V}O_{2max}$ is dependent on the mass and type of muscle involved. The $\dot{V}O_{2max}$ in arm ergometry is only 60 to 80% of leg ergometry or of combined arm and leg ergometry. The reason for the $\dot{V}O_{2max}$ limitation when smaller muscle masses such as the arm are involved has been attributed to (a) a lesser mechanical efficiency (*i.e.*, a smaller ratio of work output to caloric expenditure) or (b) a lesser degree of conditioning (which usually prevails in arm vs. leg muscles).

But regardless of the cause, there is almost invariably a greater HR and pressor response to a similar level of arm compared to leg work (Fig. 12.4). This phenomenon is usually held responsible for the oft-repeated history of the keen sensitivity of angina pectoris patients to arm exercise. Aside from the lesser mechanical efficiency of small muscle groups, there is also a lesser "myocardial efficiency." For equivalent degree of work, arm exercise induces a greater systolic pressure-HR increment than leg work. Since the pressure-rate product is a close correlate of myocardial oxygen consumption, arm work is more likely to produce myocardial ischemia in angina patients.

Figure 12.4. Systolic blood pressure and heart rate response at rest and at various levels of arm and leg ergometer exercise in patients with ischemic heart disease. At every work level the SBP and HR responses were greater during arm exercise. (Reprinted with permission from H.K. Hellerstein and B.A. Franklin. In: *Rehabilitation of the Coronary Patient*, edited by N.K. Wenger and H.K. Hellerstein. New York: John Wiley and Sons, 1978.)

Systemic Response to Exercise

With the onset of exercise, respiratory changes occur rapidly so there is increased gas exchange by the first or second breath. In the normal individual, the arterial P_{O_2} is unchanged even in severe exercise, which suggests that the factor limiting the exercise is not pulmonary ventilation. There is, however, a progressive decrease in venous O_2 saturation (Fig. 12.1) and, therefore, an increasing (A-V)o_2 difference, indicating a heightened extraction of O_2 by the tissues. The O_2 extraction, which is greater in congestive failure patients at similar work loads, is sometimes used as a rough index of decreased cardiac output in cardiac decompensation.

Important changes occur in blood chemistry. Because of the intense metabolic activity in the active muscles, the P_{CO_2}, H^+ ion concentration and blood temperature are all considerably increased in the tissues; this results in a shift of the HbO_2 dissociation curve to the right, which facilitates the release of O_2 to the tissues. The accumulation in muscle of certain metabolites, $e.g.$, K^+, lactic acid and H^+ ions, during exhausting exercise is thought to be the main factor responsible for local discomfort, muscle pain and fatigue. The increase in blood lactate reflects the anaerobic breakdown of glucose necessary to maintain the exercise; the capacity to develop an O_2 debt is important in achieving maximal work.

Both aerobic (oxidative) and anaerobic (nonoxidative) metabolism contribute to the production of ATP necessary for muscle contraction. Muscle work that requires an energy expenditure greater than that which can be supplied by the ongoing oxidative processes is termed anaerobic; this situation prevails at the onset and during the intensive stages of exercise, $i.e.$, those which exceed 50 to 60% $\dot{V}_{O_{2max}}$. This level is referred to as the "anaerobic" or "ventilatory" threshold. The lactic acid and other metabolites that accumulate during anaerobic exercise represent an oxygen debt that must be repaid during recovery in order to restore the metabolic system. Within the muscle there is, with exercise, increased glycogenolysis with increased production and release of pyruvate and lactate, increased lipolysis of muscle triglycerides and increased free fatty acid (FFA) oxidation. For sustained exercise, the muscles are supplied with increased glucose and FFA by the liver and adipose tissue. The sympathetic nervous system and various hormones (particularly insulin and glucagon) are importantly concerned with metabolic regulation.

Plasma catecholamines increase markedly depending on the intensity of the exercise and the active muscle mass involved. This is a reflection of the sympathetic hyperactivity that is characteristic of the exercise response. Plasma levels of epinephrine may increase 3- to 4-fold and norepinephrine levels 5- to 7-fold in intensive exercise. The plasma catecholamines increase only slowly during submaximal exercise but when approaching $\dot{V}_{O_{2max}}$ rise steeply. Plasma renin activity and plasma levels of vasopressin are also increased. During exercise there is an enhancement of blood coagulability and fibrinolytic activity, which is thought to be either a part of a nonspecific sympathetic response to stress or a "pseudo-immune" response.

The limitation to maximal aerobic exercise performance does not lie in the respiratory system but in the transport of O_2 to the tissues and removal of CO_2 and waste products. The specific limitation is either in the limited CO or in the enzymatic capabilities of the muscle tissue itself to extract the oxygen.

Exercise Stress Tests

The use of exercise as a screening test in cardiac disease has grown enormously in the last 10 years and has become common procedure in cardiovascular medicine. The primary purposes are (a) to reveal latent ischemic heart disease and (b) to determine the functional capacity of the circulatory system.

While there are numerous test procedures, the most common in the United States is a prescribed treadmill test with progressive levels of physical work, designed to bring the subject to his limit of work capacity. Within narrow limits, each work level requires a specific O_2 uptake per kg body weight per min; thus $\dot{V}_{O_{2max}}$ may be estimated from the stage of the test at which the subject reaches his highest work level (Fig. 12.5). For example, if the subject is forced to stop at the end of the third stage of the Bruce test, *i.e.*, at 3.4 mph at a 14% grade (Fig. 12.5) his $\dot{V}_{O_{2max}}$ will be about 35 ml O_2/kg/min which is about average for middle-aged sedentary American men. Within such a group (of sedentary healthy subjects or functional class I patients), a $\dot{V}_{O_{2max}}$ of 42 ml O_2/kg/min would be an above-average fitness level (Fig. 12.5). As previously mentioned, $\dot{V}_{O_2}$ and heart rate are closely related so that an alternate method to express physical fitness would be the work level at which the subject attains his "target HR."

Each individual has a definable HR_{max}, which declines progressively with age. The average HR_{max}, which is about 190 to 200/min at age 20, will decrease to about 165/min at age 60. By setting the mean age-predicted HR_{max} (or 90% of HR_{max}) as a reasonable end-point or "target" HR, it can be determined if the individual can achieve a normal, or near normal, HR_{max}, *i.e.*, has a normal or near normal work capacity.

The presence of cardiac disease is not always easy to distinguish from poor physical condition. Coronary disease is suggested by inability to achieve maximum HR, by abnormal increase in arterial pressure during exercise, by high values of the (A-V)$_{O_2}$ difference or by unusually high levels of plasma catecholamines for the exercise level achieved.

FUNCTIONAL CLASS	CLINICAL STATUS	O₂REQUIREMENTS ml O₂/kg/min	STEP TEST NAGLE, BALKE, NAUGHTON* 2 min stages 30 steps/min	TREADMILL BRUCE† 3-min stages mph %gr	BICYCLE ERGOMETER** For 70 kg body weight kgm/min
NORMAL AND I	PHYSICALLY ACTIVE SUBJECTS	52.5			
		49.0			
		45.5	Height (cm)	4.2 16	1500
		42.0	40		1350
		38.5	36		1200
	SEDENTARY HEALTHY	35.0	32	3.4 14	1050
		31.5	28		900
		28.0	24		
	DISEASED, RECOVERED	24.5	20	2.5 12	750
II		21.0	16		600
	SYMPTOMATIC PATIENTS	17.5	12	1.7 10	450
		14.0	8		300
III		10.5	4		150
		7.0			
IV		3.5			

Figure 12.5. Oxygen requirements (ml/kg/min) at different stages of three standard physical stress tests, *i.e.*, step test, Bruce treadmill test and bicycle ergometer test. The maximum work level achieved defines the $V_{O_{2max}}$. The left hand columns show functional classification of normal subjects or patients. (*, from F.S. Nagle, B. Balke, and J.P. Naughton. Gradational step tests for assessing work capacity. *J Appl Physiol* 20:745–748, 1965; †, from R.A. Bruce. Multi-stage treadmill test of submaximal and maximal exercise: Appendix B, *Exercise Testing and Training of Apparently Healthy Individuals: A Physician's Handbook.* American Heart Association, 1972; **, from S.M. Fox, J.P. Naughton, and W. L. Haskell. Physical activity and the prevention of coronary heart disease. *Ann Clin Res* 3:404, 1971. Figure reprinted with permission from *Exercise Testing and Training of Apparently Healthy Individuals: A Handbook for Physicians.* American Heart Association, 1972.)

However, much more specific evidence for ischemic heart disease is the characteristic anginal pain (described in Chapter 14) or a 1-mm or more displacement of the S-T segment on the exercise ECG. Even these signs, while highly suggestive, are not absolute since in both cases false positives or false negatives may occur in 10 to 15% of the cases. As shown in Figure 12.6, S-T displacement of 1 mm or more occurs in a high percentage of patients with angina but also in a significant percentage of the normal population.

One difficulty in the diagnosis of coronary disease (particularly milder disease) is that a degree of coronary sclerosis as well as some decrease in cardiac functional ability is inherent with normal aging. In this regard, Bruce and coworkers have suggested that the response alterations in maximal exercise caused by cardiovascular disease and those attributable to aging can be separated by comparison with age-predicted values for healthy subjects. Deviations from the predicted norm in HR_{max} would suggest deficiencies in $\dot{V}O_{2max}$, *i.e.*, work capacity; deviations in systolic pressure-HR (double) product values would suggest myocardial $\dot{V}O_2$ or left ventricular deficiencies (Chapter 11). Residual differences between these two values would represent peripheral circulatory impairment. These investigators have found this approach useful in separating a deficiency in circulatory delivery of oxygen into left ventricular and peripheral components.

Figure 12.6. S-T segment displacement in myocardial ischemia. *Left*, prevalence of S-T segment depression after maximal exercise in normal subjects (*N*), patients with healed myocardial infarcts (*MI*) and patients with angina pectoris (*AP*). Note the relative independence of age in angina patients but age dependence in other groups. *Right*, types of S-T changes in exercise: *A*, normal ECG; *B*, false junctional J depression due to atrial T wave; *C*, true junctional S-T depression; *D*, S-T downslope segment depression. (Reprinted with permission from E. Simonson, *Physiology of Work Capacity and Fatigue*. Springfield, Ill.: Charles C Thomas, 1971.)

A report on a five-year extensive exercise screening study in Seattle indicated four variables that were significantly associated with subsequent primary coronary heart disease events: (a) chest pain during maximal exertion; (b) duration of exercise of less than 6 minutes on the Bruce protocol; (c) a failure to attain at least 90% of the age-predicted maximal heart rate; and (d) ischemic S-T depression on the ECG.

Static (Isometric) Exercise

In static (isometric) exercise, the energy expenditure is small compared to dynamic (isotonic) work, but the hemodynamic changes are equally pronounced. Experimentally, static exercise is often induced through maintenance of a sustained handgrip contraction at 30% of maximum voluntary tension to fatigue, which for most subjects is about 4 to 7 minutes. The sustained contraction calls forth a powerful cardiovascular reflex which results in a marked increase in both systolic and diastolic pressure.

If the responses to dynamic and static exercises are contrasted, it will be seen that in both cases there are large increases in systolic pressure; however, in dynamic exercise the increase in HR is much greater and

Figure 12.7. Hemodynamic response to static and dynamic exercise. Note in dynamic exercise the much greater rise in heart rate and pulse pressure. (Reprinted with permission from A.R. Lind and G.W. McNicol, *Can Med Assoc J* 96:706, 1967.)

the response of diastolic pressure much less (Fig. 12.7). Pushing, lifting or carrying weights can elicit a hemodynamic reflex similar to the standard isometric test; *e.g.*, carrying or holding a 20-kg suitcase for 2½ minutes can induce a systolic blood pressure increase of about 45 mm Hg, a diastolic rise of about 30 mm Hg and a HR increase of about 24 beats/min. Because of the pronounced increase in diastolic pressure and therefore of afterload, static exercise greatly increases myocardial O_2 demand and therefore is commonly responsible for inciting precordial pain in angina patients.

Isometric exercise has been used as a myocardial stress test during cardiac catheterization; patients with cardiac disease but with normal ventricular function at rest, often develop ventricular pressure and wall motion abnormalities during static exercise which help to uncover latent myocardial disease.

At lower muscle tensions (30 to 40% of maximum), the blood flow to the contracting muscles is increased but at higher tensions (70% or more) the blood flow is stopped by the muscle compression. Blood flow in the exercising muscle is a compromise between the metabolically induced vasodilation and the compression of the blood vessels by the contracting muscles.

The arterial pressure increase during static exercise is due mainly to the increase in CO, which in turn is due primarily to the increase in HR. This is particularly true during strenuous static exercise when the intrathoracic pressure increase—associated with the exercise effort—impedes venous return and therefore stroke volume (Chapter 13, Valsalva Maneuver). The degree of blood pressure response is dependent on several factors but mainly on the intensity of exercise and the amount of muscle mass involved. A sustained level of 50% maximal voluntary contraction (MVC) will elicit a greater blood pressure response than a 30% MVC (Fig. 12.8).

The circulatory response to static exercise involves both central and peripheral mechanisms. The cerebral or "central command" factor is a direct effect of the motor cortex on medullary CV centers. The blood pressure increase is partially related to the intensity of the "command," *i.e.*, the subjective effort exerted, which probably affects the number of motor units recruited. The peripheral mechanisms involved are the somatic afferent fibers which activate the exercise pressor response similar to that in dynamic exercise. In static exercise there may be additional peripheral reflex factors initiated by metabolic or chemical agents, *e.g.*, K^+ ions, liberated in the muscle tissues.

In static exercise—as in dynamic exercise—plasma catecholamines and blood lactate levels are elevated.

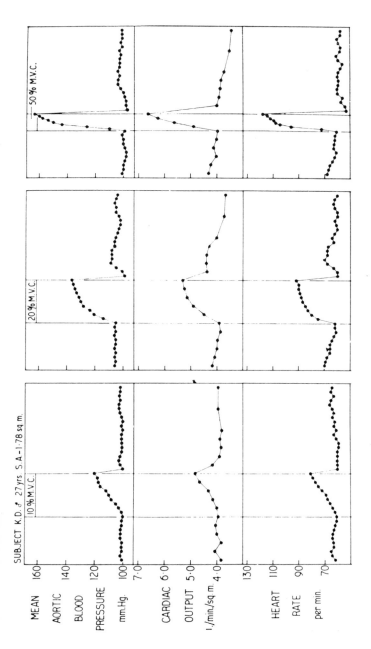

Figure 12.8. Hemodynamic response to sustained handgrip contraction. Mean aortic blood pressure, cardiac output and heart rate before, during and after different degrees of contractile tension, *i.e.*, 10, 20, and 50% of maximum voluntary contraction. The degree of tension is the main factor which significantly influences the hemodynamic response. (Reprinted with permission from A.R. Lind, S.H. Taylor, P.O. Humphreys, B.M. Kennelly, and K.W. Donald, *Clin Sci* 27:229, 1964.)

Physical Training

General

Repeated physical exercise will induce significant training effects that markedly alter the body's ability to perform work. A minimum regimen necessary to achieve such effects would involve large muscle masses continuously for at least 20 to 30 minutes, in two to three exercise sessions per week at 60% $\dot{V}O_{2max}$ for a minimum period of 8 to 10 weeks. In addition to frequency, intensity of effort is also an important determinant of the degree of training achieved. Many studies on normal people, trained athletes and animals trained to exercise, have indicated that during such "conditioning" important metabolic and circulatory adaptations are made. The changes are most marked in young adults who start training at a low fitness level. There is currently widespread interest in physical training effects with particular reference to their possible preventive and therapeutic role in certain cardiovascular disorders, especially ischemic heart disease.

British investigators in the 1950s were the first to suggest a link between exercise and heart disease when they reported fewer heart attacks in those who walked rather than remained seated on the job, *e.g.*, bus conductors vs. bus drivers and postmen vs. sedentary postal workers. Subsequent studies of large populations have shown that activity which burns about 300 calories/day—the equivalent of an hour's brisk walk—results in a markedly lowered chance for an initial heart attack, *i.e.*, such activity is effective in primary prevention. Some investigators believe that more strenuous exercise will result in even greater reduction of risk for an initial heart attack, but this is as yet not proven. The role of exercise in prevention of subsequent attacks (secondary prevention) is not yet established.

Certainly exercise physiology has emerged as one of the most important fields of study of our time. It is obvious that the human body was never meant to be sedentary and coping with the results of sedentary living poses some of the greatest health problems of our day.

Cardiovascular Changes

The enhanced ability to perform physical work is particularly evidenced by substantial increases in $\dot{V}O_{2max}$ as well as lesser accumulation of blood lactate (Fig. 12.9). The rise in $\dot{V}O_{2max}$ is due mainly to the elevation in CO (usually about 20 to 25%) and only to a limited extent to an increase in the $(A-V)O_2$ difference. The increased CO is facilitated by the decreased vascular resistance which is an important facet of the training response. There is an inverse relationship between the $\dot{V}O_{2max}$ and systemic peripheral resistance. At the same work load, the "conditioned" individual will have a lesser HR and a more rapid post-exercise

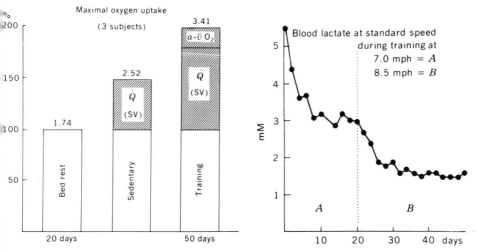

Figure 12.9. Effect of physical training on VO_{2max} (L/min) and blood lactate (mM/L) during exercise. *Left*, comparison of VO_{2max} of normal subjects after 20 days of bed rest, while sedentary and after 50 days of physical training. *Right*, progressive decrease of blood lactate for a standard exercise: *A*, during first 20 days of training, and *B*, during next 30 days of training. (Reprinted with permission from P. Astrand and K. Rodahl, *Textbook of Work Physiology*. New York: McGraw-Hill, 1977.)

HR recovery; however, his HR_{max} is usually unaffected. With training, stroke volume (SV) will be increased at rest and at both submaximal and maximal exercise. In a recent study, Paulsen et al. found that, compared with sedentary controls, trained runners also had lower rate-pressure (HR × systolic pressure) products at rest and during submaximal exercise.

There are significant differences in cardiac effects depending on the type of physical training. In endurance training (long distance runners, cyclists and rowers), there is an increase in heart volume due mainly to an increase in size of the cardiac cavities and to a lesser extent to an increase in muscle mass. There is an increase in SV/heart volume ratio and an increase in ejection fraction (EF). In power training (weight lifters, shot putters, hammer throwers), there is an increase in LV wall thickness, *i.e.*, a concentric hypertrophy similar to that seen in early hypertension. The increase in wall thickness is at the expense of volume so that end-diastolic volume is either decreased or unchanged in relation to body weight. In power athletes, there is a decrease in SV/heart volume ratio and in EF. Reports indicate no myocardial damage in either type of training.

There are conflicting reports on the effects of physical training on arterial blood pressure. Endurance athletes usually have a lower systolic pressure at rest and at various levels of exercise. The fit subject often has a lower diastolic pressure during exercise, probably as a manifestation of his greater ability to decrease the peripheral vascular resistance of the arterioles in his exercising muscles. There is some evidence, as yet only fragmentary, that prolonged physical training will reduce arterial blood pressure in hypertensive patients.

Animal studies have indicated that prolonged physical conditioning will result in increased myocardial fiber mass, increased capillary/fiber ratio, improved myocardial contractility and increased coronary artery size. The cardiac hypertrophy of the human endurance athlete also occurs in the physically trained animal, and with it there is improved hemodynamic performance. The evidence on the formation of new collateral vessels in the myocardium is conflicting; however, one definitive study indicates that the effect of ischemia on opening new capillaries is enhanced in the physically trained heart, suggesting that training plays at least an adjunctive role in promoting new capillary formation. It is, however, very significant that almost all of the above training effects occurred mainly in young animals and only to a very limited extent in older ones, suggesting that physical training, if it is to have lasting effects, might have to be started at an early age.

Systemic Responses to Training

With physical training, adaptive changes occur in many other bodily systems. Cardiac myoglobin and plasma hemoglobin both increase; the latter increase correlates well with the increase in $\dot{V}_{O_{2max}}$. Conversely, athletes with suboptimal Hb levels do not perform well in endurance events. However, sustained intensive physical training has itself been shown to induce a mild, transient "sports anemia," which usually subsides in several days. While there is disagreement among investigators, some reports indicate that endurance training may result in a decrease in plasma triglycerides and an increase in plasma high-density lipoprotein levels. Some reports have associated these changes with a lesser risk for ischemic heart disease. In addition, physical training, especially in the obese subject, reduces body weight and body fat percentage, increases lean body mass, and causes a general reduction in the "fat envelope."

The levels of plasma norepinephrine (NE) at rest and at same relative work loads (*i.e.*, at the same percentage of $\dot{V}_{O_{2max}}$) are unchanged with physical training. However, the increase in plasma NE at the same absolute work load is much less after training, which indicates a lesser sympathetic response for the same exercise level.

It has been reported that physical training also has psychological manifestations. Some studies have shown that physical fitness can attenuate emotional stress, reduce anxiety and improve social adjustment. However, only limited data is available on this question. In some endurance athletes, a euphorialike state, sometimes called a "runner's high," occurs after distance runs. Other reports indicate a diminished sensitivity to pain after endurance events and on occasion have termed distance running as a "near addiction." It has been theorized that such subjective sensations may be due to the liberation of endorphins, which are amino acid complexes released by the CNS or pituitary gland and transported to specific CNS or peripheral sites. It is believed that endorphins react with opiate receptors located within the brain and play an important role in pain modulation, sleep and stress reactions. Farrell et al. have recently reported a 2- to 5-fold increase in plasma β-endorphins after a strenuous 30-minute treadmill run in endurance athletes. However, mood state and perceptual data showed no significant relationship to the β-endorphin levels so that the role of endorphins in these psychological alterations remains speculative.

Cross Adaptation and Detraining

As indicated above, there is abundant evidence that repeated vigorous, endurance-type exercise will greatly increase cardiac output, lower resting heart rate and blood pressure, decrease body fat and improve musculoskeletal function. Some studies have indicated that physical training will lessen the risk of ischemic heart disease (IHD). But does physical fitness improve general resistance to the physical inroads of stress and disease, *e.g.*, IHD, when these occur? The answer to this interesting question is not known and investigations of this type are still in their early phases.

A few preliminary studies have indicated some degree of cross adaptation to physical training. During generalized hypoxia, *e.g.*, physically trained rats maintained significantly greater cardiac output and cardiac work performance than untrained rats even though O_2 delivery and lactate production were similar: the trained animals were capable of more efficient energy utilization for external cardiac work. Physical training also improves heat tolerance; rats that were treadmill-trained in a cool environment performed better on a work-heat tolerance test and suffered less tissue damage than untrained animals. Physically trained human subjects also have better circulatory adaptation to heat.

German investigators, on the other hand, have reported postural intolerance in some endurance athletes, *i.e.*, a lesser resistance to gravity stresses such as head-up tilt after prolonged water immersion. The mechanism of this effect is not certain but may be due to a lesser baroceptor sensitivity or to a sluggish cardioaccelerator response in the athletes.

The mechanisms for the above-described "training effects," particularly the increase in $\dot{V}O_{2max}$, are not certain but are probably due to a combination of an increased oxygen delivery to the muscles (mainly increase in CO) and an increase in the size and number of muscle mitochondria (*i.e.*, increased oxidative capacity of the muscle cell). It is interesting, however, that one training effect, *viz.*, bradycardia, if achieved with repetitive exercise of certain large muscle groups, is operative only when the same trained muscles were used and did not occur with exercise involving the untrained muscles. These findings would suggest that peripheral mechanisms were involved and that cross adaptation was minimal.

Detraining or deconditioning of the trained endurance athlete is rapid, *i.e.*, it will occur within about 12 to 20 weeks after cessation of exercise training. Bed rest, which will induce even more rapid deconditioning, will cause a substantial decrease in $\dot{V}O_{2max}$ (Fig. 12.9), shortening of exercise endurance time, and decreases in plasma volume within 2 to 3 weeks. Bed rest or exposure to zero gravity eliminate the usual relocation of venous blood to the dependent veins in the sitting or standing position. Plasma volume then tends to accumulate in the thoracic veins. A hypovolemia of 15 to 25% may result from the diuresis induced by the continued effect of this increased central blood volume on the cardiopulmonary "volume" receptors (Chapter 10). The detraining effect in these situations is also due to decreased muscle activity with a consequent diminution of muscle mass, *i.e.*, a "disuse atrophy."

Clinical Application of Physical Training

Most patients who have undergone physical training after their myocardial infarct (MI) can achieve performance levels at least equivalent to that of normal, sedentary subjects; however, the response to training is sometimes restricted in patients with more extensive infarcts, presumably because of reduced myocardial function. After physical training, MI patients will have decreased body fat and plasma triglycerides compared to nontrained control patients. In other studies performed after 8 weeks of training, MI patients performed subanginal work loads at lesser rate-pressure product levels, *i.e.*, with a lesser increase in myocardial O_2 consumption. One group of IHD patients who exercised intensively for more than one year developed a capacity for endurance exercise equal to that of trained normal subjects; these patients equaled the normal subjects in running endurance, in spite of a lower $\dot{V}O_{2max}$, by developing a higher lactate threshold. It is thus evident that some post-MI patients with limited $\dot{V}O_{2max}$ can undergo training adaptations enabling them to maintain close to a metabolic steady state during exercise that elicits $\dot{V}O_{2max}$.

The obvious beneficial effects of supervised physical exercise for coronary patients has prompted increased efforts to provide the much needed physical rehabilitation programs for such patients. It is now evident that in the case of many coronary patients, their ability to achieve a well-adjusted and productive future life will largely depend on a well-planned and well-executed physical training rehabilitation program (Chapter 14, Cardiac Rehabilitation).

Effects of Aging

Aging and the Circulation—General

There are currently about 28 million Americans over 65 years of age—more than 11% of the population. In this group, cardiovascular disease is the most frequent cause of hospitalization and death. Not only does the incidence of cardiovascular disease increase steeply with age but there is also (as mentioned previously) a striking similarity between the effects of age *per se* and early coronary heart disease. This sometimes poses a serious problem in differential diagnosis and makes it particularly important to establish norms for cardiovascular function in the aged before reaching conclusions regarding cardiovascular pathology.

At rest there are only minor changes in cardiac function with age. However, with exercise, older individuals show significant differences in their circulatory responsiveness. In adults, $\dot{V}O_{2max}$ tends to be highest at about age 27 and, thereafter, steadily decreases by about 1% per year so that at age 65 it is about 60% of the former value (Fig. 12.10).

A recent study has shown that sedentary young men have about 30% greater $\dot{V}O_{2max}$ than sedentary young women but the rate of decline with age was significantly greater in the men than in the women. The sedentary young men also had higher HR_{max}, cardiac index$_{max}$ and stroke index$_{max}$ values than the young women, but again (except in the case of the SI) the rate of decrease was greater in the sedentary men. The decline of $\dot{V}O_{2max}$ is also more rapid in the obese and in the smoker.

A number of physiological and psychological studies have separated the elderly population into the young-old (65–75 years) and the old-old (over 75 years) on the basis of degree and rate of the changes. Geriatrics, the systematic study of aging, is presently in its very early stage, and the following outline of the physiological alterations with age is based on a brief survey of the limited data available.

Circulatory System—Structural Changes

During aging there are a number of cardiopulmonary structural changes that have far-reaching physiological consequences. The decreased arterial distensibility and venous compliance with age (Chapter

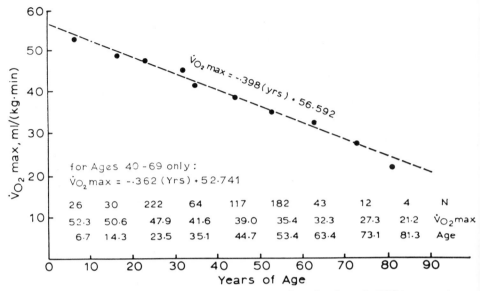

Figure 12.10. Regression of mean Vo_{2max} per decade of age in 700 boys and men, corrected for body weight showing a steady decline of oxygen uptake during maximal exercise with advancing age. (Reprinted with permission from M.M. Dehn and R.A. Bruce, *J Appl Physiol* 33:805, 1972.)

1) occurs in both man and animals and is related to a progressive increase in the collagen/elastin ratio of the vessel wall. There is increasing stiffness of the aorta and large arteries in both a radial and longitudinal direction as determined by pressure-volume curves (Fig. 1.7).

This arterial rigidity is the result of a diffuse process involving the replacement of elastin with connective tissue; the result is due to an alteration of the viscoelastic properties of the wall at large and not to atherosclerosis, which is generally a patchy and irregular process. While (as mentioned in Chapter 1) the increase in aortic volume, especially after age 60, provides some hemodynamic buffering, this is quite inadequate to offset the marked compliance changes. An arterial volume change, which induces a pressure of 100 mm Hg is, at age 70, only about one-half that at age 20 (Fig. 1.7).

The decreased aortic distensibility along with the increased peripheral resistance of the arterial bed serve to increase the mechanical impedance of the aortic bed and impose a heavier afterload on the aging left ventricle. This increased impedance to ejection is very likely an important factor in limiting the increase in left ventricular stroke volume (LVSV) during exercise in the older subject. Associated with the increased aortic impedance there is also an increase in left ventricular chamber size. The limited data available thus far indicates a decreased

LV compliance, which could be a significant factor in limiting both LV end-diastolic volume and the Starling response. There is also in older subjects increased stiffness of the heart valves and pericardium that may exert a functional handicap.

As Kenney has pointed out, aside from the alterations in the cardio-vascular system, each step in the path O_2 takes from the outer air to the metabolizing cell is vulnerable to aging. The pulmonary alveoli become smaller and more shallow so there is a steady decline in vital capacity and about a 20% decrease in alveolar surface area by age 70. There is a decrease in pulmonary elastic recoil and lung compliance, and because of the stiffened rib cage there is increasing reliance on diaphragmatic breathing. Since skeletal muscle typically shows prolonged contraction and relaxation periods, all the timed, ventilatory functions are slower.

The alveolar-arterial O_2 difference is increased with age. Although Hb concentration is maintained in the healthy older person, there is a small alteration in RBC metabolism and a resultant decreased concentration of 2,3-diphosphoglycerate. As a consequence, there is a shift of the HbO_2 dissociation curve to the left thereby making the tissue unloading of O_2 more difficult.

Age Effect on Circulation at Rest

A number of studies have shown that in addition to the decline in $\dot{V}O_{2max}$ there is, in older individuals, a gradual decline in resting values of cardiac index (CI), stroke index (SI) and (A-V)O_2 difference. There is generally a steady rise in systolic and diastolic pressure (Fig. 6.5) and in peripheral vascular resistance. With left ventricular hypertrophy there is a slowing of left ventricular contraction and relaxation and a prolongation of left ventricular ejection time (Fig. 12.11). The distribution of the diminished cardiac output is not an equitable one. Cerebral and coronary blood flow change little with age but renal and splanchnic flow decrease significantly.

It should be pointed out that the cardiovascular changes described above were average findings from large samplings of different age populations. Chronological age does not always parallel physiological age and there frequently are wide individual differences in functional capability. These may occur both at rest and during exercise in individuals of the same age and will depend mainly upon physical condition and hereditary, dietary and environmental factors.

Age Effect on Exercise Response

While the above structural changes impose relatively little handicap to the normal, older individual at rest, circulatory stresses such as exercise will uncover the depth of the physiological reserve and will

Figure 12.11. Structural changes in the rat heart during senescence. Left ventricular weight (relative to tibial length) (LVW/TL), myocardial contraction duration (CD) and ventricular wall stiffness, *i.e.*, Δ stress/Δ length (a_A) do not increase over adult life up to about 16 months. Thereafter, all parameters increase progressively (tibial length is one of the standards used for normal growth). (Reprinted with permission from E.G. Lakatta, Age-related changes in rat cardiac muscle. In: *Biological Markers of Aging*, edited by M.E. Reff and E.L. Schneider. Bethesda, Md: NIH Publication No. 82–22, USDHHS, USPHS, 1981, pp. 57–66.)

reveal significant functional deficiencies with increasing age. As mentioned above, beginning at about age 25, dynamic work capacity (*i.e.*, $\dot{V}O_{2max}$ per unit body weight) decreases steadily with age. Older men and women respond to exercise with progressively lesser increases in HR, SI, CI and (A-V)O_2 differences and greater increases in systolic pressure.

It has been consistently observed that in man, peripheral resistance at rest and at comparable work loads is increased with age and that in exercise there is a lesser dilator capability of vascular smooth muscle. It is also significant that during exercise the elderly have elevated pulmonary arterial wedge pressures and increased right ventricular end-diastolic pressure, suggesting a diminished reserve capacity in older hearts. While younger individuals usually respond to exercise with an increased ejection fraction (EF), a recent report has shown that there was a progressive decline in the LVEF response to exercise with age and further that there was also an increasing frequency of myocardial wall motion abnormalities in patients 50 years and older. Generally, the attainment of steady-state levels of HR, blood pressure and ventilatory responses are slower and the rate of recovery more prolonged with increasing age. Translated into practical terms, this would mean that the quantity of work that can be performed during a given work period is reduced in the aged and that more frequent or prolonged rest periods may be needed.

The reason for this diminishing myocardial performance in the elderly is not certain. It may be associated with (a) increased aortic impedance and the afterload limitations it imposes on LV ejection, (b) decreased responsiveness of the Frank-Starling mechanism (*i.e.*, a preload deficiency), or (c) decreased myocardial contractility, perhaps due to diminished sympathetic response of cardiac muscle, which has been shown to occur in animals. Some reports have indicated that these functional hemodynamic changes may be arrested or delayed by a well-planned program of physical training. Other investigators have expressed doubts about the degree of improvement to be expected in older subjects during training. The bulk of evidence indicates, however, that systematic and consistent physical training will result in lesser increases in VO_2, CO, SV and $(A\text{-}V)O_2$ difference at any given work level in a great majority of older subjects as well as in the other favorable adaptive changes described in the section on physical training.

Autonomic Responsiveness and Aging

As described above, the older individual generally has an impaired response to physical exercise that is associated with a heightened aortic impedance, a decreased myocardial performance and an inadequate peripheral circulatory response. It is not certain, however, to what extent these pathophysiological manifestations are due to anatomical deficiencies, defective autonomic reflexes or insufficient neurohumoral stimulation.

Autonomic stress tests in normal subjects of different ages have shown a lesser rise in heart rate and in diastolic pressure in the older subjects during head-up tilt and lesser heart rate increments to the standard Valsalva test. Whether the defect lies in the afferent or efferent limb of the autonomic reflex or in a higher integrating CNS center is not certain. Studies in animals and man indicate that the arterial baroceptors may become less sensitive with advancing age (Fig. 12.12). It has been suggested that this decreased baroceptor sensitivity may be due to increased rigidity of the aorta and carotid arteries which would result in lesser deformation of the receptors and less stimulation for equivalent pressure changes.

There have been consistent findings of increased plasma NE levels in older individuals both at rest and in response to standard stresses such as exercise or upright posture. However, there is apparently no effect of

Figure 12.12. Effect of age on baroreflex sensitivity indicating a progressive fall in the sensitivity index (pulse interval/Δ systolic pressure) with increasing age in both normotensives and hypertensives. (Reprinted with permission from B. Gribbin, T.G. Pickering, P. Sleight, and R. Peto, *Circ Res* 39:424, 1971.)

age on plasma epinephrine response, which might suggest a selective age effect on certain neurohormonal pathways.

Animal studies have shown decreased responsiveness of myocardial tissue and decreased heart rate response to β-adrenergic stimulation with increased age. This effect may be due to a diminution of β-adrenergic binding sites in the tissue.

As mentioned previously, there is some evidence (albeit limited) that the diminished performance of the left ventricle may be due to an age-related decrease in myocardial contractility. This would seem to be substantiated by the lesser response of the myocardium to β-adrenergic agonists in animal experiments. However, the important question as to whether this decreased response is due to a deficiency of neural receptor-impulse transmission mechanism or to an inherent weakness of the myocardial muscle cell itself is still unresolved.

Aging and the Circulation—Summary

From a review of available evidence it appears that from an aging standpoint, the heart and blood vessels are highly dependent for their normal function on the physical properties of distensibility, contractility and elasticity, all of which involve connective tissue as well as muscle. With increasing age there is an increasing ratio of collagen to muscle. A significant feature is that the collagen itself changes character and becomes cross-linked with calcium deposits and is thus less compliant. As a result of the anatomical and physiological changes, there are (a) a heightened aortic impedance with an increased work load on the left ventricle, and (b) a less distensible myocardium that has longer contraction and relaxation periods. Functionally these changes are associated with (c) a steadily decreasing work capacity ($\dot{V}O_{2max}$), the rate of decrease being heavily dependent on individual factors such as physical training and obesity. The decreasing work capacity is, in turn, associated with (d) an altered hemodynamic response to exercise. In particular, there is a decreased HR_{max}, SV_{max} and CO_{max} with increasing end-diastolic and arterial blood pressure.

In the healthy human subject, the structural changes that occur with normal aging produce little or no functional handicap at rest and only a minor handicap at moderate work levels in normal, physically fit elderly persons. In the healthy older subject, the main circulatory effect of the structural and physiological changes is a reduction of hemodynamic reserve and a lesser ability to cope with supervening environmental stress.

References

Exercise and Physical Training

American Heart Association: *Exercise Testing and Training of Apparently Healthy Individuals: A Physician's Handbook*, 1972.

Amsterdam EA, Wilmore JH, and DeMaria AN. *Exercise in Cardiovascular Health and Disease.* New York: Yorke Medical Books, 1977.

Astrand P and Rodahl K. *Textbook of Work Physiology*, New York: McGraw-Hill, 1977, 2nd ed.

Blomqvist CG. Cardiovascular adaptations to physical training. *Annu Rev Physiol* 45:169–189, 1983.

Bruce RA, Fisher LD, Cooper MN, and Gey GO. Separation of effects of cardiovascular disease and age on ventricular function with maximal exercise. *Am J Cardiol* 34:757–763, 1974.

Bruce RA, DeRouen TA, and Hossack KF. Value of maximal exercise tests in risk assessment of primary coronary heart disease events in healthy man. *Am J Cardiol* 46:371–378, 1980.

Christensen NJ and Galbo H. Sympathetic nervous activity during exercise. *Annu Rev Physiol* 45:139–153, 1983.

Convertino VA, Sandler H, Webb P, and Annis JF. Induced venous pooling and cardiorespiratory responses to exercise after bed rest. *J Appl Physiol* 52(5):1343–1348, 1982.

Coyle EF, Martin WH, Ehsani AA, Hagberg JM, Bloomfield SA, Sinacore DR, and Holloszy JO. Blood lactate threshold in some well-trained ischemic heart disease patients. *J Appl Physiol* 54(1):18–23, 1983.

Farrell PA and Barboriak J. The time course of alterations in plasma lipid and lipoprotein concentrations during eight weeks of endurance training. *Atherosclerosis* 37:231–238, 1980.

Farrell PA, Gates WK, Maksud MG, and Morgan WP. Increases in plasma β-endorphin/β-lipotropin immunoreactivity after treadmill running in humans. *J Appl Physiol* 52(5):1245–1249, 1982.

Froelicher VF. Techniques of exercise training. In: *The Heart, Arteries and Veins.* New York: McGraw-Hill, 1982, 5th ed., pp. 1726–1733.

Fruth JM and Gisolfi CV. Work-heat tolerance in endurance-trained rats. *J Appl Physiol* 54(1):249–253, 1983.

Hyers TM, Martin BJ, Pratt DS, Dreisin RB, and Franks JJ. Enhanced thrombin and plasmin activity with exercise in man. *J Appl Physiol* 48(5):821–825, 1980.

Judy WV. Physiology of exercise. In: *Physiology*, edited by EE Selkurt. Boston: Little, Brown, 1976.

Lind AR, and McNicol GW. Local and central responses to sustained muscle contractions and the effect of restricted arterial inflow. *J Physiol* 192:575–593, 1967.

Mark AL, Kioschos JM, Abboud FM, Heistad DP, and Schmid PG. Abnormal vascular responses to exercise in patients with aortic stenosis. *J Clin Invest* 52:1138–1146, 1973.

Mitchell JH, Kaufman MP, and Iwamoto GA. The exercise pressor reflex: its cardiovascular effects, afferent mechanisms and central pathways. *Annu Rev Physiol* 45:229–242, 1983.

Mitchell JH, Blomqvist CG, Lind AR, Saltin B, and Shepherd JT. Static (isometric) exercise: cardiovascular responses and neural control mechanisms. *Circ Res* Part II. 48:I1–I188, 1981.

Moore RL, Reidy M, and Gollwick PD. Effect of training on β-adrenergic receptor number in rat heart. *J Appl Physiol* 52(5):1133–1137, 1982.

Naughton JP, Hellerstein HK, and Mohler IC (eds.). *Exercise Testing and Exercise Training in Coronary Heart Disease*, New York: Academic Press, 1973.

Paulsen W, Boughner DR, Ko P, Cunningham DA, and Persaud JA. Left ventricular function in marathon runners: echocardiographic assessment. *J Appl Physiol* 51(4):881–886, 1981.

Peronnet P, Cleroux J, Perrault H, Cousineau D, deChamplain J, and Nadeau R. Plasma norepinephrine response to exercise before and after training in humans. *J Appl Physiol* 51(4):812–815, 1981.

Radomski MW, Sabiston BH, and Isoard P. Development of "sports anemia" in physically fit men after daily sustained submaximal exercise. *Aviat Space Environ Med* 51(1):41–45, 1980.

Reybrouck T, Heigenhauser GF, and Faulkner JA. Limitations to maximum O_2 uptake in arm, leg and combined arm-leg ergometry. *J Appl Physiol* 38(5):774–779, 1975.

Saltin B and Rowell LB. Functional adaptations to physical activity and inactivity. *Fed Proc* 39:1506–1513, 1980.

Savin NM, Davidson DM, and Haskell WL. Autonomic contribution to heart rate recovery from exercise in humans. *J Appl Physiol* 53(6):1572–1575, 1982.

Scheuer J and Stezoski SW. Effect of physical training on the mechanical and metabolic response of the rat heart to hypoxia. *Circ Res* 30:418–429, 1972.

Schwade JL, Blomqvist CG, and Shapiro W. A comparison of the response to arm and leg work in patients with ischemic heart disease. *Am Heart J* 94(2):203–208, 1977.

Seals DR, Washburn RA, Hanson PG, Painter PL, and Nagle FJ. Increased cardiovascular response to static contraction of larger muscle groups. *J Appl Physiol* 54:434–437, 1983.

Shepherd J. Behavior of resistance and capacity vessels in human limbs during exercise. *Circ Res* 20 and 21 (Suppl. I):70–82, 1967.

Stegemann J, Busert A, and Brock D. Influence of fitness on the blood pressure control system in man. *Aerosp Med* 45:45–48, 1974.

Wenger NK and Hellerstein HK (eds.). *Rehabilitation of the Coronary Patient*. New York: John Wiley & Sons, 1978.

Aging

Bassey EJ. Age, inactivity and some physiological responses to exercise. *Gerontology* 24:66–77, 1978.

Ebert TJ, Hughes CV, Tristani FE, Barney JA, and Smith JJ. The effect of age and coronary heart disease on the circulatory responses to graded lower body negative pressure. *Cardiovasc Res* 16:663–669, 1982.

Hodgson JL and Buskirk ER. Physical fitness and age with emphasis on cardiovascular function in the elderly. *J Am Geriatrics* Sec. 25:385–392, 1977.

Hossack KF and Bruce RA. Maximal cardiac function in sedentary normal men and women: comparison of age-related changes. *J Appl Physiol* 53(4):799–804, 1982.

Kenney RA. *Physiology of Aging: A Synopsis.* Chicago: Year Book Medical Publishers, 1982.

Lakatta EG. Age-related changes in rat cardiac muscle. In: *Biological Markers of Aging,* edited by ME Reff and EL Schneider. Bethesda, Md.: U.S. Department of Health and Human Services, NIH Publication No. 82:2221, 1982, pp. 57–66.

McDermott DJ, Tristani FE, Ebert TJ, Porth CJ, and Smith JJ. Age-related changes in cardiovascular response to diverse circulatory stresses. In: *Arterial Baroceptors and Hypertension,* edited by P Sleight. Oxford: Oxford University Press, 1980, pp. 361–364.

Port S, Cobb FR, Coleman RE, and Jones RH. Effect of age on response of left ventricular ejection fraction to exercise. *New Engl J Med* 303:1133–1137, 1980.

Shephard RJ. *Physical Activity and Aging.* Chicago: Year Book Medical Publishers, 1978.

Strandell T. Circulatory studies on healthy old men. *Acta Med Scand* 175(Suppl. 414): 1–44, 1964.

Weisfeldt ML (ed). *The Aging Heart: Its Function and Response to Stress.* New York: Raven Press, 1980.

Weisfeldt ML. Aging of the cardiovascular system (Editorial). *New Engl J Med* 303:1172–1174, 1980.

chapter 13

Circulatory Response to Nonexercise Stress

Stress is the result of a real or imagined threat to the well-being of the individual; it usually involves the autonomic nervous system and if sufficiently serious, there is activation of the defense center of the hypothalamus with a powerful sympathoadrenal release (Chapter 10). Individuals vary widely in their responses to stress depending upon their age, physical and emotional state and the nature and severity of the stress. The effects of physical exercise, both dynamic and static, as well as the principles of exercise stress testing were discussed in Chapter 12.

In this chapter are included brief descriptions of a few common nonexercise physical stresses and the clinical tests which are sometimes used to simulate them. Because inadequate reactions to such tests are often the first signs of impending disease, compensatory stress responses and their mechanisms will be analyzed.

Postural and Gravity Effects on the Circulation

Normal Postural Responses

For normal man, standing erect presents no problem but an inadequate orthostatic response may be an indication of a serious clinical disturbance. The upright posture requires proper functioning and coordination of the musculoskeletal system, the nervous system and the circulatory system. From a circulatory standpoint the two main elements concerned in postural abnormalities are the skeletal muscle pump and the baroceptor reflexes.

Postural changes are often simulated through use of a tilt table or by "lower body negative pressure"; in the latter procedure, air is evacuated and pressure reduced in a box enclosing the lower body below the iliac crests. These devices produce hemodynamic changes virtually identical to standing erect and have the advantage of facilitating physiological measurements. Investigations have shown that within 10 to 15 seconds after a 70° head-up tilt, there is, in the normal adult, a rapid caudal shift of about 500 to 700 ml of thoracic venous blood; this results in a decrease in venous return (about 20%), stroke volume (about 40%) and cardiac output (about 15–20%). The amount of translocated central venous blood is, therefore, roughly equivalent to that removed for a blood bank donation by a standard phlebotomy (500 ml of blood withdrawal from a peripheral vein). It has been estimated that about 80% of this displaced blood comes from the thoracic (central) blood volume. A typical hemodynamic response pattern to head-up tilt is shown in Figure 13.1.

As the central blood volume and cardiac output decrease and the arterial pressure begins to fall, there is a strong vasoconstriction, particularly of the splanchnic, renal and skeletal muscle beds, with a consequent net rise in total peripheral resistance. The increases in resistance (about 40%) and in heart rate (about 20%) not only maintain but increase the diastolic and mean arterial pressure (about 10%). Systolic pressure shows little or no change.

Although the blood pressure and heart rate changes are fairly consistent among normal individuals of similar age, other parameters show variations; e.g., in some cases blood pressure is maintained with only a small decrease in cardiac output and a modest increase in peripheral resistance; however, in other subjects there is a greater fall in stroke volume and cardiac output and a larger rise in peripheral resistance. The significance of such variations is not known at present.

With prolonged standing, the renal vasoconstriction leads to a pro-

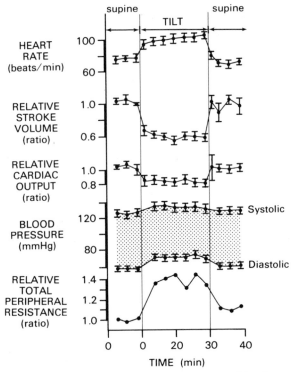

Figure 13.1. Response of normal young men to a 20-minute head-up tilt showing means and standard error of means. Note the prompt increase in heart rate, vascular resistance and diastolic pressure and the decrease in stroke volume, cardiac output and pulse pressure. (Reprinted with permission from J.J. Smith, J.E. Bush, V.T. Wiedmeier, and F.E. Tristani, *J Appl Physiol* 29:133, 1970.)

gressive decrease in renal blood flow and consequently a sharp increase in plasma renin, angiotensin and plasma aldosterone levels—hormonal changes which help to maintain plasma volume. In the upright position there is a 20% decrease in cerebral blood flow and, for reasons which are not clear, a hyperventilation, with a tendency toward hypocapnia; this combination of factors undoubtedly contributes to the 5 to 10% fainting rate usually encountered during prolonged postural tests. Cerebrospinal fluid protects the brain from excessive postural variations in blood flow as discussed in the section on hydrostatic factors and cerebral blood flow (Chapter 11). Within a few minutes of standing, plasma catecholamines are markedly elevated (norepinephrine by about 60 to 80% and epinephrine by about 20 to 30%). Plasma ADH levels increase about 6- to 8-fold.

The cardiac and resistance changes are reflex responses of the arterial and cardiopulmonary baroceptors; curiously enough, venoconstriction is transient and limited. As stated in Chapter 6 (Venous Pressure, Gravity Effect), the upright posture will not alter the pressure gradient between the arterial and venous beds but will increase the transmural pressure in vessels below the heart; *e.g.*, pressure in the foot veins will rise by 80 to 90 mm Hg when standing. As a result there may be an increased transfer of fluid into the interstitial space producing a mild edema of the feet, even in normal individuals, after several hours of standing; heat exaggerates this effect.

The skeletal muscle pump is the primary method of counteracting the tendency toward lower extremity edema during prolonged standing. Although there is little or no venoconstrictor response to the upright position, the progressively increasing muscle content in venous walls from the thigh to the foot probably helps to minimize venous dilation and dependent venous pooling. Patients with varicose veins displace more blood to the lower extremities in the upright position but usually do not have a notable postural intolerance. The total blood volume, which is often increased in varicose vein patients, may exert a partially compensating effect (Chapter 6, Venous Pressure Disturbances).

Reports indicate that in normal young adults, a change from the recumbent to the sitting position will result in diastolic pressure increases of about 90% and heart rate increases of about 55% of those occurring during the change from the recumbent to the upright position. The systolic pressure does not alter significantly in either case.

Autonomic responses are usually diminished with increasing age (section on aging, Chapter 12), which would theoretically lessen postural tolerance. While response to head-up tilt is not significantly altered in normal 50- to 59-year-old subjects, in the elderly, 75 years and older, postural intolerance becomes more common, presumably due to decreased autonomic responses, diminished skeletal muscle pump function, or both.

Abnormal Postural Responses

Decreased tolerance to the upright posture will occur if the skeletal muscle pump effect on venous return is inadequate (Chapter 6) or if the baroceptor reflexes (Chapter 10) are interrupted. As described in the section on fainting (in this chapter), loss or diminution of the muscle pump action may result in severe postural intolerance. Partial or complete loss of sympathetic vasoconstrictor responses may occur (a) in certain systemic diseases such as diabetes or syphilis, (b) in primary idiopathic hypotension, or (c) after administration of α-adrenergic blocking agents. Such patients, upon standing or being tilted, experience a rapid fall in blood pressure and often faint abruptly without the usual premonitory symptoms of pallor, sweating and nausea.

Transient postural hypotension will also occur after prolonged bed

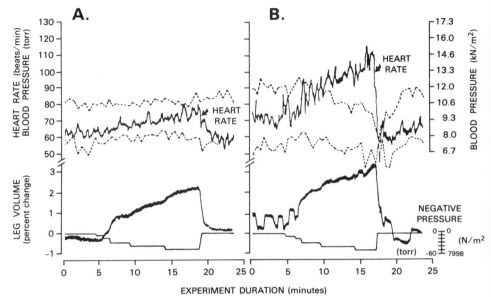

Figure 13.2. Response of Skylab commander to lower body negative pressure test before (*A*) and on 20th day (*B*) of zero gravity. In *B* there is a greater rise in heart rate and decrease in blood pressure during LBNP; with the sudden fall in heart rate, fainting was imminent and the test was discontinued. (Reprinted with permission from R.L. Johnson, G.W. Hoffler, A.E. Nicogossian, S.A. Bergman, and M.M. Jackson, *Third Manned Skylab Mission*, NASA Tech Memo TMX 58154, November, 1974.)

rest, water immersion of 6 hours or longer or exposure to the weightless or zero gravity state (Fig. 13.2). The hypotension in these situations has been attributed to the decreased plasma volume (common in these conditions) and to the lessened gravity effect on the arterial baroceptors. The latter explanation seems less likely since gravity changes affect all parts of the body equally, and theoretically should not influence the arterial stretch induced by internal pressure changes.

Cardiac patients with congestive failure may show increased tolerance to postural stress, and head-up tilt often results in an increased stroke volume and cardiac output associated with relief of dyspnea (Fig. 13.3). It has been suggested that this paradoxical effect may be associated with a leftward shift of the failing heart on the "Starling curve" to relative compensation, permitting an increased stroke volume at lesser filling pressure. Hypertensive patients may show hemodynamic alterations to head-up tilt depending on the stage of their disease. Early hypertensives tend toward orthostatic hypertension while severe hypertensives may have orthostatic hypotension (Chapter 15, Fig. 15.1).

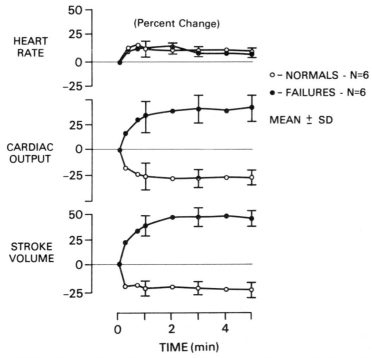

Figure 13.3. Comparison of hemodynamic response of congestive heart failure patients and normal subjects to head-up tilt. In contrast to the normal subjects, note the increased stroke volume and cardiac output in the patients. (Courtesy of Dr. W.V. Judy, University of Indiana.)

Increased Intrathoracic Pressure (the Valsalva Test)

Normal Valsalva Responses

In 1707 the Italian anatomist, Valsalva, described a maneuver in which the subject closes the mouth and nose, expires forcibly and thereby increases the pressure inside the pharynx and lung passages. The original purpose was to inflate the middle ear via the eustachian tubes; today the test is more commonly used as a means of assessing autonomic responsiveness to circulatory changes. By increasing intrathoracic pressure and thereby impeding venous return, cardiac output and arterial pressure are reduced; the resulting hemodynamic strain tests the circulatory system and particularly the integrity of the autonomic circulatory reflexes. As commonly performed, the subject blows into a mouthpiece (attached to a manometer) against a 40 mm Hg resistance for 15 seconds; there is a sudden rise in intrathoracic, intra-

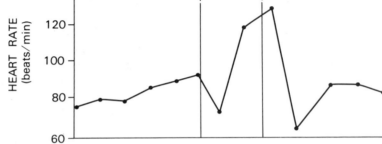

Figure 13.4.   Blood pressure and heart rate response to Valsalva test in a normal young adult. Intrathoracic pressure, 40 mm Hg. Note (*top*) the falling arterial pressure and tachycardia in phase II. The highest (phases II and III) and lowest (phases I and IV) heart rates for the respective phases are shown in the bottom figure. The pressure overshoot and bradycardia in phase IV (*top*) and the large heart rate decrement from phases III to IV (*bottom*) indicate functional baroceptor reflexes.

abdominal and cerebrospinal fluid pressure. The peripheral venous valves shut, and the blood, prevented from flowing into the vena cavae, accumulates in the peripheral veins, and venous pressure increases sharply. Central venous pressure rises about 7 mm Hg for each 10 mm Hg increase in mouth pressure. This induces a sharp reduction in venous return and as a result, aortic flow decreases to about 40 to 50% of control with rapid and profound changes in blood pressure.

The Valsalva response is classically divided into four phases as illustrated in Figure 13.4. At the start of the strain (phase I) there is a sudden rise in arterial pressure as the heightened intrathoracic pressure is transmitted directly through the aorta to the arterial tree; the heart rate usually shows a small decrease. In phase II there is diminished venous return to the right heart; cardiac filling becomes inadequate and the mean arterial and pulse pressures begin to fall; then follow a reflex tachycardia and peripheral vasoconstriction which limit the pressure drop. Mean arterial pressure may actually rise above control at the end of phase II. In phase III, immediately after release, blood pressure drops quickly because of the sudden fall in intrathoracic pressure and the heart rate increases further. In phase IV, the blood pressure rebounds as a result of the rapid surge of venous return and the ejection of the increased stroke volume into the constricted arterial system. About 5 to 6 seconds after release, the blood pressure overshoots, reflexly inducing a marked bradycardia (Fig. 13.4).

Since heart rate, a noninvasive measurement, is reportedly as valid an autonomic indicator as blood pressure, it may also be used to assess the Valsalva response; in the normal individual, the heart rate changes, as might be predicted, are roughly opposite to those of the blood pressure as shown in Figure 13.4.

The Valsalva test simulates the type of stress often associated with lifting, pushing, blowing a musical instrument, straining at stool, coughing etc. The maneuver tests the ability of the circulatory system to cope with a decreasing venous return and a falling arterial pressure and thus is a measure of the integrity of the baroceptor and cardiopulmonary reflexes. In addition to the pronounced arterial constrictor reaction, peripheral venoconstriction is a prompt response, not only to a Valsalva maneuver, but also to a deep breath or to hyperventilation. It has been suggested that the venoconstriction is mediated via sympathetic adrenergic fibers; the afferent source is probably in the chest wall, the diaphragm or in cardiopulmonary mechanoreceptors.

Abnormal Valsalva Responses

Most clinical abnormalities of the Valsalva are due either to (a) an increased intrathoracic blood volume, or (b) interruption of the baroceptor reflex arc, or (c) a combination of these two.

125 ⌉
100 ⌐   ARTERIAL PRESSURE (mmHg)
75 ⌋

Figure 13.5. "Square wave" blood pressure response to the Valsalva test in hypertensive heart failure. There is no change in pulse pressure, no pressure overshoot and very little change in heart rate. (Reprinted with permission from E.P. Sharpey-Schafer, *Handbook of Physiology*, Section 2: *Circulation*, edited by W.F. Hamilton and P. Dow. Washington, D.C.: American Physiological Society, 1965, Vol. III.)

Figure 13.6. Heart rate response to Valsalva test (40 mm Hg for 15 sec); *A*, in congestive heart failure patients (reprinted with permission from E.I. Elisberg, *JAMA* 186:200, 1963); and *B*, coronary patients not in congestive failure. Note in both cases the "flattened" response compared to control subjects. (Reprinted with permission from F.E. Tristani, D.G. Kamper, D.J. McDermott, B.J. Peters, and J.J. Smith, *Am J Physiol* 233:H694, 1977.)

Increase in intrathoracic blood volume occurs in congestive heart failure and results in a "square wave" Valsalva response in which there is little or no change in pulse pressure in phases II and III and very little or no overshoot in phase IV (Fig. 13.5). Since the blood pressure changes are diminished, the heart rate alterations are less marked.

The arterial pressure is maintained because (a) the increased central blood volume and atrial filling pressure provide a reservoir of venous return which maintains the cardiac output, and (b) the heightened peripheral venous pressure which usually accompanies the increased central blood volume, reduces venous distensibility and helps maintain a higher venous pressure gradient toward the right atrium. As the congestion lessens, the Valsalva response becomes more normal because of the abatement of these factors. In congestive heart failure, because the blood pressure changes are greatly diminished, the heart rate response is also flatter than normal (Fig. 13.6*A*).

Recent reports have indicated that ambulatory coronary heart disease patients not in congestive failure also have decreased heart rate responses to the Valsalva test (Fig. 13.6*B*); this lessened heart rate response may be due either to a subclinical intrathoracic congestion or decreased baroreflex responsiveness.

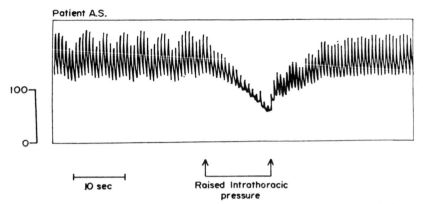

Figure 13.7.   Valsalva response in a patient with idiopathic orthostatic hypotension. There is an excessive fall in blood pressure in phase II and an absence of overshoot and bradycardia in phase IV. (Reprinted with permission from R.H. Johnson and J.M.K. Spalding, *Disorders of the Autonomic Nervous System.* London: Blackwell Scientific Publications, 1974.)

Interruption of the baroreflex arc may occur in neurological disorders involving the autonomic nervous system such as primary idiopathic hypotension. In such cases, the Valsalva test will show a continued pressure fall in phase II and no arterial pressure rebound or bradycardia in phase IV because of the failure of vasoconstriction and cardioacceleration (Fig. 13.7); these individuals, as previously mentioned, are also prone to postural hypotension.

Diving (Face Immersion) Response

This unique reflex represents the ultimate defense of the submerged vertebrate against asphyxia, *i.e.*, a gross redistribution of the circulation in order to concentrate oxygen in the brain and heart. This remarkable response enables the domestic duck to remain submerged for 15 minutes, the sea lion for 30 minutes and the whale for 2 hours. Its residual counterpart in man can be activated by diving or by immersion of the face in cold water.

Hemodynamic Changes

The three key elements of the diving response are apnea, an intense vagal bradycardia, and a powerful, extensive peripheral vasoconstriction, most marked in vessels of the muscle, kidneys, skin and splanchnic areas.

In the duck, hemodynamic changes involve a sudden decrease in cardiac output and heart rate to about 6% of the control values. Except for the coronary and cranial vessels, there is a massive vasoconstriction of the entire arterial tree so that the circulation becomes in effect a heart-brain circuit. The stroke volume and arterial pressure are relatively unchanged; when the animal surfaces, these changes are reversed within seconds with a large overshoot in cardiac output and heart rate (Fig. 13.8*A*). The face immersion reflex in man will induce a comparable but less intense response characterized by a quick reduction in heart rate (about 25%), skin blood flow (75%) and muscle flow (50%). Arterial blood pressure increases by about 20% (Fig. 13.8*B*).

Breath holding alone will cause similar but much less marked effects. The bradycardic effect is greater with cold (rather than cool) water and an attenuated response can be elicited by dry cold. An unusual feature is that the bradycardic effect of face immersion is increased during physical exercise so that paradoxically, the combination of a tachycardic stimulus (dynamic exercise) and a bradycardic stimulus (diving reflex) may yield a stronger bradycardic tendency than diving alone.

In contrast to the face immersion response, which is activated by cold receptors in the trigeminal area, cold water to other parts of the body causes reflex increases in heart rate and blood pressure; the cold pressor test (Chapter 10), involving immersion of the hand in ice water (0°C),

Figure 13.8. Diving and face immersion reflex: *A*, hemodynamic responses to 90-second head submersion in a duck (reprinted with permission from B. Folkow, N.J. Nilsson, and L.R. Younce, *Acta Physiol Scand* 70:347, 1967); *B*, responses to 30-second face immersion in normal male subjects. (Reprinted with permission from D.D. Heistad, F.M. Abboud, and J.W. Eckstein, *J Appl Physiol* 25:542, 1968.) In man the decrease in heart rate and blood flow are of lesser degree.

will stimulate pain fibers as well as cold receptors and produce a greater rise in blood pressure and heart rate than cold water (10°C).

Mechanism of Diving Response

In a series of interesting studies, Daly and his colleagues have demonstrated the role of the arterial chemoreceptors in the central modulation of this response. Stimulation of receptors of the face or upper airway initiates the reflex, inhibits the respiratory center (producing the apnea) and elicits vagal bradycardia and generalized vasoconstriction. The apnea leads to hypoxemia and hypercapnia; both of these would ordinarily induce a reflex hyperventilation, sympathetic vasoconstriction (mainly in skeletal muscle), and vagal bradycardia through the action of the arterial chemoreceptors (Chapter 10). It is theorized that during the apnea and the absence of activity of the pulmonary stretch receptors and central inspiratory neurons, the hyperventilation stimulus is suppressed; the cardiovascular limbs of the chemoreceptor reflex are retained and are responsible for the continuation and reinforcement of the existing vasoconstriction and bradycardia.

Due to the massive, generalized increase in peripheral resistance, the arterial pressure is maintained, and in the absence of coronary and cerebral vasoconstriction, the blood is made available to the heart and brain. The importance of the chemoreceptors in maintaining the response is underscored by the fact that experimental withdrawal of the chemoreceptor drive by perfusion of the carotid bifurcation region of the seal with normoxic blood during the later stages of the dive results in a reversal of the bradycardia. The integrating center for the diving reflex is not known. A cerebral connection is likely since threatening motions toward a seal will induce the reflex even before immersion.

Clinical Implications

Because of the powerful vagal action, pathological arrhythmias, such as ventricular premature contraction and idioventricular rhythm, as well as T wave inversion, commonly occur after only 30 seconds of diving in man. On the other hand, immersion of the face in a basin of cold water has been used to invoke the vagal effect to advantage in order to terminate supraventricular paroxysmal tachycardia. In certain situations the reflex apnea may be protective against the inhalation of liquids or noxious fumes. Since the response is potent in the newborn, it may serve to protect the fetus at birth.

In clinical cardiovascular studies, the face immersion response is sometimes used as a test for relatively "pure" vagal bradycardia; while sympathetic vasoconstriction is simultaneously activated, the brady-

Table 13.1.
Arterial Blood Pressure and Clinical Result of Hemorrhage

Loss of Blood Volume	Mean Arterial Pressure— Immediate Response	Likely Result
5–10%	Little change	Spontaneous recovery
15–20%	80–90 mm Hg	Moderate hypotension, spontaneous recovery
20–30%	60–80 mm Hg	Early shock—usually reversible
30–40%	50–70 mm Hg	Serious shock— irreversible in some cases

cardic effect is relatively immune to other reflex restraints, *e.g.*, by baroceptors or physical exercise. The bradycardic response decreases linearly with age and reportedly is diminished in coronary patients after myocardial infarction, while sympathetic pressor responses remain intact.

Hemorrhage

Circulatory Changes in Hemorrhage

The clinical results of blood loss depend on many factors, but particularly on the rate and degree of bleeding, the age and health of the patient and availability of treatment. The blood pressure and general response in an uncomplicated, untreated hemorrhage in a normal adult occurring within a relatively brief period (15 to 30 min) might be roughly estimated as shown in Table 13.1.

The brief description in this section refers mainly to short-term responses to moderate bleeding (less than 30% of blood volume); protracted hemorrhagic hypotension generally leads to circulatory shock, a quite different pathophysiological entity, which will be discussed in Chapter 15.

The immediate consequences of hemorrhage are (a) a decrease in blood volume, (b) a fall in venous return and cardiac output, and (c) a resultant decline in arterial and venous pressure.

Compensatory Response to Hemorrhage

Within seconds after bleeding begins, the fall in central blood volume and arterial pressure will activate cardiopulmonary and baroceptor reflexes (particularly from the carotid sinuses) and as a result, the sympathoadrenal defense system is fully mobilized. In case of a relatively small hemorrhage, *e.g.*, a standard phlebotomy of 500 ml, there is a

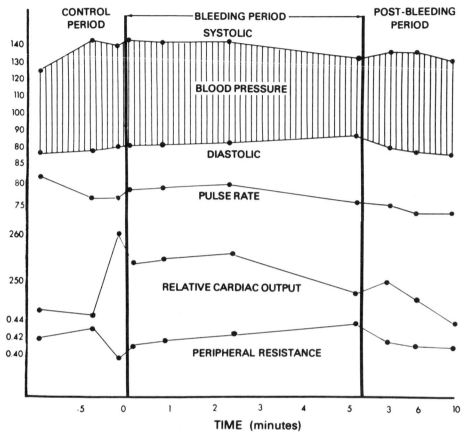

Figure 13.9. Mean hemodynamic response of normal male donors to 540 ml phlebotomy (*n* = 25). Uncomplicated hemorrhage of about 10% of blood volume. Note the preliminary fall in peripheral resistance and rise in cardiac output just after insertion of the needle and before bleeding was begun. Note also the immediate widening of the pulse pressure as the bleeding is stopped. (Reprinted with permission from J.R. Logic, S.A. Johnson, and J.J. Smith, *Transfusion* 3:83, 1963.)

modest rise in peripheral resistance and a small decrease in pulse pressure (Fig. 13.9).

With a greater blood loss and more marked hypotension, the responses will be correspondingly greater. The main compensatory changes are:

1. *Increase in Heart Rate and Contractility.* Tachycardia does not usually occur, however, in uncomplicated hemorrhage until the blood loss exceeds 700 to 800 ml.

2. *Strong Generalized Constriction of Both Resistance and Capaci-*

tance Vessels. In particular, vessels of skin (producing a marked pallor), splanchnic area (with resulting ischemia of gut and liver), skeletal muscle and kidney are affected. Cerebral and coronary beds are unaffected.

The renal vasoconstriction reduces glomerular filtration leading to oliguria and sometimes to anuria. Venoconstriction is a prominent aspect of the compensatory reaction; in the splanchnic bed for example, which contains about 20% of the total blood volume, a translocation of even half of this amount to the central veins can provide a significant autotransfusion.

Maintenance of Plasma Volume

Vasoconstriction assists the circulation in two ways: (a) by decreasing the circulatory capacity so the remaining blood volume will create a greater venous filling pressure; and (b) by lowering the general capillary hydrostatic pressure and thus promoting fluid transfer from tissues to the plasma. Certain hormonal mechanisms are also activated during hemorrhage to help maintain the plasma volume (Fig. 13.10). Renal vasoconstriction reduces glomerular filtration and urine formation; renin and angiotensin production is increased via renal ischemia. The decreased atrial stretch causes reflex release of vasopressin (ADH) and

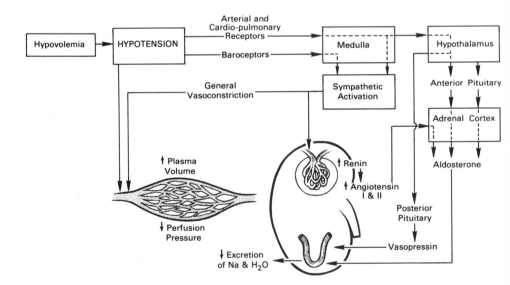

Figure 13.10. Schema of factors tending to restore plasma volume and extracellular fluid during and after hemorrhage. Reduced general capillary pressure and renal vasoconstriction are key elements in maintaining plasma volume; increased vasopressin and aldosterone levels are helpful adjuncts.

(along with other factors) is responsible for the release of aldosterone from the adrenal cortex. These two hormones maximize H_2O and Na^+ reabsorption from renal tubules and help conserve plasma volume.

Other Responses to Hemorrhage

There is a pronounced increase in plasma catecholamines; epinephrine is responsible for the hyperglycemia in hemorrhage but it is unlikely that any of the circulatory hormones, i.e., catecholamines, angiotensin or vasopressin contribute significantly to the general vasoconstriction. There is a decrease in RBCs, hematocrit and plasma protein concentration in blood because of the dilution by the absorbed tissue fluid. After the hemorrhage, the plasma proteins are usually replaced in about 3 to 6 days and the RBCs in about 4 to 6 weeks. Therapy is logically directed at fluid replacement, whole blood if the hematocrit is low but if not available, plasma or plasma substitutes.

Fainting (Syncope)

Fainting is the loss of consciousness due to cerebral ischemia; clinically a differentiation is usually made between "organic" and "functional" causes. Among the more common "organic" causes, i.e., those in which an apparent known disease process is involved, are cerebrovascular syncope (usually associated with cerebral arteriosclerosis), orthostatic hypotension (often associated with central or peripheral disorders of the sympathetic nervous system) and cardiac syncope.

The most common causes of cardiac syncope include supraventricular tachycardia, disorders of the His-Purkinje system, Stokes-Adams syndrome (complete heart block, see Chapter 4), carotid sinus hypersensitivity and intrinsic sinus node dysfunction. Fainting tendencies are also a frequent accompaniment of α-adrenergic blockade, the latter occurring, e.g., as a side effect of antihypertensive therapy. As previously mentioned, these patients usually faint abruptly upon standing without showing the usual preliminary symptoms.

Functional syncope or ordinary fainting (also called vasodepressor or vasovagal syncope) has multiple causes. It may occur in unusually sensitive individuals after a purely psychic stimulation such as emotional shock or the sight of blood; on the other hand practically everyone will faint during extreme somatic stress such as a 1,500-ml phlebotomy or a 30- to 40-minute passive, suspended tilt. However, clinical fainting in the healthy individual is usually due to a combination of stresses; the most common predisposing factor is decreased circulating blood volume induced, e.g., by a previous blood withdrawal, excessive physical exercise, diarrhea, protracted bed rest or prolonged standing in the heat.

Figure 13.11. Hemodynamic response of blood donor (53-year-old healthy male) to a 580-ml phlebotomy. Toward the end of the bleeding, subject developed pallor, nausea and abdominal discomfort. Blood pressure just before end of bleeding was 46/25. Note the sharp fall in mean and pulse pressure, peripheral resistance and heart rate. Cardiac output was maintained. (Reprinted with permission from J.R. Logic, S.A. Johnson, and J.J. Smith, *Transfusion* 3:83, 1963.)

Circulatory Responses during Fainting

The usual preliminary symptoms of extreme pallor, nausea, sweating and abdominal discomfort are sometimes stated as being due to sympathoadrenal activation but are more likely due to the liberation of vasopressin. These symptoms are usually accompanied by a decreasing systolic and pulse pressure, a rapid heart rate and decreasing right atrial pressure. At the moment of vascular failure, there is a sudden sharp decrease in mean arterial and pulse pressure, a marked bradycardia, cerebral ischemia and loss of consciousness—all occurring very rapidly, sometimes within seconds (Fig. 13.11).

The right atrial pressure usually falls further but cardiac output remains relatively unchanged. The key defect is a powerful vagal stimulation accompanied by a sudden loss of peripheral vascular resistance, primarily in skeletal muscle; the mechanism is probably a massive sympathetic inhibition from the hypothalamic cardioinhibitory center (Chapter 10). Cholinergic vasodilators do not seem to be involved.

Mechanism of Vasodepressor Syncope

While it is generally agreed that the immediate prelude to fainting is cerebral ischemia, there are little data and no unanimity of opinion regarding the final common pathway through which the circulatory collapse is brought about. Because of the unusual autoregulatory ability of cerebral vessels, signs of cerebral ischemia usually do not occur until arterial pressures reach very low levels, *i.e.*, about 40 mm Hg. However, a heightened cerebral arterial tone decreases autoregulatory ability so that cerebral ischemia develops at higher arterial pressures than is usually the case. Two conditions which increase cerebral vascular tone are hypocapnia and hypertension.

Hyperventilation and its resultant hypocapnia commonly occur not only in emotional strain but during hemorrhage and postural stress; the hypocapnia will, in turn, induce tachycardia and increased cardiac output. However, the most striking effect of hypocapnia is the cerebral vasoconstriction which can reduce cerebral flow by 40% after only 1 or 2 minutes of active hyperventilation. Although uncomplicated hyperventilation rarely causes syncope in normal subjects, it can be an important contributing factor. Similarly, certain hypertensive patients develop cerebral ischemia at higher than normal levels of arterial pressure and have fainting tendencies in spite of increased arterial perfusion pressures; the cause is not certain but it is probably due to cerebral arteriosclerosis or decreased autoregulatory capability of cerebral vessels.

For fainting to occur consistently, both hypotension and an adjunct factor are necessary. For example, a moderate hemorrhage (10% of blood volume), a Valsalva maneuver or prolonged standing will all cause a decrease in cardiac output and a modest hypotension but none will, by itself, ordinarily produce fainting. However, in all of them, a fainting tendency may be precipitated by an unnoticed hyperventilation.

While practically all individuals have one or two fainting episodes in their lifetime, there is a small but consistent fraction of the adult population, without apparent organic disease, which is prone to repeated fainting episodes. About 5% of blood donors, *e.g.*, have such fainting tendencies; reports indicate that such "fainters," compared to control subjects, experience a greater fall in arterial pressure and a greater decrease in alveolar P_{CO_2} to a standard 500-ml phlebotomy. Psychological tests further showed that the fainters also had a greater tendency toward hypochondriasis and depression than did control subjects; such studies suggest an interrelationship between psychic factors and hemodynamic response to stress which might account for the tendency toward circulatory collapse in these individuals. As described in Chapter 10, such psychogenic fainting may involve the depressor area of the hypothalamus.

References

Abboud FM, Heistad DD, Mark AL, and Schmid PG. Reflex control of the peripheral circulation. *Prog Cardiovasc Dis* 18:371–403, 1976.

Angell-James JE and Daly MD. The diving response: some possible clinical implications. In: *Advances in Psychological Sciences*, Vol. 20: *Advances in Animal and Comparative Physiology*, edited by G Pethes and VL Frenyo. Oxford: Pergamon Press, 1981, pp. 277–284.

Daly MD and Angell-James JE. The diving response: its possible clinical implications. *Int Med* 1:12–19, 1979.

Ebert TJ, Hughes CV, Tristani FE, Barney JA, and Smith JJ. The effect of age and coronary heart disease on the circulatory responses to graded lower body negative pressure. *Cardiovasc Res* 16:663–669, 1982.

Fox IJ, Crowley WP, Grace JB, and Wood EH. Effects of the Valsalva maneuver on blood flow in the thoracic aorta in man. *J Appl Physiol* 21:1553–1560, 1966.

Frey MAB and Kenney RA. Changes in left ventricular activity during apnea and face immersion. *Undersea Biomed Res* 4:27, 1977.

Gauer ON and Thron HL. Postural change in the circulation. In: *Handbook of Physiology*, Section 2: *Circulation*, edited by WF Hamilton and P Dow. Washington, D.C.: American Physiological Society, 1965, Vol. III, pp. 2409–2440.

Heistad DD, Abboud FM, and Eckstein JW. Vasoconstrictor response to simulated diving in man. *J Appl Physiol* 25:542–549, 1968.

Klein LJ, Saltzman HS, Heyman A, and Sicker HO. Syncope induced by the Valsalva maneuver. *Am J Med* 37:263–268, 1964.

Korner PI, Tonkin AM, and Uther JB. Reflex and mechanical circulatory effects of graded Valsalva maneuvers in normal man. *J Appl Physiol* 40:434–440, 1976.

Logic JR, Johnson SA, and Smith JJ. Cardiovascular and hematologic responses to phlebotomy in blood donors. *Transfusion* 3:83–93, 1963.

McHenry LC, Fazekas JF, and Sullivan JF. Cerebral hemodynamics of syncope. *Am J Med Sci* 241:173, 1961.

Robertson D, Johnson GA, Robertson RM, Nies AS, Shand DG, and Oates JA. Comparative assessment of stimuli that release neuronal and adrenomedullary catecholamines in man. *Circulation* 59:637–643, 1979.

Ruetz PD, Johnson SA, Callahan R, Meade RE, and Smith JJ. Fainting: a review of the mechanisms and a study in blood donors. *Medicine* 46:363–384, 1967.

Ryan C, Hollenberg M, Harvey DB, and Gwynn R. Impaired parasympathetic responses in patients after myocardial infarction. *Am J Cardiol* 37:1013–1018, 1976.

Sharpey-Schafer EP. Effect of respiratory acts on the circulation. In: *Handbook of Physiology*, Section 2: *Circulation*, edited by WF Hamilton and P Dow. Washington, D.C.: American Physiological Society, 1965, Vol. III, pp. 1875–1886.

Shepherd JT. Role of the veins in the circulation. *Circulation* 33:484–491, 1966.

Smith JJ, Bonin ML, Wiedmeier VT, Kalbfleisch JH, and McDermott DJ. Cardiovascular response of young men to diverse stresses. *Aerospace Med* 45:583–590, 1974.

Tristani FE, Kamper DG, McDermott DJ, Peters BJ, and Smith JJ. Alteration of postural and Valsalva responses in coronary heart disease. *Am J Physiol* 233:H694–699, 1977.

chapter 14

Pathophysiology: Ischemic Heart Disease and Congestive Heart Failure

Circulatory Pathophysiology—General

The next two chapters are intended to show in a limited sense how disease may alter the physiology and how the disordered state often helps us to better understand the normal. An understanding of the pathophysiology often requires basic investigation as well as observation of the patient. Dr. Carl J. Wiggers, one of our truly great cardiovascular physiologists, was fond of saying that the mistakes of nature, *i.e.*, disease, can best be solved by shuttling the problems back and forth between the clinic and the experimental laboratory. In these chapters, in which we present capsule descriptions of four of the more common cardiovascular diseases, we have, therefore, also included accounts of basic studies and animal experiments insofar as they relate to the disease process.

In the following discussions of pathophysiology, the term *anoxia* refers to a complete absence of an oxygen supply, local or general. *Hypoxia* denotes a state of reduced oxygen supply. *Ischemia* is a condition of reduced perfusion of blood, local or general. Hypoxia (or anoxia) is classically subdivided into four types, *i.e.*, hypoxic, anemic, stagnant and histotoxic.

Hypoxic hypoxia is a condition in which there is a reduction of P_{O_2} of arterial blood; this may be caused by an inadequate partial pressure of oxygen in inspired air (*e.g.*, by ascent to altitude), by hypoventilation, or by lung disease in which there is an inadequate transfer of oxygen from the alveoli to the pulmonary capillary blood. *Anemic hypoxia* is the result of an inadequate amount of hemoglobin to carry the oxygen, *i.e.*, a reduced oxygen carrying capacity, such as may occur in anemia or carbon monoxide poisoning. *Stagnant hypoxia* is a condition in which blood flow is so diminished that insufficient oxygen is delivered to the tissues despite a normal blood P_{O_2} and normal hemoglobin concentration; this commonly occurs in low-flow states such as circulatory shock or congestive heart failure.

In *histotoxic hypoxia,* both the oxygen carrying capacity of blood and the tissue perfusion are adequate but the oxygen is denied to the cells because of the presence of a toxic agent. This may occur as a result of cyanide poisoning in which cellular hypoxia is produced through paralysis of the electron transfer function of cytochrome oxidase. *Cyanosis* is a bluish discoloration of the tissues due to reduced hemoglobin. The discoloration becomes evident particularly in the nail beds of the fingers, lips and mucous membranes when the blood concentration of reduced hemoglobin exceeds 5 g/dl; it commonly accompanies states of severe heart failure and advanced lung disease.

Asphyxia is a simultaneous decrease in P_{O_2} (hypoxic hypoxia) with an increase in P_{CO_2} (hypercapnia) of the blood produced by a restriction or cessation of respiratory ventilation. With acute, complete asphyxia, there follows in sequence and within a matter of minutes unconsciousness, failure of the respiratory center with respiratory arrest, failure of the vasomotor center with a consequent fall in arterial pressure, and finally, ventricular ischemia and fibrillation. While pure hypoxia is usually painless and may even induce euphoria (*e.g.*, in high altitude flying), asphyxia, because of the associated hypercapnia, usually evokes extreme discomfort and panic.

Ischemic Heart Disease (IHD)

Epidemiology—Risk Factors and Diagnosis

Since not all coronary artery disease results in cardiac ischemia and since cardiac ischemia can result from noncoronary diseases, ischemic heart disease (IHD) is the preferable term to designate changes occurring in the myocardium from reduction of blood flow (ischemia) or reduction of oxygen supply (hypoxia). Beginning in 1968, the annual mortality from coronary heart disease has shown a progressive and modest decline for reasons that are not yet certain. However, in spite of this decline, IHD is the leading single cause of mortality in the western world and in the United States alone accounts for over 600,000 deaths annually; obviously, it is a clinical and social problem of the highest magnitude. It primarily affects males in their forties or older. Unfortunately, the disease is usually "silent" in the sense that symptoms appear late and early diagnosis is at present very difficult.

IHD's insidious nature is illustrated by the fact that approximately two-thirds of coronary deaths occur outside the hospital, usually without preceding symptoms and with little or no warning. The great majority of these acute deaths are precipitated by ventricular fibrillation, and at autopsy over three-fourths of the victims show advanced coronary disease. Curiously, only a minority of these patients appeared to have their ventricular fibrillation as a consequence of acute myocardial infarction and most did not have antecedent chest pain. The instigation of disordered impulse conduction by aberrant autonomic reflexes has been suggested as a mechanism in these cases. The cardiac "sudden death" syndrome is currently the subject of intensive clinical investigation. The increasing therapeutic capabilities, which could now be applied if the existence of the disease were known, make it abundantly clear that one of the great deficiencies in modern preventive medicine is the lack of an adequate method for the early diagnosis of ischemic heart disease.

The primary factor contributing to IHD is coronary arteriosclerosis, a general term for thickening and hardening of the arterial wall. Atherosclerosis, the most prevalent type of arteriosclerosis, is the basic lesion, not only in coronary heart disease but in cerebrovascular disease and most renal and peripheral vascular diseases as well. Atherosclerosis apparently begins with the deposition of cholesterol beneath the arterial intima; why the process accelerates in IHD is not certain but appears to be related to hyperlipidemia, *i.e.*, increased triglyceride and low density

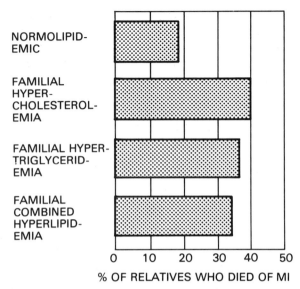

Figure 14.1.   Predisposition of familial hyperlipidemic subjects to myocardial infarct (MI). MI death rates in adult, first degree relatives of hyperlipidemic MI patients were twice as high as relatives of normolipidemic patients. (Reprinted with permission from J.L. Goldstein, *The Myocardium: Failure and Infarction.* New York: HP Publishing Co., 1974.)

lipoprotein but most importantly, increased cholesterol levels of plasma. The tendency of hyperlipidemic subjects to coronary disease is illustrated in Figure 14.1.

Hypercholesteremia, hypertension and cigarette smoking have been established as major risk factors in coronary artery disease. In addition to these major factors, diabetes mellitus, obesity, physical inactivity and a positive family history of atherosclerosis are contributing risk factors for IHD. Recently, emotional stress has been added to this select group, specifically a hyperactive behavior pattern termed "Type A." Studies have shown that aggressive, competitive, impatient and sometimes hostile "time-fighters" may be statistically twice as apt to develop heart problems as are more passive individuals. It is believed that the common pathophysiological denominator in these individuals is catecholamine overdrive; although catechol levels at rest or during sleep are not distinctive, Type A individuals reportedly exhibit a much greater increase in arterial pressure and plasma catechols than do Type B individuals in competitive or harassing situations. Of the many recent developments in cardiovascular research, none is more important than the clear demonstration that different cultural patterns, life styles and personal characteristics carry different degrees of risk of eventual heart attack or stroke.

Only when the arteriosclerotic process has progressed sufficiently to produce at least a 70% luminal narrowing of one or more of the three primary coronary arteries (or one of their larger branches) is the disease apt to manifest symptoms. Two of the most common clinical manifestations of ischemic heart disease are angina pectoris and myocardial infarction. Both are characterized by precordial chest pains which may radiate to the left shoulder, arm and back. During periods of angina, the ECG may show S-T and T wave changes and in myocardial infarction, abnormal Q waves.

The diagnosis of IHD is generally made on the basis of a history of angina or myocardial infarction and is confirmed by noninvasive studies such as ECG, exercise stress tests, nuclear and ultrasonic imaging techniques and invasive procedures such as cardiac catheterization and angiography. Angiography involves the injection of radioopaque dye into the cardiac chambers (ventriculography) and the coronary arteries (arteriography) with the subsequent filming of the fluoroscopy for later review. From ventriculograms are determined end-diastolic volume (EDV), end-systolic volume (ESV), ejection fraction (EF), and, very importantly, any defects in ventricular wall motion such as akinesia (defective contraction) or asynergy (nonuniform contraction); these defects might indicate ischemia or a previous infarction. The arteriography allows visualization of the obstructive lesions. The diagnostic approach chosen is tailored to the needs of the individual patient.

Angina Pectoris

Angina pectoris is a condition featured by attacks of sudden substernal discomfort or pain that may be described as "dull" or "burning" or as a "tightness"; it may last several minutes and is the result of a transient, reversible, myocardial ischemia. The chest pain—sometimes severe—is associated with a temporary reduction of cardiac output, stroke volume and ventricular contractility. It may be accompanied by dyspnea (shortness of breath) or other signs of early heart failure. Angina pectoris is the result of a temporary disparity between myocardial oxygen demand and supply and is classically associated with the clinical sequence of "exertion-pain" and "rest-relief." Prompt cessation of the pain usually follows administration of nitrites.

Angina may be induced by exertion, emotional stress, cold, isometric exercise or by a meal. However, in some patients the attack may develop without any evident prior physical or emotional strain or other apparent inciting cause. Patients with angina may remain "stable" for many years with only an occasional attack; on the other hand the condition may become progressive so that the attacks will become increasingly severe. While most angina patients have evidence of narrowing of the coronary arteries, a small percentage have, on angiography, anatomically normal coronary arteries.

In such cases, two possibilities exist. The first is that coronary arterial spasm is responsible for the myocardial ischemia. One form of this condition is "Prinzmetal's angina" in which arterial vasospasm may (but not necessarily) be superimposed on atherosclerotic coronary disease. In this variant, the patients develop chest pains at rest rather than during exertion and S-T segment elevation is more common than S-T depression. A second possible explanation of the occurrence of angina without apparent narrowing of coronary arteries is that the patient may have disease of the smaller vessels which are difficult to visualize. In any event, angina pectoris patients are more prone than normal subjects to an eventual myocardial infarct.

Myocardial Infarction

Pathogenesis

MI is a sudden, irreversible, ischemic injury due to coronary arterial narrowing or occlusion with sustained damage to a segment of the myocardium; it is associated with electrocardiographic, metabolic and hemodynamic changes which depend on the size and location of the ischemic area. If the SA or AV nodes or a vital part of the conduction apparatus is affected, bradycardia, arrhythmia or conduction defects such as AV block may result. If as much as 20 or 25% of the left ventricular mass ceases to contract, there is usually hemodynamic evidence of left ventricular failure. Involvement of 40% or more results in severe pump failure with cardiogenic shock or death.

It is thought that complete obstruction is initiated at the damaged inner surface of an already partially occluded vessel, probably by accumulation of fibrin or platelets at the site. The exact sequence of events, however, is not certain and some investigators believe that the thrombosis actually occurs after the infarct rather than preceding it.

Metabolic Changes in MI

Myocardium is dependent on aerobic metabolism for sufficient energy in the form of ATP to provide for the continuous contraction of the heart. As previously mentioned (Chapters 1 and 5), the myocardium contains very little reserve high-energy phosphate (HEP). ATP, together with creatine phosphate and adenosine diphosphate, supplies only enough to support about a minute of left ventricular contractile activity. This extraordinary dependence of myocardium on aerobic or mitochondrial metabolism is reflected in the fact that about 30% of the volume of a normal left ventricular myocyte is occupied by mitochondria.

Glucose and amino and fatty acids can be oxidized to CO_2 and water with equal facility and yield large quantities of HEP. However, when substrates are equally available to the heart, fatty acids are preferentially oxidized and are the dominant mitochondrial substrate. The entry of glucose—the next most common substance— into the cell is facilitated by insulin. Amino acids are only a minor energy source.

Experimental studies have shown that if oxygen is cut off or perfusion is stopped in an isolated ventricle or working heart, depression of myocardial contractility begins within 15 seconds. Tissue Po_2 decreases and when it falls below 5 mm Hg, HEP concentration (mainly creatine phosphate) decreases and myocardial energy metabolism promptly shifts to anaerobic glycolysis. The metabolic and functional consequences of this transition occur within seconds of the onset of the oxygen deficiency. Anaerobic glycolysis generates lactate at a high rate of speed during the first minute of ischemia but the rate then quickly slows; the slowed rate is unable to provide enough HEP. If the ischemia is prolonged, the tissue ATP in the affected zones is reduced to a low level and when anaerobic glycolysis ceases, the process becomes irreversible and myocyte death occurs. At this time, electron microscopy reveals intracellular edema and swelling of sarcoplasmic reticulum and mitochondria. While these metabolic and ultrastructural changes occur quite rapidly during the first few minutes, they progress relatively little during the next 10 to 24 hours. After the death of the myocytes there is phagocytosis, gradual removal of the dead fragments and replacement with connective tissue, a process that takes about 30 to 40 days for completion.

Ischemia and hypoxia produce very different biochemical and pathological effects. During ischemia, the acid products of glycolysis are not washed out, lactic acid concentration rises, intracellular pH falls quickly and the necrobiotic process is more rapid. Both oxidative metabolic and anaerobic production of ATP are diminished and eventually glycolysis is inhibited and lactate production falls off. This lower glycolytic flux probably results from the acidotic inhibition of phosphofructokinase (PFK), a key enzyme in the glycolytic chain. Upon sudden experimental occlusion of a major coronary artery in the dog, a transmural gradient of ischemia results. Residual collateral flows are very low in the inner myocardium but are considerably greater in the outer layer. As might be expected, there are also lateral zones of tissue damage. Although the entire ischemic tissue is acontractile and may exhibit electrical abnormalities, cell death occurs quickly in inner zones of severe ischemia, more slowly in zones of moderate ischemia, and often does not develop at all in zones of mild ischemia. The result depends primarily on the collateral circulation.

The critical objective in clinical treatment is to limit the severely ischemic zone and salvage as much as possible of the border zones. Studies in experimental animals have suggested that the transition from reversible to irreversible ischemic injury occurs within 20 to 40 minutes after coronary occlusion. While this time limit is not certain, at least in the human heart, and obviously depends on the degree of cellular hypoxia, it appears very likely that significant salvage can only be achieved within the first few hours. Such studies have provided the basis for the occasional application of certain invasive treatment methods such as coronary artery bypass surgery, intracoronary infusion of fibrinolytic enzyme preparations or PCTA (described later), shortly after acute myocardial infarction.

Myocardial Enzymes

Normally lactate is taken up by the heart and oxidized so that the coronary arterial concentration exceeds the coronary venous concentration. With the acceleration of glycolysis in hypoxia and ischemia, this lactate gradient is reversed. Furthermore, when MI occurs, the damaged cells become permeable to macromolecules so that large molecular weight proteins and enzymes escape from their normal intracellular location and enter the circulation through either venous drainage or cardiac lymphatics. Consequently, there is an increased output of lactate as well as a release of certain enzymes such as glutamic oxaloacetic transaminase (SGOT), lactic dehydrogenase (LDH) and creatine kinase (CK) from the infarcted myocardium. Elevated serum levels and the time-concentration course of these enzymes (or their isoenzymes) are diagnostically useful in MI. The tests are sensitive but not specific and the false positive rate may be as high as 15%.

Effect on Ventricular Contractility

As mentioned in Chapter 11, the greater net perfusion pressure to epicardial coronary vessels is generally offset by the greater metabolic vasodilation (autoregulation) in the subendocardial vessels. In the presence of restricted coronary blood flow and hypotension, coronary autoregulation declines and the subendocardium is further underperfused so that necrosis of subendocardium is much more common than that of the subepicardium. Thus, after coronary occlusion, contractility of the epicardium is better preserved than the endocardium, apparently as a manifestation of this preferential perfusion of the outer wall.

After severe hypoxia or ischemia, the deterioration of myocardial function is abrupt and profound. In the early ischemic state, this functional decline occurs while high energy phosphate is still present in adequate amounts, so the latter does not appear to be the critical

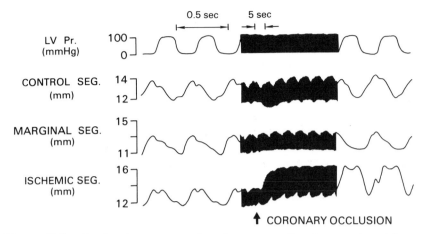

Figure 14.2.   Regional responses of canine myocardium to experimental coronary occlusion. Occlusion was produced at the arrow; the degree of shortening (or lengthening) of muscle is indicated in the bottom three tracings. Within 15 seconds after occlusion, the ischemic segment bulged and remained expanded both in systole and diastole. The marginal segment showed some increase in end-diastolic length and decrease in systolic shortening. The control non-ischemic segment shows an initial increased shortening with a later increase in end-diastolic length and degree of shortening, a compensatory response of the uninvolved muscle. The left ventricular pressure *(top)* remained unchanged. (Reprinted with permission from P. Theroux, D. Franklin, J. Ross, Jr., and W.S. Kemper, *Circ Res* 35:896, 1974.)

initiating factor. The metabolic, electrical and contractile activities cease as necrosis develops and the myocardial changes are generally permanent with eventual scar formation. The critical factors in the prognosis are the size of the infarct, the ability to limit its spread, the general condition of the heart and the assistance that can be rendered to the uninvolved myocardium.

Experimental ischemia of cardiac muscle usually results in a decrease or loss of contractile power with reduced contraction in the adjacent or marginal zones. In the uninvolved areas there are increased systolic, diastolic and stroke volume excursions as these segments assume a greater share of the contractile burden (Fig. 14.2).

If more than about 25% of myocardial mass is involved, there is usually a decrease in left ventricular stroke volume, stroke work and V_{max}. There is also an increase in ventricular EDV and EDP and a decrease in ventricular EF. With the loss of contractile power, the center of the ischemic zone may become immobile and, at first, bulges passively during ventricular systole, thus exhibiting "paradoxical" motion or dyskinesis.

Figure 14.3. Left ventricular angiograms showing normal contraction pattern (*left*) and impaired contraction (*right*) because of hypokinesis of apical inferior area, with a fall in ejection fraction (EF). (Reprinted with permission from E.A. Amsterdam, R.R. Miller, D.H. Foley, and D.T. Mason, *Peripheral Circulation*, edited by R. Zelis. New York: Grune & Stratton, 1975.)

However, shortly after the coronary occlusion, cellular swelling, edema and fibrocellular infiltration take place so that now the infarcted, noncontracting myocardial segment becomes stiff and contributes to the rise in EDP. These changes may produce abnormalities in cardiac sounds and ventricular wall motion; accentuated presystolic sounds and large "a" waves become evident on the phonocardiogram and on the apex cardiogram. Because a part of the myocardium is not functioning, asynergy of the ventricular muscle may appear on the ventriculogram (Fig. 14.3).

At a later time in the postinfarct period, the systolic tension generated by the contracting myocardium may possibly stretch and eventually disrupt and weaken the tissue of the noncontracting segment with accentuated bulging during systole and aneurysm formation. In accord with Laplace's law (Chapter 1), the wall stress will increase progressively and may further enlarge the ischemic zone.

Hemodynamic Response to MI: Autonomic Effects

The result of a myocardial infarct on systemic hemodynamics is not always predictable; sometimes a systemic pressor and sometimes a depressor response results. Randall and others have pointed out that this variability may be due to cardiopulmonary baroceptors and specifically to the cardiocardiac reflexes that are important in self-regulation of the heart. The role of the autonomic nervous system in determining the result of MI is indicated by the fact that experimental coronary occlusion in dogs after cardiac denervation resulted in a near zero incidence of ventricular ectopic activity and fibrillation and a reduced infarct size compared to normally innervated animals.

Upon coronary occlusion in experimental animals, there follows within 30 to 60 seconds bradycardia and frequently arrhythmia, efferent sympathetic inhibition with hypotension, and a prolonged renal vasodilation with inhibition of secretion of renin and ADH. This response is due to ischemia and bulging of the infarcted myocardial wall with a resultant chemical and mechanical stimulation of the ventricular sensory receptors whose fibers travel in the vagus nerve. Vagotomy will abolish the response (Chapter 10, Ventricular Receptors). Ischemia of the inferoposterior myocardium will produce a more pronounced cardioinhibitory and vasodepressor response than a comparable anterior myocardial ischemia, perhaps because of a denser population of these receptor endings in the inferoposterior cardiac region. Clinical studies have shown that bradyarrhythmias are seen more often in posterior than in anterior infarcts suggesting that a comparable reflex mechanism exists in the human. This inhibitory reflex overrides that of the arterial baroceptors which would be expected to induce a strong sympathetic stimulation in response to the reduced cardiac output and decreased arterial pressure that occur after coronary occlusion.

As mentioned in Chapter 10, there are chemosensitive endings not only in the ventricles but also in the atria and lungs that can be activated by veratrine, nicotine and other chemicals; such activation will induce bradycardic and cardioinhibitory responses similar to those induced by ventricular mechanoceptors.

Afferent *sympathetic* fibers in the ventricles will also be stimulated following coronary occlusion but their precise role is less clear; they may be important in the generation of some cardiac arrhythmias, in the induction of cardiac pain and perhaps in some cases in causing the tachycardic and hypertensive response sometimes seen in MI.

Patients who have recovered from MI or who have chronic angina pectoris have shown altered circulatory responses to certain autonomic stresses. Recent reports have indicated that in such patients there was a lesser heart rate slowing during phase IV of the Valsalva maneuver and a lesser vasoconstrictor response to upright tilt with a greater decline in systolic pressure. It is suspected that such changes in sympathetic and parasympathetic responses may be due to a decrease in sensitivity of arterial or cardiopulmonary baroceptors; however, the underlying cause is not known. Investigations are currently underway to explore the possibility that these altered autonomic reflexes may be useful as adjunctive tests for the diagnosis and characterization of IHD.

Treatment of IHD

The general term, IHD, includes a wide spectrum of disease entities such as stable and unstable angina, MI, heart failure, pulmonary edema and sudden death. Obviously, the therapy will be tailored to the needs of the individual patient. The following is intended to be only an outline of some physiological principles in the treatment of IHD and not a treatise on clinical management. The immediate treatment objectives are (a) to relieve symptoms, (b) to detect and promptly treat any life-threatening complications such as arrhythmia or shock, and (c) to limit infarct size by reducing myocardial O_2 demand and increasing the supply.

As previously described (Chapter 5), the main work of the heart is expended in pressure energy, which is used to eject the stroke volume against the aortic afterload. Since aortic pressure is a key component of aortic impedance or afterload, an effective way to reduce cardiac work, and therefore myocardial oxygen demand, is through a reduction in mean arterial pressure consistent with maintenance of an adequate coronary perfusion pressure. An increase in myocardial oxygen supply must be achieved mainly by increasing coronary flow since myocardial oxygen extraction is normally at a high level. Since the pressure-rate (double) product is a close correlate of myocardial $\dot{V}_{O_2}$ demand (Chapter 5), it is a useful clinical measure of cardiac work requirements.

Nitrates and Nitrites

Nitrates and nitrites (*e.g.*, nitroglycerin) are widely used to relieve anginal attacks by reducing venous tone and peripheral resistance and thereby lowering preload and afterload as indicated by aortic pressure. This, in turn, reduces myocardial O_2 requirements. The resulting decrease in left ventricular end-diastolic volume and myocardial tension override the disadvantages of the slight tachycardia, and increased cardiac contractility, which result from the baroceptor response to the mild induced hypotension. The direct coronary dilator action of these agents is a secondary and less important one compared to the above effects.

β-Adrenergic Blockade

β-adrenergic blockade as induced, *e.g.*, by propranolol or timolol, exerts a beneficial effect by minimizing the increase in heart rate and myocardial contractility, which may occur during stress. Its effectiveness in IHD is indicated by the fact that many patients receiving this drug will have less release of myocardial lactate during activity. This medication, however, is contraindicated in heart failure since it would deprive the myocardium of the compensatory sympathetic stimulation, which is a support of the weakened muscle in failure. Since it also decreases the atrial-ventricular conduction rate, it is also contraindicated in patients who have some conduction abnormalities, *e.g.*, heart block.

Calcium Antagonists

The recently introduced slow channel inhibitors (calcium antagonists) are proving to be important aids in the treatment of heart disease. Studies thus far indicate that agents such as verapamil, nifedipine or diltiazem exert their effects by inhibiting transmembrane influx of extracellular calcium into cardiac and vascular smooth muscle. In isolated cardiac tissues, these drugs produce a depression of SA and AV node function and a negative inotropic effect. The peripheral effects consist mainly of an inhibition of excitation-contraction coupling in vascular smooth muscle and varying degrees of coronary and peripheral vasodilation. In patients, these drugs protect the myocardium (a) by a direct relaxant action on vascular smooth muscle, which increases blood flow through coronary and other beds, (b) through reduction of peripheral resistance, arterial pressure and, therefore, of left ventricular afterload, and (c) through prevention or reversal of coronary spasm. The inotropic action is countered by the afterload reduction so that cardiac index is usually not decreased. The different agents have varying degrees of cardiac and peripheral vascular effects, and so the specific drug chosen depends on the individual hemodynamic problem.

Percutaneous Transluminal Coronary Angioplasty (PCTA)

This recently introduced technique consists of the percutaneous (through the skin) introduction of a dilating balloon catheter (via a brachial or femoral artery) into a stenosed coronary artery under fluoroscopic control. When the part of the slender catheter containing the balloon straddles the stenosis, the balloon is briefly inflated while balloon pressure and volume are carefully monitored. Successful dilation is indicated by enlargement of the coronary lumen and diminution of the pressure gradient across the stenosis. Patients with proximal, symmetrical, uncalcified coronary artery lesions are the best candidates for this procedure. In skilled hands, the technique has proven successful and complications have been minor.

Direct Myocardial Revascularization

The surgical construction of a bypass venous graft around the obstructed vessel is done in certain cases to reduce pain, alleviate anginal symptoms and preserve the myocardium. It is also reported to increase ventricular performance and contractility. For treatment of left main coronary artery occlusion, surgical treatment seems established. However, the relative effectiveness of medical vs. surgical treatment of one or two vessel coronary artery disease is still an unsettled question.

PCTA and coronary artery bypass are at present the only treatment modalities that increase coronary artery blood flow. The other therapeutic maneuvers work by decreasing myocardial O_2 requirements. In any event, all methods have the common objective of improving the ratio of myocardial O_2 supply to needs.

Cardiac Rehabilitation

For the recuperating IHD patient, the most important part of therapy is this long-term, carefully planned program of cardiac rehabilitation. This includes: (a) early ambulation; (b) periodic exercise stress-testing; (c) a subsequent prescriptive exercise program; and (d) the coordinated, interdisciplinary efforts of psychosocial, educational and vocational counseling aimed at returning the patient to a normal or near-normal life style.

Early ambulation is intended to prevent the detrimental effects of prolonged immobilization (deconditioning) such as the decrease in physical work capacity, hypovolemia, the decrease in pulmonary ventilation, and a negative nitrogen and protein balance. In order to achieve the "training effect," there must be a minimum of two to three exercise periods per week lasting 30 to 40 minutes each, including warmup and cool down. The goal is to reach 70 to 85% of the exercise intensity level (as indicated by heart rate) that was safely achieved during the previous exercise testing.

A successful exercise training program will result in a decrease in the resting heart rate and increases in $\dot{V}O_{2max}$ and maximal cardiac output. As a result, there is a lesser increase in heart rate and systolic pressure (lower double product), less angina, fewer ischemic ECG changes and a more rapid slowing of the heart rate at any given level of submaximal work. The exact mechanism of this improved circulatory performance is not certain but appears to involve peripheral adaptation since there is increased peripheral oxygen extraction. Whether or not there is improved myocardial contractility is uncertain. There is evidence, however, that a certain number of coronary patients are able with high intensity training to achieve endurance capacities almost equal to those of trained normal subjects.

Since many occupations involve arm work, consideration should be given in the exercise prescription to the lack of adaptability transfer of leg to arm training and also the greater tachycardic and hypertensive effect of arm work vs. leg work. It should also be recalled that isometric exercise has a relatively greater hypertensive effect than dynamic exercise and therefore will invoke a much greater cardiac workload.

There is currently little evidence that exercise training alters the natural history of atherosclerotic coronary artery disease or increases myocardial perfusion, but further study is required on these important issues. However, there is little question but that the great majority of patients who follow a planned rehabilitation regimen after MI are greatly benefitted by improved working capacity, greater emotional stability and a distinctly more productive and satisfying life. Exercise stress testing, physical training, detraining, arm vs. leg exercise and isometric exercise are discussed in Chapter 12.

Congestive Heart Failure

Etiology

Congestive failure is a condition in which the heart is unable to pump blood at a rate commensurate with systemic metabolic requirements. It is not a single disease but rather a symptom complex with many causes. Although there is still a considerable knowledge gap, our understanding of the pathophysiology of this disorder has been greatly advanced in recent years. Some of these developments will be discussed in outline form in this section.

The basic cause of the cardiac output deficiency in congestive failure may be *cardiac* or *extracardiac.* The *cardiac* disturbance may be (a) a myocardial contractile failure due to ischemic heart disease, myocarditis or cardiomyopathy (degeneration of the myocardium) or (b) a disorder which prevents proper filling or emptying of the heart such as a valvular stenosis, valvular regurgitation or pericardial disease. *Extracardiac* disorders which may cause congestive failure are high-pressure overloads such as hypertension, or high-output overloads such as renal failure, anemia, AV fistula or thyrotoxicosis. The apparent paradox of a heart failing because of increased output is the result of myocardial work demands in excess of coronary flow capabilities.

From a therapeutic standpoint it would be important to know whether the failure is due to an extracardiac, valvular or pericardial disorder, which may be remediable, in contrast to a basic myocardial, contractile weakness, which is not.

Hemodynamic Mechanisms in Congestive Failure

Theory of the Failure

Controversy has long centered on the question of whether this disorder was primarily a *backward cardiac failure;* in this case the decreased ventricular output and the rising ventricular EDP produced, through retrograde action, increased venous and capillary pressures. The resulting fluid transudation into the tissue spaces contracts the plasma volume which presumably "signals" an increase in tubular reabsorption of sodium and water. It was theorized that this combination of heightened capillary pressure and renal "hyperfunction" resulted in pulmonary and peripheral congestion and edema.

In contrast, the *forward-failure theory* held that the symptoms and signs stemmed from an inadequate left ventricular output with a reduction of renal perfusion pressure and glomerular filtration, and as a consequence, increased sodium and water reabsorption through the renin-angiotensin-aldosterone mechanism. Because it is now known that both mechanisms operate to varying degrees, this classification is not currently useful and has been generally abandoned.

The signs and symptoms of the failure are ascribable to three main hemodynamic changes, *i.e.*, *decreased cardiac output* with hypoperfusion of the peripheral bed, *increased left atrial pressure* with resulting pulmonary congestion and *increased right atrial pressure* with resultant systemic and splanchnic congestion.

Decrease in Cardiac Output

Decreased cardiac output is primarily responsible for the limitation of physical activity, the renal hypoperfusion, the sodium and water retention and the chronic fatigue which is characteristic of this condition; fatigue may precede the other symptoms by many months. The *increased left atrial pressure*, the aftermath of the increased LVEDV and LVEDP, results in increased size of the atrium, increased pulmonary venous and capillary pressure, pulmonary congestion and edema and, if continued, decreased pulmonary air space and pulmonary compliance with resultant dyspnea and orthopnea. In addition to decreasing the available air space, congestion stiffens the lung and increases the work of breathing, leading to a feeling of breathlessness. In the upright position, some of the thoracic blood volume is displaced footward and central venous pressure is decreased. Thus, the patient may be able to breathe comfortably only when upright or propped up with several pillows (orthopnea). This is particularly true at night when, in the supine position, the dependent edema that has developed because of the gravity effect on the circulation (Chapter 6, Venous Pressure) tends to be reabsorbed into the circulation. This increases the central venous volume and congestion of the thoracic veins and leads to nocturnal dyspnea.

As described in Chapter 13, heart failure patients, unlike normal individuals, may show an increased stroke volume and cardiac output in the erect position (Fig. 13.3). If pulmonary capillary pressure becomes sufficiently high, fluid may transude from the plasma into the alveoli (pulmonary edema). The patient then becomes extremely breathless and may produce frothy sputum tinged with blood that has escaped from the capillaries.

Increase in Right Atrial Pressure

This will produce comparable changes in the systemic circulation, *i.e.*, increased volume and pressure in the vena cavae, peripheral veins and capillaries with peripheral edema, particularly of the feet and ankles. There is also increased hepatic venous pressure with hepatic congestion and, if continued, liver dysfunction and intraperitoneal accumulation of fluid (ascites). Hepatic congestion, because of stretch of the liver capsule, may cause aching and tenderness in the region of the liver. Persistent hepatic congestion may also cause hepatic lobular necrosis. Increased right atrial pressure may develop from pulmonic valve stenosis or regurgitation but more commonly is a backward extension of left ventricular failure and pulmonary venous congestion.

In some cases, only one or two of these hemodynamic changes may occur, but all three frequently develop in the same patient. Signs and symptoms may vary considerably depending on the severity and rate of development of the underlying disorder. As mentioned earlier, a myocardial infarct involving over 40% of the myocardium will probably

Figure 14.4. Length-tension curves for normal (O), hypertrophied (□) and failing (△) ventricular muscle in the cat. *Bottom curves* show resting, passive tension and *top curves* show peak contractile tension. Tension is corrected for cross-sectional area. In heart failure, maximum tension is clearly depressed but in hypertrophied muscle, depression is borderline. (Reprinted with permission from J.F. Spann, R.A. Buccino, E.H. Sonnenblick, and E. Braunwald, *Circ Res* 21:341, 1967.)

cause a hemodynamic collapse and cardiogenic shock. On the other hand, a patient may, from a lesser lesion, be in "compensated failure" for many years without severe disability.

Pathophysiological and Compensatory Changes

The most important manifestations of congestive failure are those involving (a) the myocardium, (b) fluid balance, (c) bioenergetics, and (d) the peripheral circulation. These will be discussed in the following sections.

Myocardial Failure and Compensatory Responses

In congestive failure, both clinical and experimental, there is usually a deficit in ventricular contractility as evidenced by depressed length-tension and ventricular function curves (Fig. 14.4, *curve c*).

In addition the myocardium usually shows a decreased force-velocity curve, thus clearly indicating inotropic inadequacy of the myocardium. This contractile defect may arise from a primary myocardial lesion such as MI or from a secondary ischemia resulting from a ventricular pressure or output overload.

The *ejection fraction* (EF) is an important measure of cardiac function in heart failure. The EF generally shows a positive correlation with the cardiac index, although this relationship may not hold in certain conditions such as mitral regurgitation or congestive heart failure. With the decline in left ventricular performance, the EF decreases from its normal value of about 50 or 70% and in severe failure may be as low as 10 to 20%.

The two compensatory mechanisms available to improve myocardial performance, *i.e.*, the *Starling effect* and the *sympathetic inotropic effect* (Chapter 6) are both activated in congestive failure; in addition, *ventricular volume and hypertrophy* changes also occur. These adaptions are discussed in the following.

Starling Effect. The decrease in cardiac output, aided by the increased sodium and water retention (discussed below), leads to progressive elevation of EDV and EDP. This increased diastolic stretch results in increased ventricular performance so long as the ventricle functions on the rising portion of the length-tension curve (Fig. 14.4, *curve c*). However, this improved ventricular performance is achieved at the price of pulmonary congestion in the case of the left ventricle, and systemic venous congestion in the case of the right. As the failure progresses, the heart is operating on a depressed ventricular function curve that is shifted down and to the right (Fig. 14.4).

Increased emphasis has been given recently to another effect of the increased EDV, namely the adverse influence of heightened EDV on ventricular diastolic compliance and the effect of the latter on the hemodynamics of congestive failure.

It will be noted in Figure 14.4 that as the ventricle fills and EDV and resting tension increase, the tension/length ratio, or stiffness, which under normal circumstances is considerably greater than that of skeletal muscle, increases disproportionately. This means that the diastolic or resting compliance (*i.e.*, the reciprocal of stiffness or the length/tension ratio) decreases sharply as the EDV rises. This decreased compliance, coupled in the case of MI with the decreased compliance incident to stiffening of the ischemic segment of the myocardium (mentioned earlier) tends to perpetuate the congestive state. Some investigators have suggested that in some cases the reduced diastolic compliance, *i.e.*, diastolic dysfunction, may be as important a factor in producing congestion as the impaired ventricular systolic contractility, *i.e.*, systolic dysfunction.

Ventricular Volume and Hypertrophy. If a cardiac chamber is subjected to continued distension from an increased preload or afterload stress, its internal capacity will increase; if it is required to consistently produce increased muscular work, either by a volume or pressure overload, it will hypertrophy, *i.e.*, the number of sarcomeres will increase, the wall becomes thicker and the muscle will increase in mass. Pressure overload, *e.g.*, in hypertension or aortic stenosis, produces an increase in muscle mass and relatively little change in ventricular volume in the absence of heart failure. Volume overloads (*e.g.*, those resulting from abnormal shunts, such as atrial septal defects or incompetent valves as in aortic regurgitation) result mainly in ventricular dilation. Ordinarily, they would cause thinning of the wall but because some hypertension almost always develops, the wall thickness is maintained. In most cases, such as occurs physiologically in the endurance athlete and pathologically in congestive failure, there is an increase in both ventricular volume and mass. But changes in myocardial volume and mass are different phenomena and exert independent effects.

As the left ventricular chamber enlarges during early failure, it assumes a more spherical shape and the increased EDV, as described above, has a compensatory, supportive action. However, a continued EDV increase eventually becomes self-defeating because in an expanding, more spherical ventricle, the total force required for an equivalent systolic ejection against a comparable afterload will also increase as the radius increases (Laplace's law). Since myocardial VO_2 is closely correlated with the ventricular wall stress which generates the cardiac force (Chapter 11), the oxygen demand becomes disproportionately greater than the stroke work produced and the process becomes inefficient. This effect on wall stress is only partially offset by the fact that at a larger ventricular size, a given fraction of circumferential shortening will result in a larger stroke volume.

Hypertrophy, *i.e.*, increased mass, is a compensatory mechanism which increases the force-generating capacity of the ventricle. But does hypertrophy lead to improved muscle function? The answer is not clear at present and seems to depend on the individual circumstances. The contractility of the hypertrophied muscle is reportedly only slightly less than that of a normal muscle (Fig. 14.4, *curve b*). Hypertrophy causes the increased pressure load to be distributed over a greater number of sarcomeres, and wall tension (T) becomes more normalized since the increase in pressure (P) is balanced by the increase in wall thickness (μ) (Laplace's theorem, Chapter 2). Therefore in conjunction with the Starling and other compensatory effects, hypertrophy helps to maintain overall circulatory compensation.

However, there is also a limit to this adaptive process, imposed mainly by an already borderline coronary perfusion pressure supplying a growing tissue mass. The net benefit will depend on the ability of a limited hypertrophy to establish compensation. Unfortunately, increased wall thickness will also decrease wall compliance and in the case of failing heart, increased wall stiffness is an added disadvantage.

Gradually developing ventricular hypertrophy produced by intermittent volume overload (*e.g.*, the hypertrophy of endurance athletes engaged in sports that involve largely isotonic activity such as running or swimming) results in improved cardiac functioning. Abrupt pressure overload usually (but not inevitably) leads to depressed ventricular performance. Clinical and experimental studies have shown that myocardial hypertrophy is at least to some extent reversible. For example, in experimental animals a 50% increase in left ventricular mass was induced by 10 weeks of gradually developing experimental hypertension; reversal of this pressure overload resulted (in 10 more weeks) in the regression of all the mechanical and biochemical abnormalities. Recent animal studies have shown that aside from arterial pressure reduction, decline of myocardial mass also depends on sympathetic stimulation. Decrease of myocardial catecholamines favors regression of myocardial hypertrophy.

Bioenergetics of Congestive Failure

The biochemical changes accompanying muscle contraction may be divided into three sequential processes: energy production or the conversion of substrates to high energy phosphates; energy utilization, *i.e.*, the translation of high energy phosphates to contractile activity; and excitation-contraction coupling, the mechanism by which the myocardial action potential results in calcium movement, which in turn mediates the contraction and relaxation (Chapter 6).

Studies have shown that even in severe failure, mitochondrial function is not disturbed so that energy production appears adequate. ATP is converted to ADP primarily during the interaction of myosin and actin to produce shortening; the rate of this reaction correlates well with contractility. It has been shown that there is a deficiency in the myofibrillar-ATPase system in severe failure and some reduction of function in myocardial hypertrophy without failure, but the full implications of these defects are not yet known.

In some types of congestive failure, the ATP-dependent calcium pump of the isolated sarcoplasmic reticulum is defective. Both the amount and the rate at which calcium is pumped into the sarcoplasmic reticulum are deficient and with the development of hypertrophy, the content of sarcoplasmic reticulum per muscle unit is reduced; thus there may be a dilution of sarcoplasmic reticulum incident to the hypertrophy process itself. It is, therefore, evident that biochemical defects do exist in the failing muscle, but which are the critical ones is not yet known.

Fluid Balance in Congestive Failure

✝As cardiac output decreases in congestive failure, the reduced renal arterial hydrostatic pressure as well as the reflex renal vasoconstriction (described below) combine to reduce renal blood flow, particularly in the outer renal cortex. There results a reduction in glomerular filtration rate which leads to salt and water retention and eventually, if continued, to edema. The mechanism resembles the response to hemorrhage described in Chapter 13; the reduced renal blood flow leads to the liberation of renin, the elaboration of angiotensin II and ultimately to the production of aldosterone by the zona glomerulosa of the adrenal cortex.

The hepatic dysfunction which accompanies severe congestive failure is responsible for a reduced catabolism of aldosterone so that aldosterone plasma levels are higher and more sustained, thus accentuating the fluid retention. Renal venous congestion plays a variable but generally limited role in the fluid balance disturbance.

Thus patients with congestive failure usually have increased blood volume, interstitial fluid volume and increased total body sodium levels; however, this may be associated with normal or even decreased serum Na^+ concentrations. Increased physical activity, because it causes increased sympathetic stimulation and heightened plasma norepinephrine, will result in further lowering of renal blood flow and the glomerular filtration rate and will increase the salt and water retention. Thus, during the decompensated phase of congestive failure, rest and restricted activity are an important part of therapy.

Figure 14.5. Norepinephrine levels in arterial blood are higher in severe heart failure patients (class III and IV) at rest and after exercise than in normal subjects or in patients with milder heart failure (I and II). (Reprinted with permission from E. Braunwald, *The Myocardium: Failure and Infarction*. New York: HP Publishing Co., 1974.)

Autonomic Reflexes in Congestive Failure

On the basis of experimental studies and clinical findings, Abboud et al. have suggested that in the early hypervolemic stage of heart failure there is a suppression of the renin-angiotensin-aldosterone system due perhaps to the increased cardiac distension and firing of cardiac vagal afferent fibers. It is further theorized that in the later stages of hypervolemia and cardiac distension the cardiac vagal endings adapt and there is a decrease in discharge frequency in these cardiac afferent nerves thereby resulting in the increased neurohormonal drive seen in chronic heart failure in animals and humans (Chapter 10, Cardiopulmonary Reflexes). This result is associated with increased sympathetic outflow and elevated plasma norepinephrine, renin, aldosterone and ADH. This increased sympathetic outflow is responsible for an increased inotropic effect on the myocardium and an increased peripheral vasoconstriction described below.

Sympathetic Inotropic Effect: Myocardial Response. During congestive failure, there is augmented sympathetic activity and increased concentration of plasma norepinephrine at rest and during exercise (Fig. 14.5). The resultant increase in force and velocity of myocardial contraction exerts a considerable functional support for the heart. However, with continued sympathetic overactivity, the myocardial catecholamine stores become depleted, due mainly to a reduction of myocardial tyrosine hydroxylase, which is the rate-limiting step for the conversion of tyrosine to norepinephrine. This depletion is apparently not involved, however, in the pathogenesis of failure; it may be that the residual catecholamines from the adrenal medulla and other sources remain effective because of the *de facto* denervation of the myocardium and the consequent hypersensitivity response to catechols (Chapter 9).

Sympathetic Vasoconstriction Effect. The vasoconstriction results in a significant redistribution of left ventricular output, which, like hypervolemia and the inotropic effect, is an important compensatory mechanism (Fig. 14.6).

This redistribution diverts the renal and cutaneous portions of an already reduced cardiac output to the more critical cerebral and coronary beds. This occurs even at rest but is intensified in the presence of exercise, fever or other stresses. There is a general increased tone of peripheral arteries and veins and with only modest physical activity, a marked vasoconstriction of mesenteric and renal vascular beds as well. The heightened tone of the peripheral vessels is partially due to an increased infiltration of sodium and water into the arterial walls. The net result is a reduced ability of the vessels to dilate with increased activity so that oxygen extraction is limited (Fig. 14.7). Exercise or increased metabolic states will, therefore, produce lactic acidemia and an inability to dissipate heat. Consequently, the heart failure patient frequently has a heat intolerance.

The cause of the heightened sympathetic activity is not certain; it may be due—as mentioned above—to a lessened cardiac receptor activity (because of adaptation) or to a lessened arterial baroceptor stimulation secondary to a decrease in arterial pressure. An increased arterial chemoreceptor stimulation from an elevated PCO_2 and lowered pH may also contribute to the sympathetic activation. Heart failure is also associated with a marked deficiency of parasympathetic function as shown, *e.g.*, by a marked reduction of the bradycardic reflex response to both arterial hypertension and to the pressure overshoot phase of the Valsalva test.

As previously mentioned, the decreased ability to alter peripheral blood flow is of considerable functional significance to heart failure patients. Equally disadvantageous is the reduced ability to alter heart rate. Since these patients already have severe limitations in their ability to adjust stroke volume, the added rate limitation is an appreciable further handicap in meeting cardiac output needs.

Treatment of Congestive Failure

Therapy will depend on the severity and rate of development of the disease and will be directed first of all toward the specific cause of the failure. The treatment of the congestive failure itself usually has three objectives: (a) reduction of cardiac work load, (b) enhancement of cardiac contractility and (c) control of excessive fluid retention.

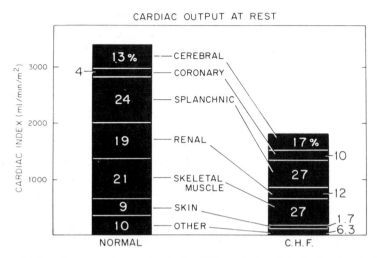

Figure 14.6.   Decrease in cardiac index (CI) and alteration in fractional distribution of CI in congestive failure patients (CHF). (Reprinted with permission from A.C. Hseih, *The Peripheral Circulation*, edited by R. Zelis. New York: Grune & Stratton, 1975.)

Figure 14.7.   Forearm blood flow in congestive heart failure patients (CHF) increased less during handgrip exercise than that of normal subjects at all exercise levels showing inability of peripheral vessels to dilate properly to metabolic stimulus. (Reprinted with permission from A.C. Hseih, *The Peripheral Circulation*, edited by R. Zelis. New York: Grune & Stratton, 1975.)

Reduction of Cardiac Work. This is done mainly by reducing afterload through rest, lessening of physical and emotional stress and sometimes through modest doses of vasodilators. The latter agents reduce peripheral vessel resistance and preload thereby reducing ventricular EDV, EDP and myocardial O_2 demands while increasing stroke volume and cardiac index. The reduction in EDV is highly beneficial since it is mechanically more advantageous to increase SV by increasing ejection fraction than by increasing EDV.

The objective is to reduce the cardiac work with a minimal reduction in aortic pressure. In attempting to manipulate aortic pressure, a balance must be struck between a relatively low value to reduce afterload and cardiac work while maintaining a sufficiently high level to insure reasonable perfusion of the coronary bed and peripheral tissues. As previously mentioned, the autoregulatory capacity of the coronary bed is often compromised in heart failure so that flow is more directly dependent on perfusion pressure.

In some cases, the above forms of treatment will also relieve fluid retention. If not, more specific therapy is used in the form of (a) *thiazide diuretics* which reduce tubular reabsorption of sodium and thus increase its excretion, or (b) agents such as furosemide or aldactone (the latter because of its aldosterone-antagonist activity), which also exert powerful diuretic action.

Therapy must be carefully controlled. Although it is a pathological condition, hypervolemia is a compensatory change with a purpose. Rapid loss of fluid without improved cardiac performance might trade the edema for the increased fatigue of inadequate cardiac output. Overzealous use of diuretics with resultant hypovolemia must be particularly avoided.

Vasodilators. These unloading agents exert their effect through their ability to dilate arteries and veins. Some agents (*e.g.*, hydralazine) are primarily arteriolar vasodilators and help to reduce afterload while other agents (*e.g.*, nitrates) act mainly to dilate veins and help to reduce preload stress. Nitroprusside and prazosin have both arterial dilating and venous pooling effects. A recently introduced afterload reducing agent, captopril, an inhibitor of the enzyme that converts angiotensin I to angiotensin II, has also been reported as effective in congestive failure.

Glycosides. Digitalis and other glycosides have the fortuitous property of producing a more effective positive inotropic action in the failing rather than the normal heart; this is probably due to a combination of its direct myocardial effect with an arteriolar and venular dilation action. Positive inotropic agents shift the ventricular function curve upward, permitting reestablishment of some cardiac reserve and improvement of ejection fraction.

References

Ischemic Heart Disease

Abboud FM, Fozzard HA, Gilmore JP, and Reis DJ. *Disturbances in Neurogenic Control of the Circulation.* Bethesda, Md.: American Physiological Society, 1981.

Bosnjak ZJ, Zuperku EJ, Coon RL, and Kampine JP. Acute coronary artery occlusion and cardiac sympathetic afferent nerve activity. *Proc Soc Exp Biol Med* 161:142–148, 1979.

Braunwald EA, Ross J, and Sonnenblick EH. *Mechanisms of Contraction of the Normal and Failing Heart.* Boston: Little, Brown, 1976, 2nd ed.

Brooks H, Holland R, and Al Sadir J. Right ventricular performance during ischemia: an anatomic and hemodynamic analysis. *Am J Physiol* 233:H500, 1978.

Cobb LA, Werner SA, and Trobaugh GB. Sudden cardiac death. *Mod Concepts Cardiovasc Dis* 42:31–42, 1980.

Elliot RS. *Stress and the Major Cardiovascular Disorders.* Mt. Kisco, N.Y.: Futura Publishing Co., 1979.

Ellrodt G, Chew CYC, and Singh BN. Therapeutic implications of slow channel blockade in cardiocirculatory disorders. *Circulation* 62:669–679, 1980.

Gross GJ. Antianginal drugs. In: *Modern Pharmacology*, edited by CR Craig and RW Stitzel. Boston: Little, Brown, 1982.

Gruntzig AR. Percutaneous transluminal dilation of chronic coronary stenosis. In: *Advances in Heart Disease*, edited by DT Mason. New York: Grune & Stratton, 1980, Vol. III.

Heart Book. American Heart Association. New York: EP Dutton, 1980.

Herman MV and Gorlin R. Pathophysiology of ischemic heart disease. In: *Clinical Cardiovascular Physiology*, edited by HJ Levine. New York: Grune & Stratton, 1976.

Hillis LD and Braunwald E. Coronary artery spasm. *N Engl J Med* 299:695–702, 1978.

Kirk ES and Jennings RB. Pathophysiology of myocardial ischemia. In: *The Heart, Arteries and Veins*, edited by JW Hurst. New York: McGraw-Hill, 1982, 5th ed., pp. 976–1008.

Ogawa T, Wyden JK, Rose HB, Kanazana M, Seino V, and Swan HJC. Peripheral circulatory changes after physical conditioning in coronary artery disease patients. *J Cardiac Rehabil* 1:269–275, 1981.

Pantridge JF, Webb SW, Adgey AAJ, and Geddes JS. The first hour after the onset of acute myocardial infarction. In: *Progress in Cardiology*, edited by PN Yu and JF Goodwin, Philadelphia: Lea & Febiger, 1974, Chap. 5, Vol. 3, pp. 173–188.

Pollack ML and Schmidt DH.: *Heart Disease and Rehabilitation.* Boston: Houghton Mifflin, 1979.

Randall WC. *Neural Regulation of the Heart.* New York: Oxford University Press, 1977.

Shand DG. Beta adrenergic blocking drugs after acute myocardial infarction. *Mod Concepts Cardiovasc Dis* 51:103–106, 1982.

Thames MD, Klopfenstein HS, Abboud FW, Mark AL, and Walter JL. Preferential distribution of inhibitory cardiac receptors with vagal afferents to the inferoposterior wall of the left ventricle activated during coronary occlusion in the dog. *Circ Res* 43:512–519, 1978.

Tristani FE, Kamper DG, McDermott DJ, Peters BS, and Smith JJ. Alteration of postural and Valsalva responses in coronary heart disease. *Am J Physiol* 233:H694–H699, 1977.

Wenger NK and Hellerstein HK. *Rehabilitation of the Coronary Patient.* New York: John Wiley & Sons, 1978.

Congestive Heart Failure

Abboud FM, Thames M, and Mark AL. Role of cardiac afferent nerves in regulation of circulation during coronary occlusion and heart failure. In: *Disturbances in Neurogenic Control of the Circulation*, edited by FM Abboud, HA Fozzard, JP Gilmore and DJ Reis. Bethesda, Md.: American Physiological Society, 1981, pp. 65–86.

Braunwald E, Ross J, and Sonnenblick EH. *Mechanisms of Contraction of the Normal and Failing Heart.* Boston: Little, Brown, 1976, 2nd ed.

Brenner BM, and Rector FC. *The Kidney.* Philadelphia: WB Saunders, 1976.

Capasso JM, Strobeck JE, Malhotra A, Scheuer J, and Sonnenblick EH. Contractile behavior of rat myocardium after reversal of hypertensive hypertrophy. *Am J Physiol* 242:H882–889, 1982.

Langer GA. Myocardial force development in health and disease. In: *Pathophysiology of the Heart,* edited by G Ross. New York: Masson Publishing Co., 1982, pp. 1–39.

Levine HJ and Gaasch WJ. Diastolic compliance of the left ventricle. *Mod Concepts Cardiovasc Dis* 47:95–102, 1978.

Mason DT, Zelis R, and Wikman-Coffelt J. Symposium on congestive heart failure. *Am J Cardiol* 32:395, 1973.

Sen S and Tarazi RC. Regression of myocardial hypertrophy and influence of the adrenergic system. *Am J Physiol* 244:H97–101, 1983.

Spann JG and Hurst JW. The recognition and management of heart disease. In: *The Heart, Arteries and Veins,* edited by JW Hurst. New York: McGraw-Hill, 1982, 5th ed., pp. 407–451.

Tillisch JH. Pump failure and cardiogenic shock. In: *Pathophysiology of the Heart,* edited by G Ross. New York: Masson Publishing Co., 1982, pp. 225–256.

Zelis R, Flaim SF, Liedke AS, and Nellis SH. Cardiocirculatory dynamics in the normal and failing heart. *Annu Rev Physiol* 43:455–476, 1981.

Zucker IH and Gilmore JP. Atrial receptor modulation of renal function in heart failure. In: *Disturbances in Neurogenic Control of the Circulation,* edited by FM Abboud, HA Fozzard, JP Gilmore and DJ Reis. Bethesda, Md.: American Physiological Society, 1981, pp. 1–16.

chapter 15

Pathophysiology: Hypertension and Circulatory Shock

Hypertension

Definitions and Classification

About 20% of the adult population are afflicted with hypertension, the most common single disorder seen in the office of an internist. It is a major risk factor for coronary artery disease and a common cause of heart failure, kidney failure, stroke and blindness. As Pickering has pointed out, the designation of a single dividing line between normotension and hypertension is somewhat artificial. The diagnosis is usually based on repeated resting levels of $\geqq 140/90$ mm Hg in adults 18 to 49 years of age and $\geqq 160/95$ mm Hg in adults over 50 years of age. It is more common among males than females and far more common among blacks than whites.

Systolic hypertension, *i.e.*, the condition in which the systolic rise is more prominent, increases with age, and in men over 45 years is considered a greater risk factor for coronary heart disease (CHD) than diastolic hypertension. Obesity is a strong predisposing factor and hypertension is 10 times more common in persons 20% or more overweight. About 10% of adult hypertension is due to a specific, identifiable cause and is termed *secondary hypertension*. The remaining 90%, in which the cause cannot be determined, is classified as primary or *essential hypertension* (EH). The latter develops more often between the ages of 35 to 50 years. Hypertension developing during infancy or childhood or after the age of 50 is often of the secondary variety.

There are multiple ways in which arterial blood pressure can be raised and for almost each pressor mechanism, there is a representative example of a clinical type of hypertension. Only EH and a few of the more common types of secondary hypertension will be considered in this chapter. The renal circulation, which is closely involved in the pathogenesis of hypertension, was reviewed in Chapter 11.

Secondary Hypertension

Renovascular Hypertension

Renal diseases are the most frequent cause of secondary hypertension and include two clinical entities, *renovascular hypertension*, a disease of the renal arteries, and *renal parenchymal hypertension*. While kidney disease and hypertension have long been clinically associated, the relation between the two was obscure until Goldblatt showed that persistent hypertension could be produced experimentally by constriction of the renal arteries.

Renovascular hypertension is the result of stenosis of one or both renal arteries, usually caused by atherosclerosis or fibromuscular hyperplasia. Although these patients frequently have evidence of increased adrenergic drive to the circulatory system (*e.g.*, increased heart rate, cardiac output, left ventricular ejection, venoconstriction, increased autonomic responsiveness) the underlying cause of the hypertension is the increased production and release of renin and angiotensin II (Fig. 11.13). Angiotensin II raises arterial pressure through (a) its very potent systemic vasoconstrictor effect and (b) through stimulation of aldosterone secretion with a resultant sodium retention and increase in interstitial fluid volume and plasma volume. Because β-adrenergic blockade can reduce renin activity, it is sometimes used in the treatment of renovascular hypertension.

Renal Parenchymal Hypertension

This occurs in a variety of acute and chronic renal parenchymal diseases such as pyelonephritis (inflammation of the renal pelvis) or chronic glomerulonephritis. It is thought that the underlying cause is a decreased renal perfusion due to inflammatory and fibrotic changes. In contrast to renovascular hypertension, patients with volume-loading hypertension, such as renal parenchymal hypertension, aldosteronism or Cushing's syndrome (described below), usually have a normal cardiac output associated with elevated peripheral resistance and increased heart rate.

Endocrine Hypertension

Clinically and experimentally, it is known that when about 70% of the kidney mass has been destroyed and fluid and sodium intake increased, a "volume-loading hypertension" will be produced. It is basically the sodium which is responsible, since a persistent hypertension will not result if only water is retained. Similar types of hypertension will occur in certain endocrine disorders such as *primary aldosteronism*, a condition due to an adrenal tumor with excessive aldosterone secretion and increased sodium reabsorption; there is frequently an associated muscle weakness due to potassium depletion.

Hypertension will also occur in *Cushing's syndrome* which is characterized by excessive secretion of glucocorticoids and sodium retention. Another cause of hypertension is *pheochromocytoma*, an adrenal medullary tumor in which there is increased secretion of epinephrine and norepinephrine associated with chronic peripheral vasoconstriction and myocardial hyperkinesis; in this disorder, heightened sympathetic tone rather than volume expansion is the main characteristic. *Mineralocorticoid hypertension* is characterized by low plasma levels of renin and aldosterone but elevated secretion of deoxycorticosterone (DOCA) or DOCA analogues, often associated with hypokalemia. In some of these patients, the administration of an aldosterone antagonist such as spironolactone will result in a loss of sodium and a lowering of the blood pressure.

Other Types of Hypertension

There are other varieties of hypertension in which the inciting cause is known but the mechanism is uncertain. These include hypertension due to drugs such as oral contraceptives or monoamine oxidase and those due to hypercalcemia and to the toxemia of pregnancy. Hypertension, primarily systolic in nature, can also be caused by coarctation of the aorta, hyperthyroidism and decreased distensibility of the aorta.

Essential Hypertension

Hemodynamic Changes

Arterial pressure can rise because of an increase in cardiac output or vascular resistance or both. The fundamental defect in essential hypertension (EH) is the failure of the pressure-regulating mechanisms, although exactly where the failure lies is not yet known. The hemodynamic changes as well as the ensuing clinical picture depend on the stage and type of the disease.

Borderline, mild or labile hypertension include almost three-quarters of hypertensives. Most of these patients have increased heart rate, stroke volume (SV), cardiac output (CO) and increased rate of ventricular ejection but normal or only slightly elevated total peripheral resistance (TPR). In some patients, there is evidence of increased venomotor tone and decreased systemic venous compliance, which are undoubtedly responsible for the migration of blood toward the thorax with a resultant increased central blood volume (CBV). Since the total blood volume (TBV) is usually normal, these patients have an increased ratio of central to total blood volume (CBV/TBV). The increased CBV in turn, via the Starling mechanism, is probably responsible for the increased stroke volume and cardiac output, as suggested by clinical reports which show a highly significant, positive correlation between the CBV/TBV ratio and the cardiac output. These patients usually have elevated plasma renin activity (PRA) levels.

These hemodynamic findings indicate a hyperkinetic circulation with increased adrenergic drive to the heart and peripheral vessels. During head-up tilt, mental arithmetic and other stresses, borderline hypertensives frequently respond with a greater rise in blood pressure than normal subjects. These increased autonomic reflex reactions are undoubtedly further manifestations of the sympathetic hyperkinesis that exists during this stage of EH.

About one-fourth of hypertensives fall into the *moderate, severe or accelerated hypertension* classification. In these patients the pathophysiology depends on the level of the arterial pressure and the degree of TPR and cardiac enlargement. As the disease progresses, TPR rises. The left ventricular ejection rate and cardiac output decrease to normal or

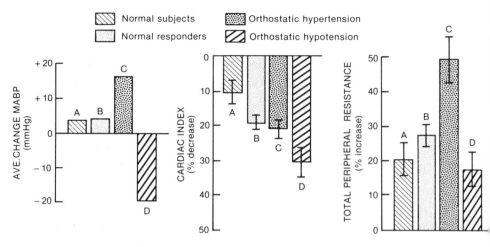

Figure 15.1. Responses of mean arterial blood pressure (MABP) (*left*), cardiac output (*middle*), and total peripheral resistance (*right*) to 50° head-up tilt in hypertensive patients. Normal subjects (*A*) and moderate hypertensives (*B*) showed similar arterial pressure changes. Patients with mild or early hypertension (*C*) showed increased arterial pressure (orthostatic hypertension) characterized by a moderate fall in cardiac output and a marked elevation in peripheral resistance—a hyperkinetic reaction. Severe hypertensives (*D*) had orthostatic hypotension which was the result of a marked fall in cardiac output and a lesser rise in vascular resistance. (Reprinted with permission from E.D. Frohlich et al.: Tilt test for investigating a neural component in hypertension. *Circulation* 36:387, 1967.)

subnormal levels and the left ventricle enlarges progressively in response to the increased afterload. Peripheral resistance rises in all vascular beds but most notably in the kidney. Plasma volume is reduced and PRA values are often elevated although, for reasons not yet clear, some hypertensives have low PRAs.

In contrast to mild hypertension, there is in this stage little evidence of adrenergic stimulation; autonomic responses to baroceptor stimulation, to the Valsalva test and to head-up tilt (Fig. 15.1) are diminished in advanced hypertension. Postural disturbances are further discussed in Chapter 13.

The atherosclerotic process is widespread and very closely linked to the pathology of EH. With continued pressure elevation, the atherosclerosis will be progressive regardless of the cause of the hypertension. Because of atherosclerosis, the hypertension, if unchecked, predisposes to ischemic heart disease, cerebrovascular accident or renal disease with uremia (accumulation of urea and other protein metabolites in the blood). In some cases, for unknown reasons, the process becomes accelerated (malignant hypertension).

Pathogenesis

Only a brief outline will be given here of the immense investigative effort which continues to go into the etiology of EH. In this search, two features of the disease have loomed prominently, *viz.*, the strong genetic susceptibility and the self-perpetuating nature of the disease. The hereditary predisposition is polygenetically transferred as is evident not only from a study of clinical records but also from the emergence through inbreeding of spontaneously hypertensive rats (SHR) whose disease strongly resembles EH. In other genetic studies, rat strains have been developed which are supersensitive to salt feeding, *i.e.*, strains in which hypertension will occur on salt diets which are innocuous to normal rats.

The concept of the almost inevitable progression of the disease is fostered by the evidence that hypertension begets arteriosclerosis, which in turn begets further pressure elevation. But what starts the process and why the arterial pressure regulating system breaks down are not known. Among the many explanations for the initiation of EH are the *neurogenic theory*, proposed by Folkow and others, the *arterial pressure-urinary output theory* of Guyton and the *regulatory imbalance* or mosaic theory of Page.

The *neurogenic theory* is supported in part by the considerable evidence that the nervous system is much involved in the regulation of arterial pressure. For example, hypertension can be induced in experimental animals by transection of arterial baroceptor nerves, by lesions of the nucleus tractus solitarius (NTS) or lateral anterior hypothalamus or by chronic stimulation of the posterior hypothalamus (Fig. 15.2). Normal animals can become chronically hypertensive when exposed to stressful learning situations, prolonged noise or long-term psychogenic, emotional-frustration experiments. A recent interesting report indicates that carefully placed lesions in the preoptic region of the anterior hypothalamus will prevent a number of forms of experimental hypertension. Such a lesion will, *e.g.*, protect rats against subsequent development of renal hypertension, against deoxycorticosterone hypertension and also against experimental hypertension produced by arterial baroceptor denervation or NTS lesions. Obviously considerable investigation is still required to unravel the basic role of the hypothalamus and other higher centers in the production of neurogenic hypertension.

The *arterial pressure-urinary output theory* suggests a relationship that has long been suspected between elevated levels of body sodium and hypertension. In countries where Na^+ intake is high, so is the frequency of hypertension and, as mentioned above, genetic strains have been developed in which ordinarily innocuous high salt diets will cause

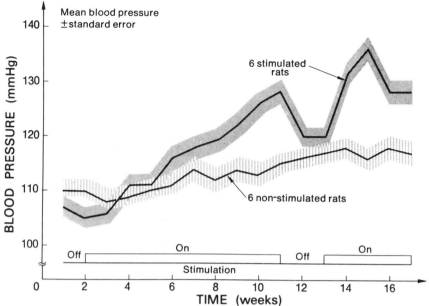

Figure 15.2. Enduring hypertension resulting from chronic stimulation of the hypothalamic defense area in the conscious rat. Stimulation was stopped during the 11th to 13th weeks. (Reprinted with permission from B. Folkow and E.H. Rubinstein, *Acta Physiol Scand* 68:48, 1966.)

hypertension. As previously described, certain types of renal pathology will induce persistent hypertension but the mechanism is not known.

From an extensive application of computer techniques to renal and arterial pressure control systems, Guyton has developed a theory (previously described in Chapter 10) for the role of the kidney in blood pressure control. This theory proposes that the predominant long-term influence on the height of the arterial pressure is the urinary output of sodium and water, particularly the former. He suggests that even a minor disturbance in renal function can lead to a progressive increase in extracellular fluid and plasma volume with a continued elevation in arterial pressure because of the infinite gain of the system. Guyton's theory holds, therefore, that EH begins as a renovascular deficiency and continues because of an obligatory arterial pressure-urinary output relation.

Page's *regulatory imbalance theory* assumes that a steady state exists among a number of factors which regulate blood pressure (Fig. 15.3). The different factors contribute, in varying degrees, to the maintenance of balance. One or more of these variables may be changed in an independent manner to produce hypertension. The theory assumes that

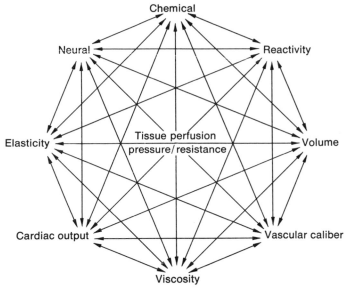

Figure 15.3.   Mosaic octagon illustrating multiple factors underlying the pressure/resistance control of tissue perfusion. (Reprinted with permission from I.H. Page, *Circ Res* 34:133, 1974.)

EH is a "multifactorial disease of regulation" and that no single underlying cause is to be expected since no one mechanism dominates the regulatory process.

Page's theory has gained recent adherents among a number of investigators who have gradually abandoned the unitary theory. Folkow, *e.g.*, believes that aside from the undoubted hereditary influence, the two paramount environmental factors are: (a) psychoemotional (neurogenic) overstress and (b) high salt intake. He believes that either of these—or other factors—may initiate the hypertension but that the arteriosclerotic process perpetuates it. Folkow suggests that the early hypertrophy of the media layer of precapillary resistance vessels (induced by the beginning hypertension) increases internal wall thickness (w), which has been shown to decrease the internal vessel radius (r_i). According to Laplace's law, T (wall tension) = P (transmural pressure) $\times$ r_i/w. If P is increased, the quotient r_i/w tends to decrease in order to maintain equilibrium (Chapter 2). However, because of the 4th power effect of radius change on vascular resistance, any r_i change instigated by the hypertension will induce an amplification effect on resistance. Thus further wall thickening and encroachment on r_i will lead to a nonspecific hyperreactivity of the vessel to constrictor stimuli; this will, in turn, trigger a progressive structural adaptation (thickening) of the vascular muscle. It is theorized that in predisposed individuals, this positive feedback phenomenon may be the basis for enduring hypertension.

Treatment of Hypertension

Among cardiovascular disorders, there are few that require greater skill in differential diagnosis or more diligent, constant attention to achieve successful treatment. Yet there are also very few in which the available treatment is as effective and the outlook as promising, provided the patient is cooperative. Because the symptoms are often minimal and the side effects of the drugs sometimes unpleasant, patients are frequently unwilling to follow their regimen.

The therapy for secondary types of hypertension is first of all directed at the specific cause. In the large exclusion group, *i.e.*, EH, general measures would be instituted such as reduction of internal and external stress (so far as possible), moderate restriction of calories, cholesterol, saturated fat and salt, and finally regular physical exercise within the limits of the patient's age and cardiovascular status. For specific therapy, it is sometimes possible to select antihypertensive medication with a mechanism of action that specifically fits the pressor mechanism involved. This usually means a combination of diuretics, sympathetic inhibitors, vasodilators and converting enzyme inhibitors.

Thiazide and related diuretics frequently form the basis of antihypertensive drug therapy. Thiazides, the most commonly used diuretics, lower arterial pressure by blocking sodium reabsorption at the distal nephron and thus cause salt and water depletion. Furosemide—a less commonly used diuretic—acts primarily to inhibit active chloride transport at the ascending loops of Henle. Diuretics are usually begun at moderate doses, the results followed, the dosage regulated and other agents added to achieve specific effects in individual patients. Careful attention is given to side effects, which include potassium loss, alkalosis and elevated uric acid, glucose and triglycerides.

Sympathetic inhibitors act at multiple sites through diverse mechanisms but affect particularly the heart, kidney and vascular smooth muscle. Clonidine is an imidazoline derivative that stimulates the α_2-receptors in the brain stem, thereby diminishing the sympathetic outflow to the vascular system. Prazosin produces its relaxing effects on vascular smooth muscle through selective blockade of postsynaptic α_2-receptors in the peripheral vascular beds. Propranolol and other β-blockers act at multiple sites and also serve to reduce the renin secretion, thus inhibiting the renin-angiotensin-aldosterone (RAA) system. "High renin" and "normal renin" hypertensives respond better to propranolol while "low renin" hypertensives respond better to diuretics. Some investigators have therefore advocated "renin-sodium profiling" in order to improve therapy selection for the hypertensive patient.

A side effect of diuretic agents and sympathetic blockers is orthostatic hypotension induced partly by the decreased plasma volume and partly (in the case of the sympathetic inhibitors) because of the reduction in cardiac output and peripheral resistance. Elderly patients are often particularly vulnerable to orthostatic hypotension so that treatment should start at lower doses and the blood pressure should be reduced very gradually over a period of one to three months.

Vasodilating agents such as hydralazine and minoxidil, which relax vascular smooth muscle, cause fluid retention and reflex tachycardia. For this reason, they are not used alone but mainly as adjuncts. Captopril, an angiotensin-converting enzyme (ACE) inhibitor, is now being used increasingly in controlling hypertension. Calcium antagonists such as verapamil and nifedipine are also proving useful in the treatment of hypertension.

The mortality in hypertension, which results mainly from myocardial failure, stroke or renal failure, has in the last years been markedly reduced with the advent of effective antihypertensive drugs. Yet there is recent disconcerting evidence that while the lives of hypertensive patients are being prolonged, arteriosclerosis is still the cause of a high percentage of deaths; thus antihypertensive therapy is apparently blunting the disease but not preventing the eventual development of atherosclerosis. These findings are being further investigated.

Circulatory Shock

General Characteristics and Classification

Circulatory shock is a failure of the circulation with decreased perfusion and/or inadequate oxygenation of the vital organs and cells of the body. It is due to trauma, blood loss, myocardial failure, infection or other serious bodily insult, and if untreated, has a tendency to progress toward general circulatory failure and death. Although the causes of circulatory shock are multiple, there are three main clinical types, *i.e.*, hypovolemic, cardiogenic and septic shock.

In *hypovolemic shock*, a decrease in circulating blood volume is responsible for the fall in arterial pressure; in *cardiogenic shock* it is myocardial failure, *e.g.*, as a result of myocardial infarction, which causes the circulatory collapse. *Septic shock* often occurs incident to a massive infection, in which cardiac output and arterial pressure are usually normal or above normal, but the vital organs, because of a metabolic defect, are unable to extract adequate oxygen from the circulating blood.

While there are important clinical differences between the various types of shock, there are also many common features. A previously untreated patient after a severe trauma or blood loss will usually have a characteristic profound pallor of the skin and mucous membranes, there will be a cold sweat and a rapid, almost imperceptible, "thready" pulse (rate ≥ 140/min). The arterial pressure will be low (perhaps 85/60), the rectal temperature is often decreased to about 96 or 97°F and respiration is feeble. The patient may be restless yet apathetic, and often semirational. Without early and proper treatment such a circulatory failure will frequently progress to irreversibility and death.

Among the earliest systematic investigations into the mechanism of circulatory shock were those of Dr. George W. Crile, a surgeon, who in 1899 reported his studies on shock in animals and the effect of different types of therapy. He described the low central venous pressure, the failure of venous return and cardiac output and the response to infusion. He believed the ultimate failure of the circulation to be due to sympathoadrenal exhaustion.

In 1918 Cannon and his colleagues studied shock in wounded soldiers in France; later in an extensive monograph they emphasized the correlation between low blood pressure and arterial acidosis as well as the beneficial effects of sodium bicarbonate infusion. These authors concluded that a histaminelike toxin, liberated from the traumatized cells, was the primary causative agent of the circulatory failure.

During the last 40 years, spurred particularly by the need for improved treatment of military casualties, extensive studies have been made of the pathogenesis and treatment of shock. As a result, shock therapy has improved dramatically; treatment is more "aggressive" with early and vigorous infusion of blood or blood substitutes and more reliable autonomic and inotropic agents have become available. Particularly effective has been the segregation of these patients into a special intensive care unit (ICU) or coronary care unit (CCU) with trained personnel and facilities for continuous on-line recording of vital cardiopulmonary parameters. As a consequence, the recovery rate in severe shock has been greatly improved.

In studies of severely shocked patients, it has been noted that in order to achieve hemodynamic stability, it is frequently necessary to infuse much greater amounts of fluid or blood than would be anticipated (Fig. 15.4). This is because of excessive fluid loss through hemorrhage, sequestration into certain capillary beds, diffusion into interstitial tissues, or failure of venomotor tone (as described below).

Hypovolemic Shock

The pathophysiological changes and, therefore, the clinical picture, will vary somewhat in the different types of shock. In this section,

Figure 15.4. Posttraumatic shock. A 77-year-old male patient with a crushing injury of both legs and bilateral fractures of the femur, tibia and fibula; the patient, who had very little external blood loss, required blood infusions totaling 8,000 ml over 7 hours. (Reprinted with permission from L.D. MacLean, J.H. Duff, and A.P. McLean, *Can Med Assoc J* 105:78, 1971.)

hypovolemic shock, which is in a sense a prototype of clinical shock, will be described; later in the chapter some of the specific features of cardiogenic and septic shock will be discussed. Hypovolemic shock may result from hemorrhage, trauma, burns, excess radiation or any other injury which involves severe loss of body fluids, plasma or blood. In many of these conditions, *e.g.*, in burns or acute pancreatitis, the loss is not external but into the interstitial tissues; nonetheless it becomes unavailable to the cardiovascular system as circulating fluid.

Cardiovascular Changes

The circulatory alterations are due to the hypovolemia, and also, as will be noted later, to the compensatory changes resulting from the hypovolemia. The initial alterations are very similar to those seen early in hemorrhage, which were described in Chapter 13. In typical hypovolemic shock, the main circulatory effects are: (a) decrease in central and peripheral venous pressure, in circulating blood volume and in venous return; (b) decrease in stroke volume and cardiac output, with particular reduction in flow to the skin, splanchnic area and kidney; (c) decrease in arterial blood pressure (mean, systolic, diastolic and pulse pressure); (d) increased heart rate and myocardial contractility; (e) generalized vasoconstriction and venoconstriction with stagnant hypoxia; (f) hemodilution, with increased $Paco_2$ and decreased pH. Within a few hours there follows a leukocytosis, a nonspecific stress response whose mechanism is not known.

The typical progression of the circulatory changes can be illustrated in an experimental animal as shown in Figure 15.5. In this experiment, hypovolemic shock and hypotension were induced by hemorrhage; after a two-hour interval, the blood was reinfused and additional periodic transfusion given. In spite of this, the circulation failed progressively and the animal died. Whether the shock becomes irreversible is mainly dependent on the degree and duration of the hypotension and the adequacy of treatment; the possible causes of this irreversibility will be discussed later.

Compensatory Responses

The reactions to the stress—most of them reflex in nature—are an important part of the shock syndrome. The initial responses are directed particularly toward restoration of the two main deficiencies—the hypovolemia and the hypotension.

Almost immediately, the decreased central venous volume (and pressure) will initiate autonomic cardiopulmonary reflexes, and the falling arterial and pulse pressure will induce strong arterial baroceptor responses (Chapter 10); these reflexes will result in tachycardia, increased myocardial contractility, widespread vasoconstriction and venoconstric-

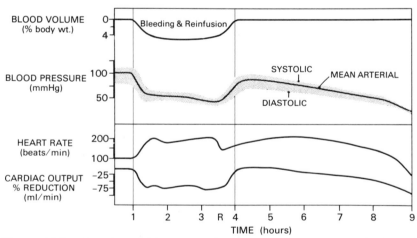

Figure 15.5. Experimental hemorrhagic shock. Two-hour hypovolemia and hypotension. Note the sharp fall in cardiac output (CO) and arterial pressure (AP), and rise in heart rate. With reinfusion of the withdrawn blood (at *R*), CO and AP recovered but later declined in spite of subsequent transfusion. (Reprinted with permission from C.J. Wiggers, *Physiology of Shock*. Cambridge: Harvard University Press, 1950.)

tion, release of adrenal medullary catecholamines and hyperventilation. When acidosis becomes evident, the arterial chemoceptors will also be activated and add an additional pressor effect; in deep shock the CNS ischemic reflex will provoke a still more intense sympathetic vasoconstriction (Chapter 10).

These reflex responses will tend to restore both cardiac output and arterial pressure but they will not be maintained equally. As increasing fractions of blood volume are removed, the cardiac output will tend to fall, while arterial pressure may be temporarily maintained if the bleeding is not too rapid (Fig. 15.6).

Several important points should be noted in Figure 15.6. First, the maintenance of pressure at the expense of flow is the classic definition of resistance and the ratio of the two is a measure of the extent to which total vascular resistance is being mobilized, as was discussed in Chapter 2. However, while the mean arterial pressure is being maintained, the pulse pressure steadily declines; if the heart rate is not changing greatly, this would suggest (if cardiac output determinations are not available) that stroke volume and cardiac output are declining. The graph also indicates that with about 15% of the blood volume removed, the bleeding still continuing and the cardiac output declining, the mean arterial pressure may still be relatively normal; thus in such a situation,

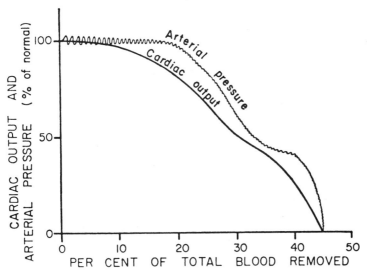

Figure 15.6. Effect of graded hemorrhage on cardiac output and arterial pressure. Early in the bleeding, cardiac output (CO) falls but arterial pressure (AP) is maintained. After withdrawal of about 20% of the blood volume both AP and CO decline rapidly. (Reprinted with permission from A.C. Guyton, *Textbook of Medical Physiology*, 6th ed. Philadelphia: W.B. Saunders, 1981.)

with circulatory collapse imminent, the mean arterial pressure is not a good index of the state of the circulation. For this reason, pulse pressure, heart rate, central venous pressure, urine output and other clinical signs must also be carefully monitored during shock.

Finally, the graph illustrates that when the arterial pressure reaches very low levels, *e.g.*, about 40 to 60 mm Hg, there is a temporary arrest in the decline of the arterial pressure and cardiac output resulting from a massive intensive sympathetic vasoconstriction—the CNS ischemic reflex (Chapter 10). This "last ditch" compensatory effort to maintain arterial pressure is thought to be initiated by ischemia of the brain stem.

Systemic vascular resistance is approximately doubled and pulmonary vascular resistance is increased about 5-fold in severe shock. As mentioned earlier, the sympathetic vasoconstriction is selective; constriction of the skin is responsible for the pallor and the renal vasoconstriction reduces glomerular filtration pressure, resulting in oliguria (decreased urine flow) or, if severe, anuria (cessation of urine output). The vasoconstriction in skeletal muscle and in the splanchnic area and the widespread venoconstriction will mobilize blood from these "reservoirs"; this mobilization and the simultaneous shrinking of the general vascular capacity are very important aids to venous return and cardiac output.

Within minutes after hemorrhage or trauma, there is also a prompt tendency to restore *vascular volume*, mainly through: (a) influx of interstitial fluid into the capillaries through reduction of intracapillary hydrostatic pressure (Chapter 8); (b) renal vasoconstriction, which will not only reduce glomerular filtration pressure and urine output, but will also activate the renin-angiotensin-aldosterone mechanism (Chapter 11, Renal Circulation) and thus increase sodium and therefore also water reabsorption from the renal tubules; and (c) the release of vasopressin (ADH) from the posterior pituitary gland, which will increase the reabsorption of water from the renal tubules. ADH release will be instigated by (a) decrease of atrial pressure and lesser stimulation of the cardiopulmonary receptors in the atria and (b) stimulation of osmoreceptors in the posterior pituitary gland by the increased osmolality of the blood (see Renal Blood Flow, Chapter 11). Some of the changes in circulatory shock are shown graphically in Figure 15.7.

The above responses are compensatory and protective. In severe and continued shock, decompensatory changes may supervene and lead to irreversibility and death. The relative importance of these various pathophysiological changes is discussed later in this chapter. There is evidence that venomotor tone, both in small and large vessels, fails in late shock; the resultant increased compliance in the large capacity venous bed may be partly responsible for the excessive infusions of fluid often needed to restore central blood volume and pressure (Fig. 15.4).

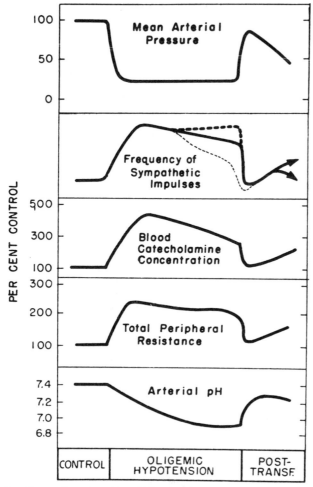

Figure 15.7.   Sympathoadrenal and blood pH responses to experimental hemorrhagic shock. The experimental procedure was similar to that shown in Figure 15.5 with reinfusion of the blood after the hypotensive period. In late shock, the frequency of sympathetic impulses may take different time courses as shown. Note the gradual decline in impulse frequency, catecholamine concentration and vascular resistance and the progressive development of acidosis. (Reprinted with permission from S. Chien, *Physiol Rev* 47:252, 1967.)

Metabolic and Endocrine Changes

While the cardiovascular fluctuations in shock are dramatic and because of their urgency receive more attention, the metabolic and endocrine changes are in the long run, equally if not more significant since it is likely that irreversibility is due primarily to metabolic failure. The primary metabolic changes in moderate or severe hypovolemic shock are as follows.

1. Decreased metabolic rate and body temperature.

2. Alteration in carbohydrate metabolism: (a) an initial hyperglycemia, due to release of epinephrine; later in shock, hypoglycemia may occur because of depletion of hepatic glycogen and failure of gluconeogenesis; (b) anaerobic glycolysis with increase in blood lactate and pyruvate. There is also depletion of high energy phosphates, especially in the liver and kidney; however, those of brain and heart are well maintained.

3. Protein catabolism: (a) increase in blood amino acid nitrogen indicating increased protein catabolism due to the stagnant hypoxia; (b) decrease in blood urea associated with a decline in deamination function of the liver due to hepatic ischemia; (c) increase in liver and blood ammonia.

4. Blood: increase in Pa_{CO_2} and decrease in pH, but the Pa_{O_2} is usually well maintained; hemodilution, except in burns and in some cases of severe trauma, in which the hematocrit is high; increase in plasma catecholamines, 17-hydroxyketosteroids and blood K^+.

The metabolic changes are mainly the result of (a) a generalized stagnant hypoxia, during which the intracellular P_{O_2} becomes very low with a resultant peripheral anaerobiosis, and (b) increased neuroendocrine activity, particularly of the sympathoadrenal and anterior pituitary-adrenal cortical systems.

Cardiogenic Shock

Cardiogenic shock usually denotes insufficient output of the heart despite an adequate ventricular filling pressure. While such a situation results primarily from myocardial infarction (MI), this type of shock can and does occur from a mechanical cardiac defect such as a large pericardial effusion (cardiac tamponade), a sudden valve failure or as a later development in septic or hypovolemic shock.

In the classical case, however, it will result from an MI. Significant arterial hypotension and shock will develop if the myocardial damage is sufficient (about 30 to 40% of the myocardial mass) and if the systemic vascular resistance is not adequate to maintain the arterial pressure. The net result will depend mainly on (a) the effect of the MI on myocardial pump function, and (b) the reflex response to the myocardial injury.

The reflex sympathetic vasoconstrictor response is of paramount importance for survival. As described in Chapter 14, the vascular impulses from cardiac receptors traveling via the vagus nerves may induce either pressor or depressor responses. Recent studies have also shown that experimental ventricular ischemia in the dog and monkey will result in afferent impulses carried via the dorsal sympathetic chain. These fibers can carry pain sensation but even more important, they can apparently inhibit sympathetic vasoconstrictors (Chapter 10, Ventricular Receptors).

Obviously the vasomotor and cardiac centers of the medulla are subjected to varied and sometimes conflicting influences; aside from the afferent cardiac impulses which are unpredictable (but generally depressor), the remaining cardiopulmonary afferents and the arterial baroceptors are strongly pressor. The net response is the result of the integration of these (and other) impulses by the medullary centers. An interesting recent finding is that efferent constrictor impulses to upper and lower limb skeletal muscle may elicit different responses, raising the possibility of more specific efferent control of vascular resistance than has been ordinarily visualized.

Septic Shock

Septic shock is usually the result of a severe infection and bacteremia, often with Gram-negative organisms. The patient frequently has an increased central venous pressure (CVP) and cardiac output, hyperventilation and alkalosis along with hypotension, tachycardia and a low peripheral vascular resistance. The hyperventilation is an important, early and often unrecognized sign of impending septic shock.

In contrast to this hyperdynamic state, there is also a form of hypodynamic septic shock in which there is a decreased CVP and cardiac output, increased peripheral resistance and cold, cyanotic extremities.

There is in septic shock a lactacidemia with a low arterial-mixed venous oxygen gradient indicating inadequate delivery of oxygen to the tissues. The cause of this deficiency is not certain but apparently involves a basic metabolic defect, perhaps due to a circulating toxin which interferes with cellular oxygen utilization. While septic shock is frequently the direct result of infection, it may also occur as an aftermath of cardiogenic or hypovolemic shock, perhaps because of the temporary deleterious effect of the latter on the body's bacterial defense mechanisms. Unlike the preceding forms of shock, septic shock is often associated with other pathological complications such as acute respiratory failure with pulmonary edema or disseminated intravascular coagulation (DIC); the latter is an extensive disorder of the blood clotting mechanism characterized by frequent occurrence of microemboli.

Pathogenesis of Circulatory Shock

The hemodynamic and metabolic changes in early hypovolemic and cardiogenic shock are the result of the low cardiac output, hypotension and generalized stagnant hypoxia. However, in many cases of septic shock the cardiac output is normal or even elevated but the cellular damage leads to similar metabolic results.

The search for the mechanism of the later changes in shock, particularly the irreversibility, has been unsuccessful in spite of enormous research efforts. Two special difficulties complicate the shock problem; first, as Wiggers has pointed out, shock not only stops the machine, but wrecks the machinery; so many processes are simultaneously affected that it is difficult to determine which is the primary disorder. The result has been innumerable theories concerning the irreversibility with the evidence frequently being only circumstantial. The second difficulty lies in finding a common denominator for a process which can be initiated in many different ways and in which the only endpoint is a fatality. However, while a single cause has not yet been found, our understanding of circulatory shock has been considerably advanced in recent years.

Site of the Failure in Shock

From the standpoint of etiology, many investigators have been concerned with the question of which organ or system initiates the irreversibility; others have concentrated on which process might be responsible. In earlier studies, the excessive splanchnic vasoconstriction and hepatic ischemia, especially in dogs, drew attention to the liver as a possible critical site. However, this approach has limited application to clinical medicine since the pronounced hepatic congestion and intestinal necrosis, which characterize irreversible canine shock, are not usually found at autopsy in fatal human shock.

The role of other organs has also been studied. The main issue of the failure site has, however, revolved around the question of whether it is basically of cardiac or peripheral circulatory origin. Jones et al. have advocated the primary role of the heart; Zweifach and Froneck, in their extensive analysis of shock mechanisms, stated that in their opinion, the issue was unsettled but favored the view that peripheral failure was responsible. Undoubtedly one of the reasons for the conflicting evidence on the role of the heart is the great difficulty—if not impossibility—of achieving with present methods the conditions necessary for making a valid assessment of cardiac contractility during severe circulatory shock.

There is considerable evidence to implicate peripheral vascular mechanisms as critical factors in shock survival. Stekiel and his colleagues have reported adrenergic neurotransmitter depletion in mesenteric arteries in hemorrhagic shock and believe that loss of such compensatory vasoconstriction may be a key defect. Rothe and Selkurt emphasized the role of skeletal muscle vascular failure in irreversible shock in dogs and recently Bond et al. found that the terminal decompensatory skeletal muscle vasodilation was probably caused by the inhibitory action of locally released prostaglandins on the peripheral sympathetic endings. Kovach and his group have found marked reduction of blood flow and loss of responsiveness in the hypothalamus and reticular formation of dogs in hypovolemic shock and have indicated the potential importance of this central neurogenic influence on irreversibility.

Metabolic Processes and Irreversibility

Some investigators have focused their efforts not on a target organ but on a basic metabolic process in order to study its role in shock development. While a number of metabolic deficiencies have been identified, none of these have thus far been proved to be an instigating factor in the irreversibility. Studies by Filkins and coworkers and Hinshaw and others have emphasized the importance of certain aspects of carbohydrate metabolism, particularly in endotoxin shock.

Irreversibility is usually characterized by a marked hypoglycemia and a profound depression of gluconeogenesis; shock mortality is also found to be increased in situations of enhanced insulin secretion, suggesting an important role for hyperinsulinemia as well as hypoglycemia in endotoxin and perhaps septic shock.

Reticuloendothelial System (RES) in Shock

In early studies, Zweifach and others noted a correlation between RES function and the mortality from trauma, as well as increased shock mortality following RES blockade. Filkins et al. demonstrated that administration of zymosan, a yeast extract with potent RES-modulating properties, significantly lowered the mortality of rats to traumatic shock. Loegering and Saba have reported that in experimental shock, there was a depression of RES phagocytic function; the evidence indicates that both humoral and cellular factors may be involved in the decreased functional capacity of the RES in shock. It has been suggested that such a decline in the body defense mechanism may play a role in septic shock and particularly in its occurrence as a sequela to other types of circulatory failure. There is also recent evidence that the RES is concerned with the depression of gluconeogenesis and the hyperinsulinism characteristic of late endotoxin shock.

Toxic Factors in Shock

A number of circulating toxins have been proposed as causative agents for the irreversibility in shock. Fine and his colleagues were the first to suggest that bacterial endotoxins absorbed from the ischemic gut might play a role in the pathophysiology of shock. This view was given support by the finding that very small doses of endotoxin could produce in experimental animals a circulatory failure resembling hypovolemic and traumatic shock. While the overall role of endotoxins in shock is uncertain, some investigators believe they are concerned in the circulatory failure in bacteremia, particularly of the Gram-negative type.

Lefer and coworkers have accumulated considerable evidence for a

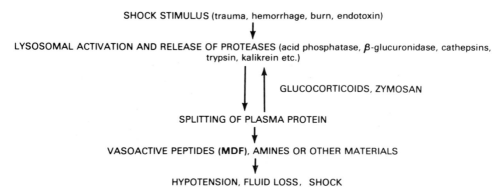

Figure 15.8. Schema illustrating possible mechanism for the development of irreversible shock. Glucocorticoids and zymosan (an extract of brewers' yeast) have both been shown to lower mortality in experimental shock, presumably through their ability to stabilize lysosomal membranes.

causal relationship between a myocardial depressant factor (MDF) and mortality in experimental shock. MDF is a low molecular weight, dialyzable polypeptide apparently produced in the pancreas and recoverable from the blood of animals suffering shock; further studies indicate that this agent has a strong myocardial depressant effect. These investigators believe MDF to be a key factor in the circulatory failure of shock.

Lysosomes in Shock

Lysosomes are cytoplasmic granules present in almost all body cells; they contain a variety of potent hydrolytic enzymes enclosed within a relatively impermeable membrane. Following the pioneer work of De Duve on the role of lysosomes in cellular function, investigations have been made of their possible role in shock. Studies have indicated that hypoxia and mechanical trauma cause disruption of lysosomes *in vitro*; furthermore after hemorrhage, endotoxin injection or trauma, lysosomal proteases escape from ischemic cells and are found in high concentration in the plasma. Some investigators have ascribed the role of the RES in shock to the fact that RES tissue is rich in lysosomes. The interaction of proteases from disrupted lysosomes with certain plasma proteins is thought to be the source of several biologically active protein derivatives, *e.g.*, the myocardial depressant factor (MDF) described above. These lines of evidence have led a number of investigators to propose that lysosomes may play a key role in the etiology of lethal shock as outlined in Figure 15.8. However, the important question of the cause of irreversibility in human shock is still unanswered.

Treatment of Shock

Fluid Replacement and Central Venous Pressure

Because in the great majority of shock patients, there is a fluid deficit, treatment is first of all directed toward replacement therapy with crystalloids, colloids, plasma, blood substitutes or whole blood depending on individual needs. The monitoring of such therapy is often done via central venous pressure (CVP). Clinical CVP monitoring usually refers to central vena caval or right atrial pressure and therefore is a general index of *right* ventricular filling pressure and *right* ventricular end-diastolic pressure (RVEDP).

As discussed in Chapter 2, pressure in the central veins (as in any blood vessel) depends on the distensibility (or compliance) of the vessel and the volume contained. Heightened sympathetic tone will decrease the distensibility; however, at any given distensibility level, CVP will be dependent on the contained volume which will, in turn, reflect the balance of inflow and outflow. If there is no abnormality of right ventricular function nor of intrathoracic pressure, CVP will be an index of venous return and serve as a rough guide to circulating blood volume and the need for fluid replacement therapy. CVP is normally about 5 to 10 cm saline and in shock usually is less than 3 to 4 cm saline. The goal is to achieve about 8 to 10 cm saline CVP with additional fluid, provided other signs do not contraindicate such treatment. The general objective is to improve ventricular function through greater diastolic filling (the Starling effect).

Monitoring of Ventricular Function in Cardiogenic Shock

In cardiogenic shock, in contrast to the above, factors other than circulating blood volume will influence ventricular filling pressure and, therefore, must be taken into consideration. As mentioned in Chapter 14, after an MI with left ventricular involvement, there will be a gradual decrease in LV compliance with a concomitant rise in LVEDP. The latter development is generally beneficial since it improves ventricular function, but it has two potential disadvantages. Since the ventricular diastolic curve rises steeply (Fig. 14.4), diastolic volume and, therefore, stroke volume will be limited. The second additional factor is that a rising LVEDP increases the possibility of pulmonary congestion.

In such a situation, left ventricular monitoring obviously becomes of prime importance in the treatment of cardiogenic shock. However, CVP is a poor reflection of LVEDP. Fortunately, Swan, Ganz and their colleagues reported in 1970 the development of a double-lumen, flow-directed catheter which could be guided via a peripheral vein into the pulmonary artery without fluoroscopy. This permits the monitoring of pulmonary arterial pressure for the detection of any developing pulmonary congestion and by gently "wedging" the catheter into a pulmonary arterial branch, also provides a reasonable estimate of left atrial pressure and thus of left ventricular filling pressure.

Using this technique, clinical studies have indicated that fluid replacement therapy can safely be continued up to left ventricular filling pressures of about 20 to 24 mm Hg. This will provide a reasonable level for improvement of ventricular function via the Starling effect without undue risk of inducing pulmonary congestion. Thus in cardiogenic shock, a pulmonary artery catheter as well as a central venous catheter is usually employed. In this way both right and left sides of the heart may be monitored.

Specific Therapy

The treatment of metabolic acidosis in shock is best accomplished by restoring tissue perfusion, rather than simply by loading with buffer. In severe acidosis (arterial blood pH under 7.2) sodium bicarbonate should be given intravenously. Shock patients usually are administered oxygen by mask to improve ventilation.

Drug therapy will depend on the type of shock and the hemodynamic and metabolic condition of the patient. If there is evidence of diminished myocardial contractility, *e.g.*, in cardiogenic shock, inotropic agents such as dopamine or dobutamine may be given. The intent is to enhance arterial pressure by increasing left ventricular ejection rather than increasing peripheral resistance. Dopamine is reasonably effective in this regard since at low doses its β-adrenergic effect is more prominent than its α-adrenergic action. However, dobutamine is theoretically preferable in this regard since it is exclusively a β-agonist, but experience with this drug has been rather limited thus far. The renal vasodilation effect of these β-adrenergic agents may be useful in increasing urine flow.

α-Vasoconstrictors, such as methoxamine or norepinephrine, are sometimes given for short periods in hypovolemic shock if severe hypotension persists; its disadvantages are that it further restricts peripheral tissue perfusion and increases cardiac afterload. Vasodilator agents—formerly believed to be contraindicated in shock—are now used selectively in some cases of cardiogenic shock. One of the factors limiting ventricular ejection is afterload, *i.e.*, aortic pressure. The success of a vasodilator, such as nitroprusside which has a direct relaxant effect on vascular smooth muscle, is based on the expectation that the reduced cardiac pressure work and the increased cardiac index that results will override the disadvantage of a somewhat lower aortic perfusion pressure. Obviously, such medication must be carefully monitored and controlled. Reports have indicated, however, that combinations of inotropic agents and vasodilators have proven effective in selected cases of circulatory shock. Because of its sometimes fulminating nature and high mortality, septic shock is challenging and often difficult to treat. Selection of the proper antibiotic in adequate doses is the cornerstone of treatment. Corticosteroids are widely used in septic shock on the basis that these agents are known to stabilize cellular and subcellular membranes and thus may prevent the escape of lysosomal hydrolases into the circulation.

Intraaortic Balloon Counterpulsation (IABC)

In very severe shock in which arterial pressure cannot be maintained despite all available methods, additional circulatory support is sometimes given by introduction via catheter of an inflatable balloon into the upper thoracic aorta (Fig. 15.9). The balloon is inflated during diastole and rapidly deflated at the end of diastole. Thus central diastolic pressure is increased which assists coronary flow, and systolic peak pressure is decreased which reduces the afterload work of the left ventricle. With this procedure, cardiac output is increased with relatively little change in mean arterial pressure. Counterpulsation has proven helpful in certain circumstances in achieving hemodynamic stability.

It should be emphasized that the treatment of shock is highly complex. The few general principles described above are intended only to illustrate some of the pathophysiology involved and not to serve as a guide to therapy.

Figure 15.9. Effect of intraaortic balloon counterpulsation (IABC) on aortic and left atrial pressure and left ventricular stroke work index. *Left*, values immediately before and after IABC; *right*, the relationship of mean pulmonary artery wedge pressure (MPAWP) and left ventricular stroke work index (LVSWI) before and after IABC. In a critically ill patient, MPAWP is equivalent to left atrial filling pressure. Note the improved ventricular function during IABC. (Reprinted with permission from R.L. Berger, V.K. Saini, T.J. Ryan, D.M. Sokol, and J.F. Keefe, *J Thorac Cardiovasc Surg* 66:906, 1973; and R.D. Weisel, R.L. Berger, and H.B. Hechtman, *N Engl J Med* 292:682, 1975.)

References

Hypertension

Brod J, Fencl V, Hejl Z, and Jirka J. Circulatory changes underlying blood pressure elevation during acute emotional stress. *Clin Sci* 18:269, 1959.

Brody MJ, Haywood JR, and Touw KB. Neural mechanisms in hypertension. *Annu Rev Physiol* 42:441–453, 1980.

Brody MJ and Johnson AK. Role of forebrain structures in models of experimental hypertension. In: *Disturbances in Neurogenic Control of the Circulation*, edited by FM Abboud, HA Fozzard, JP Gilmore and DJ Reis. Bethesda, Md.: American Physiological Society, 1981; pp. 105–117.

Chobanian AV. Pathophysiology of systemic hypertension. In: *Clinical Cardiovascular Physiology*, edited by HJ Levine. New York: Grune & Stratton, 1976, pp. 563–596.

Coleman TG, Cowley AW Jr., and Guyton AC. Experimental hypertension and the long-term control of arterial pressure. In: *Cardiovascular Physiology, MTP International Review of Science*, edited by AC Guyton and CE Jones. Baltimore: University Park Press, 1974, Vol. I, pp. 259–298.

Dustan HP. Pathophysiology of hypertension. In: *The Heart, Arteries and Veins*, edited by JW Hurst. New York: McGraw-Hill, 1982, 5th ed., pp. 1171–1181.

Folkow B. Physiological aspects of primary hypertension. *Physiol Rev* 62:347–504, 1982.

Frohlich ED. Cardiovascular pathophysiology of essential hypertension. In: *The Peripheral Circulations*, edited by R Zelis. New York: Grune & Stratton, 1975, pp. 261–282.

Gauer OH and Henry JP. Circulatory basis of fluid volume control. *Physiol Rev* 42:423–481, 1963.

Harder DR, Contney SJ, Willems WJ, and Stekiel WJ. Norepinephrine effect on in situ venous membrane potential in spontaneously hypertensive rats. *Am J Physiol* 240:H837–842, 1981.

Itskovitz HD, Kochar MS, Anderson AJ, and Rimm AA. Patterns of blood pressure in Milwaukee. *JAMA* 238:864–868, 1977.

Kochar MS. Hypertension. In: *Textbook of General Medicine*, edited by MS Kochar. New York: John Wiley & Sons, 1983, pp. 442–454.

Laragh JH, Letcher RL, and Pickering TG. Renin profiling for diagnosis and treatment of hypertension. *JAMA* 241:151–156, 1979.

Mancia G, Ludbrook J, Ferrari A, Gregorini L, and Zanchetti A: Baroceptor reflexes in human hypertension. *Circ Res* 43:170–177, 1978.

Page IH. Arterial hypertension in retrospect. *Circ Res* 34:133–142, 1974.

Pickering G. Hypertension—definitions, natural histories and consequences. *Am J Cardiol* 52:570–583, 1972.

Safar ME, Weiss YA, Levenson JA, London GJ, and Milliez PL. Hemodynamic study of eighty-five patients with borderline hypertension. *Am J Cardiol* 31:315–319, 1973.

Symposium on Hypertension and Antihypertension Drugs: NR Kaplan, Chairman. *Fed Proc* 40:2250–2294, 1981.

Circulatory Shock

Abboud FM. Pathophysiology of hypotension and shock. In: *The Heart, Arteries and Veins*, edited by JW Hurst. New York: McGraw-Hill, 1982, 5th ed., pp. 452–463.

Altura BM. Reticuloendothelial cells and host defense. *Adv Microirc* 9:252–294, 1980.

Beckman CB, Geha AS, Hammond GL, and Bave AE. Results and complications of intra-aortic balloon counter-pulsation. *Ann Thorac Surg* 24:550–559, 1977.

Bond RF, Bond CH, Peissner LC, and Manning ES. Prostaglandin modulation of adrenergic vascular control during hemorrhagic shock. *Am J Physiol* 241:H85–90, 1981.

Cohn JN. Recognition and management of shock and acute pump failure. In: *The Heart, Arteries and Veins*, edited by JW Hurst. New York: McGraw-Hill, 1982, 5th ed., pp. 463–476.

Filkins JP. Role of RES in the pathogenesis of endotoxic hypoglycemia. *Circ Shock* 9:269–280, 1982.

Goldfarb RD. Cardiac mechanical performance in circulatory shock: a critical review of methods and results. *Circ Shock* 9:633–653, 1982.

Guntheroth WG, Jacky JP, Kawabori I, Stevenson JG, and Moreno AH. Left ventricular performance in endotoxin shock in dogs. *Am J Physiol* 242:H172–176, 1982.

Hinshaw LB, Beller-Todd BK, and Archer LT. Current management of the septic shock patient: experimental basis for treatment. *Circ Shock* 9:543–553, 1982.

Hinshaw LB. Concise review: the role of glucose in endotoxin shock. *Circ Shock* 3:6–10, 1976.

Jones CE, Smith EE, and Crowell JW. Cardiac output and physiological mechanisms in circulatory shock. In: *Cardiovascular Physiology, MTP International Review of Science*, edited by AC Guyton and CE Jones. Baltimore: University Park Press, 1974, pp. 233–258.

Kostreva DR, Hess GL, Zuperku EJ, Neumark J, Coon RL, and Kampine JP. Cardiac responses to stimulation of thoracic afferents in the primate and canine. *Am J Physiol* 231:1279–1284, 1976.

Kovach AGB and Sandor P. Cerebral blood flow and brain function during hypotension and shock. *Physiol Rev* 38:571–596, 1976.

Lefer AM and Spath JA. Pharmacologic basis for the treatment of circulatory shock. In: *Cardiovascular Pharmacology*, edited by M Antonaccio. New York: Raven Press, 1977.

Loegering DJ and Saba TM. Hepatic Kupffer cell dysfunction during hemorrhagic shock. *Circ Res* 3:107–113, 1976.

Lombard JH, Loegering DJ, and Stekiel WJ. Effects of prolonged hemorrhagic hypotensive stress on catecholamine concentration of mesenteric blood vessels. *Blood Vessels* 14:212–228, 1977.

McLean LD. Shock: causes and management of circulatory collapse. In: *Textbook of Surgery*, edited by DC Sabiston. Philadelphia: W.B. Saunders, 1981, 12th ed., pp. 58–90.

Rothe CF and Selkurt EE. Cardiac and peripheral failure in hemorrhagic shock in the dog. *Am J Physiol* 207:203–214, 1964.

Smith JJ, Loegering DJ, McDermott DJ, and Bonin ML. The role of lysosomal hydrolases in the mechanism of shock. In: *Neurohumoral and Metabolic Aspects of Injury*, edited by AGB Kovach, HB Stoner and JJ Spitzer. New York: Plenum, 1973, pp. 535–543.

Swan HJ, Ganz W, Forrester J, Marcus H, Diamond G, and Chonette D. Catheterization of the heart in man with use of a flow-directed balloon-tipped catheter. *N Engl J Med* 283:447–450, 1970.

Tillisch JH. Pump failure and cardiogenic shock. In: *Pathophysiology of the Heart*, edited by G Ross. New York: Masson Publishing Co., 1982, pp. 225–256.

Zweifach B and Froneck A. Interplay of central and peripheral factors in irreversible hemorrhagic shock. *Prog Cardiovasc Dis* 18:147–180, 1975.

Index

Page numbers in **boldface** indicate more definitive discussions of the topic.

Page numbers in **boldface** indicate more definitive discussions of the topic.

Page numbers in **boldface** indicate more definitive discussions of the topic.

Page numbers in **boldface** indicate more definitive discussions of the topic.

Page numbers in **boldface** indicate more definitive discussions of the topic.

Page numbers in **boldface** indicate more definitive discussions of the topic.

Page numbers in **boldface** indicate more definitive discussions of the topic.

Page numbers in **boldface** indicate more definitive discussions of the topic.

Page numbers in **boldface** indicate more definitive discussions of the topic.

Page numbers in **boldface** indicate more definitive discussions of the topic.

Page numbers in **boldface** indicate more definitive discussions of the topic.

Page numbers in **boldface** indicate more definitive discussions of the topic.

Page numbers in **boldface** indicate more definitive discussions of the topic.